A
DEEPER
SICKNESS

A
DEEPER
SICKNESS

JOURNAL
OF AMERICA
IN THE
PANDEMIC YEAR

MARGARET PEACOCK AND
ERIK L. PETERSON

BEACON PRESS · BOSTON

BEACON PRESS
Boston, Massachusetts
www.beacon.org

Beacon Press books
are published under the auspices of
the Unitarian Universalist Association of Congregations.

25 24 23 22   8 7 6 5 4 3 2 1

This book is printed on acid-free paper that meets the uncoated paper
ANSI/NISO specifications for permanence as revised in 1992.

Text design and composition by Kim Arney

Library of Congress Cataloging-in-Publication Data
Names: Peacock, Margaret, author. | Peterson, Erik L., author.
Title: A deeper sickness : journal of America in the pandemic year /
Margaret Peacock and Erik L. Peterson.
Description: Boston : Beacon Press, [2022] | Includes bibliographical
references and index. | Summary: "An unflinching daily account of how a
viral pandemic unmasked two centuries of American disease, poverty,
violence, and disinformation"—Provided by publisher.
Identifiers: LCCN 2021036495 (print) | LCCN 2021036496 (ebook) |
ISBN 9780807040294 (hardcover) | ISBN 9780807040300 (ebook)
Subjects: LCSH: United States—Social conditions—2020 |
COVID-19 Pandemic, 2020—United States.
Classification: LCC HN59.3 .P43 2022 (print) | LCC HN59.3 (ebook) |
DDC 306.0973—dc23/eng/20211004
LC record available at https://lccn.loc.gov/2021036495
LC ebook record available at https://lccn.loc.gov/2021036496

To the essential workers of 2020,
in harm's way to keep the economy running but
without adequate protection and paid too little.
And to future generations of Americans:
learn the right lesson from our mistakes.

A companion archive holding thousands of images, videos, documents, stories, and other bonus content can be found at http://www.deepersickness.com.

In any event, the sloppy and fatuous nature of American good will can never be relied upon to deal with hard problems. These have been dealt with, when they have been dealt with at all, out of necessity — and in political terms, anyway, necessity means concessions made in order to stay on top.

—JAMES BALDWIN, "Down at the Cross" (1963)

INTRODUCTION

This journal recounts in detail the four pandemics—disease, disinformation, poverty, and violence—that charged through the United States like the proverbial horsemen of the apocalypse in the year 2020. During this calendar year, nearly four hundred thousand Americans died of COVID-19, the disease caused by a novel coronavirus. Beginning in April, the country erupted into protest, some opposing public health restrictions, others marching to stop the slaughter of Black men and women by white authorities. The experience changed how we learned, ate, shopped, worked, socialized, practiced medicine, grieved, celebrated, and died. We saw bright spots, moments of great heroism and sacrifice. And yet, in the United States, 2020 will long be known as a time of grief, frustration, confusion, loneliness, and even rage.

Could it have turned out differently?

Journalists and scholars are already uncovering the missteps made by those in power in early 2020 that failed to contain SARS-CoV-2 once it appeared in the US. In this book, in which we follow America as eyewitnesses to the tumult of the entire year, we are after a different question: Is there something in the character of the place, the bones of America, that made the layers of tragedy that unfolded in 2020 practically unavoidable?

. . . .

As professional historians, we spend our lives trying to make sense of the past, in part so that we can better understand the present. For a full year, we turned our attention to daily events and the historical contexts of this year's multiple pandemics in the hope of understanding both how we got here and how we might prevent ever returning. In January, Erik L. Peterson, a historian and philosopher of science and medicine, began following the outbreak of this new coronavirus, collecting primary sources for his course on the global history of epidemics at the University of Alabama. Independently, Margaret Peacock, an expert on propaganda, Russia, the Middle East, and the Cold War, decided to do the same for a course on the history of media and propaganda. An incidental conversation in the spring after our university moved courses online inspired us to merge projects.

We constructed this book as a journal, written mostly in real time as the year unspooled. Each day, we tracked hundreds of news stories, reports, tweets, posts, blogs, speeches, and videos from across the political spectrum, intent on capturing how people encountered these moments and what historical factors informed their understandings of the events unfolding around them. Of course, no one could describe a singular "American experience of 2020." Instead, we set out to provide a wide range of glimpses into individual, subjective encounters with the chaos of this year by recruiting and interviewing a large and diverse group of people from different races, ethnicities, classes, political beliefs, and geographic regions willing to share their expertise and experiences. Dozens of scholars, politicians, activists, physicians, epidemiologists, attorneys, nurses, and public health experts helped us make meaning of the headlines. We also received invaluable insights from "regular folks," who unpacked their unique perspectives and made this book the expansive, heart-wrenching project that it became.

This canvassing of 2020 required an effort larger than ourselves, and we are forever grateful for the work of so many. We acknowledge the ways this story is deeply subjective, shaped by our own expertise as historians and educators living and working far from the media hubs on both coasts. As such, we wrote this chronicle in the first person. When we need to speak about ourselves, it is with one collective "I," with each entry reflecting a thorough braiding of each of our experiences and each of our years of training and research leading up to this moment.

One point we want to underscore in this book is how difficult it often was to understand what was happening around us during the pandemic. We want to show how mistaken we were at times, how distorted time felt, how surprisingly powerless and ignorant we all turned out to be, despite our best efforts to stay informed and empowered. We researched and wrote all day, every day, frenetically, yet lived in a state of focused confusion for most of that exhausting year. We had to, of course. Contrary to how most academic histories are composed, including our own work, there could be no "outline," no "thesis." We could not know which events would turn out to be mundane, which would become historic—they all felt like both, all the time. So, we took each day as it came, reading and watching and writing, as frantic days rolled one into another, crescendos piling on top of each other. Inevitably, we made mistakes. Rather than fixing them in the editing process, we preserved them here as a testament to the tumult of the year. We see value in them. For, while historians in the next decade or century will no doubt shed more dispassionate clarity on 2020, they will not be able to grasp the messy immediacy of documenting it while living it, that constant sense that the ground under us was quicksand.

We constructed an expansive digital museum as a companion to the book at deepersickness.com. It displays the thousands of sources we curated over the year, the hundreds of pages of additional content we wrote that did not fit into the printed book, a collection of eyewitness narratives from contributors recounting their experiences with this year, and an exhibit space highlighting original research on 2020 from scholars and students around the country. We encourage you to engage with our voluminous research and add your stories to the historical record. We created this digital museum for three reasons. First, we wanted to preserve the anxieties, sorrows, pains, fears, angers, boredom, and even unexpected joys of this experience, including as many voices as we can. We collected many and hope to collect more. These stories take up more space than a printed book allows, but they are invaluable, nonetheless, and worth saving. Second, we built this site to preserve our sources before they disappear. Too many of the internet-based materials we used to construct the project are ephemeral. We like to imagine that our modern data is saved forever somewhere in the "cloud," but tweets, Facebook/Instagram posts, even news stories, disappear like individual raindrops into a river. On deepersickness.com, we have saved as much as we could. Third, we preserved our sources for readers to view because the recounting of history is a perennial battlefield. How we remember the past shapes everything we do. It defines us in the present and shapes what choices we will make in the future. Inevitably, some readers will disagree with our analyses of these events. In hindsight, we might disagree with ourselves in 2020 as well. Please, readers, examine the sources for yourselves. Preserving sources from 2020 makes it more difficult for people in the future to ignore or gloss over certain realities about this experience. Americans, as we found, too often substitute folklore for history.

. . . .

As we heard story after story of grief and loss, the question *Was the tragedy of 2020 inevitable, and, if so, why?* kept reoccurring. Tracing day after day, certain preexisting conditions that shaped this year came into focus—the way a physician armed with a family medical history might see a chronic illness behind a patient's present symptoms.

Three historical factors, in particular, made America sicker than we should have been in 2020: (a) entrenched racial hierarchies; (b) an economic structure dependent on individual accumulation of wealth and widespread consumption of ephemeral goods and entertainment; (c) distraction, cognitive dissonance, and an intentional historical amnesia that prevented the majority of comfortable, well-intentioned, middle-class, white Americans like ourselves from doing anything about the first two issues.

These factors channeled seventy-four million people—nearly 47 percent of all votes cast—to nearly reelect a narcissistic, predatory charlatan who accumulated immense power by repeating age-old, bigoted, malevolent, and dishonest tropes. Millions more disregarded health and safety guidelines, refusing to wear masks or avoid gatherings in poorly ventilated spaces or with large numbers of people, resulting in higher rates of disease and death in the United States than in most other countries. These factors justified ongoing official and vigilante violence toward Black citizens, whether they were jogging, bird-watching in a park, sitting in their cars, sleeping in their homes, or protesting peacefully in the streets. And in the background, these factors drove many millions of people into increasing states of socioeconomic precarity.

The American 2020 experience was so bad not because coronavirus itself was worse here, but because disease is social and cultural as well as biological. And the causes of that social and cultural disease are historical. In other words, the country's underlying disorders limited the possible outcomes of the American pandemic year. Despite our prolific technology and our deep-seated belief in progress, we Americans have not broadly diagnosed, let alone treated, the moral failings of our past. Instead, too much of white America remains willfully ignorant, manufacturing and adhering to a *false* past, preserved in the monuments that adorn our cities and public buildings, constructed in order to distract from the most deeply unequal, unpatriotic, and immoral portions of our present existences. This is among the worst of our preexisting conditions, our deeper sickness.

Through the year, we heard another question echoed time and again: *Will 2020 be recognized as a turning point*—a 1968, for instance? The answer depends not just on our politicians but on Americans in 2021 and 2031 and 2121. "Apocalypse" is not just another word for cataclysm; it originally meant a revealing of what lies beneath. True to that original meaning, the apocalypse of 2020 revealed the deep, historical deformities in the American body politic. If we allow our amazement that heavily funded biotech corporations were able to create a coronavirus vaccine in record-breaking time to distract us from addressing our deeper sickness, then 2020 will not be a turning point in anything but the most superficial, historically uninteresting way.

A
DEEPER
SICKNESS

WEDNESDAY, JANUARY 1, 2020

Sharon Sanders of Winter Haven, Florida, has been tracking global disease outbreaks on her site, FluTrackers.com, since 2006. It was the first public forum to note the H1N1 influenza (swine flu) pandemic when it appeared in North America. I came across the site in 2013 after it was the first Western media outlet to report on the H7N9 avian influenza (bird flu) outbreak in China. The very next year, they broke the story about eight hemorrhagic fever deaths in Guinea that eventually became the terrifying 2014 Ebola virus outbreak. Sanders has mobilized health experts and volunteers from around the world to translate esoteric news on disease from Arabic, Chinese, Dutch, French, German, Hindi, Indonesian, Spanish, Vietnamese, and several other languages.

What Sanders saw last night concerned her. "In the 2013 H7N9 avian flu pandemic," she tells me, "the earliest reports were that one to four people had the virus."[1] Now, she is seeing two brief media reports out of China identifying twenty-seven people sick with an unknown respiratory infection connected to an open-air market in Wuhan. Twenty-seven—a high number for a first report! She thought about calling Michael Coston, a colleague who runs the *Avian Flu Diary* blog, but it was the middle of the night. "In fourteen years, I have *never* called him late at night." Still, long ago, they had agreed that if it was *"very* significant," they would be in touch, no matter the time. So she called him.

Coston confirmed her concerns. It fit the profile of a viral outbreak. Sanders posted the stories to FluTrackers.com and slept for a few hours. Part of her worry came from knowing that news of this sort normally doesn't pass through the Chinese government internet firewall. "A single outbreak of any disease involving twenty-seven humans that was being widely broadcast means something serious is going on," she says. Overnight, others posted additional info out of China.[2] The Wuhan city government claims there has been no human-to-human transmission of this new virus.

This morning, Sanders checked again. Nothing on the American news sites. Nothing from the Centers for Disease Control and Prevention (CDC).

FRIDAY, JANUARY 10, 2020

Anthony Fauci, an American immunologist and director of the National Institute of Allergy and Infectious Diseases (NIAID), reports that the United

States has reached peak levels of influenza a month early.[3] There have been four hundred confirmed flu deaths, with larger-than-usual numbers of children being hospitalized.[4] It could be a bad year.

Meanwhile, the World Health Organization (WHO) announces a disease cluster with an unspecified illness in Hubei Province, exactly as Sanders and others at FluTrackers.com are reporting. The CDC issues a Level 1 advisory, meaning Americans should avoid live animal markets overseas and stay home if they feel sick.[5] Cases in China have grown to fifty-nine, including some in Hong Kong, which is worrying because Hong Kong is a good distance from Hubei Province.[6] China's medical and scientific community now suggest there could be human-to-human transmission.

Posts to FluTrackers.com show a run on face masks in China. Ever since the SARS (severe acute respiratory syndrome) outbreak two decades ago, it has become customary in China to wear face masks during disease outbreaks. In 2002, SARS started as a mystery pneumonia from the interior of China. By the spring of 2003, SARS was on every front page in the world—the next calamity after the 9/11/2001 terrorist attacks and the anthrax scare that followed.[7] At the time, the Chinese government clamped down on news about the outbreak, jeopardizing lives. The virus killed fewer than one thousand people globally, and fear of SARS faded.[8] When MERS (Middle East respiratory syndrome) appeared ten years later, there was even less concern in Western countries, though it was a deadlier coronavirus.

It might feel like a SARS moment for disease trackers like Sanders, but WHO takes a "wait and see" approach. We in the United States, at least, are in no danger.[9]

The real worry is that we are on the brink of war with Iran. Last week, the US government killed Iranian major general Qasem Soleimani in Baghdad, which infuriated the Iranians. People are protesting in the streets both here and in Iran. Just two days ago, Iranian ballistic missiles hit the Al Asad Air Base in Iraq, possibly injuring American soldiers. Now we hold our breath to see if tensions will escalate.

TUESDAY, JANUARY 14, 2020

WHO reports the sickness in China is a new kind of coronavirus, much like SARS or MERS. Disease trackers around the world might be unnerved by this. I've seen the American media report on it, yet the rest of the American public isn't giving it much attention.

That's no surprise. Adam Smith, the economist and moral philosopher, wrote long ago about how easy it is to detach ourselves from disasters in faraway places that are beyond many Westerners' imaginations.[10] Even in the Information Age when you can communicate with someone in China in seconds, the actual people there are abstract, too far away, and far too easy to stereotype. The reports say that this new coronavirus came from a "wet market." It is a strange term, but it just means a place where animals are often butchered and sold. Many Americans have never heard of a wet market and have no idea how it could help spread a virus. It is too remote to matter.

I have resolved to document this pandemic if it comes to the United States. As historians have long noted, disease outbreaks reveal the fault lines and weaknesses of a society. We are living on the eve of a polarizing presidential election, amidst rising income inequality, housing insecurity, underfunded education systems, continued race violence, and brutal school shootings. We inhabit a world where one's media popularity often matters more than one's commitment to speak the truth. How would we handle such a crisis if it came to our shores? Would the constant movement of populations around the globe enable a disease that started in China to spread to my front door? Could the American healthcare system, which is based on a structure of profit-driven, acute care, respond adequately to keep me safe? Given our nation's long history of violence, nativism, and racism, and given how divided we are on matters ranging from environmental protection to immigration to notions of freedom and liberty, would we be able to put aside our political differences and join forces in the face of a national crisis to protect ourselves and one another? What are the odds that our acrimonious, outrage-driven, twenty-four-hour media landscape would politicize a pandemic and prevent collective mobilization? Hopefully, we can avoid these questions. Hopefully, the virus stays in China.

WEDNESDAY, JANUARY 22, 2020

The CDC reports the new coronavirus is *already* in the United States. Two days ago, a man in his thirties checked himself into a clinic in Snohomish County, Washington, with body aches and labored breathing. The office staff gave him a mask to wear and left him waiting for twenty minutes in the front room—standard procedure. Four days earlier, on January 16, he had flown home from visiting his family in Wuhan. He had *not* been to the Huanan Seafood Market, where Chinese authorities suspect the new coronavirus originated, nor had he spoken to anyone who was sick during his travels. He hadn't felt ill until the day before going to the clinic. Healthcare workers in Snohomish County sent him home to quarantine while awaiting the test results. Later, officials in hazmat suits showed up at his house and whisked him off to an airborne-isolation unit at Providence Regional Medical Center in Everett, Washington.

This man's illness is pretty terrifying, given that Chinese scientists have confirmed rumors that the virus can spread through human-to-human contact. Sanders suspected this when she wrote on January 20 that healthcare workers in China were getting sick: "Always a bad sign." And she noted that videos from China show unconscious people lying on the streets and sidewalks, healthcare workers in full protective gear, packed hospital waiting rooms, bodies being stacked in vans outside a hospital. It looks much grimmer than most American reporting reveals.

In response to the outbreak in China, the CDC and Customs and Border Protection (CBP) of the Department of Homeland Security (DHS) decided five days ago to assign about a hundred government employees to LAX, SFO, and JFK—the three airports that handle most of the flights from Wuhan. Around two hundred million passengers travel through these three airports each year. What are one hundred government workers tracking self-reported illness going to be able to do? And what about entry from other Chinese cities?

Thankfully, today the CDC says they plan to "step up screening," though it's not clear what that means. Nancy Messonnier, director of the CDC's National Center for Immunization and Respiratory Diseases (NCIRD), maintains the risk to Americans remains low. But the novel coronavirus is certainly spreading outside Wuhan.[11] The CDC has begun contact tracing from the sick man in Washington State to anyone he may have interacted with during the four-day span between arriving from China and seeking medical attention.[12]

For what it's worth, President Trump, who is awaiting his impeachment trial in the Senate, seems unconcerned. Asked in an interview today if there is reason to worry about the pandemic, he said, "It's one person coming in from China, and we have it under control. It's going to be just fine." President Xi's China, he intimates, is going to stop it. Indeed, the Chinese government is taking unprecedented measures, shutting down airports and train stations in central China during the busiest travel time of the year. Just yesterday, January 21, China quarantined the eleven million inhabitants of the city of Wuhan in Hubei Province.[13] The Chinese government has initiated street spraying. I sympathize with the people of Wuhan, and I'm really glad not to be there right now. It is hard to imagine what the lockdown of a whole city would look like. WHO still does not consider this a public health emergency. Only seventeen people have died from the virus, after all. Sanders and the folks at FluTrackers.com, on the other hand, say that spraying means this new coronavirus is worryingly contagious.

The viral pneumonia from Wuhan is regularly reported in the American news now, but only gets a fleeting mention. The cases are relatively low still. Researchers at Imperial College London insist these low numbers are deceptive; their models suggest there could be *triple* the publicized number currently infected.[14]

FRIDAY, JANUARY 24, 2020

China has locked down a second city in Hubei Province, Huanggang, with a population of eight million. The nearby city of Ezhou shuts down its train stations. These restrictions take place during Chunyun, the forty-day period when people in China go home to celebrate the Lunar New Year with their extended families—truly the busiest travel season on Earth each year. A shutdown of these proportions will be exceedingly difficult for families and, by extension, the Chinese economy. Japan, Taiwan, Macau, Vietnam, South Korea, Thailand, and Singapore also report cases. Nevertheless, Trump tweets, "It will all work out well."[15]

The US reports its second case of the new virus today: a Chicago woman in her sixties who recently flew home from China.[16] She saw her physician for respiratory issues. The doctor immediately admitted her to a Chicago-area hospital and placed her in isolation before her test came back positive. (Her blood sample had to be sent to the CDC in Atlanta, since the US hasn't approved a test for distribution.)

Scientists measure the spread of a virus by its reproductive ratio—Ro; "R-naught" as the British say it—an estimate of how many people are likely to be infected by a single individual. If one person infects two people, then the Ro is 2.0. If the Ro is larger than 1.0, the virus will spread rapidly. Even a low-virulence disease can be scary if it spreads quickly. Influenza plus pneumonia has a lethality rate of around 0.1 percent. So, if this new coronavirus has a Ro over 1.0 for very long—and kills like the flu plus pneumonia—China, and maybe all of east Asia, could be looking at many thousands of deaths before it's contained.

These are scary numbers, but the odds seem good this time won't be as bad as the SARS epidemic two decades ago, when 774 people died.[17] Health experts are already running tests and conducting contact tracing for this new virus. In addition, significant scientific and technological advances have taken place since the 2002–03 outbreak. Genetic sequencing is inexpensive and easy now. Chinese scientists sequenced the genome of this new virus two weeks ago and shared it with the world.[18] American scientists did their own sequencing this week.[19] In contrast, when SARS appeared in Canada seventeen years ago, scientists operated more or less in the dark.

According to Michael B. A. Oldstone, professor of immunology and microbiology at Scripps Research in La Jolla, California, scientists know this virus relatively well. They are called coronaviruses because they have "crowns" around the outside that act as grappling hooks, allowing coronaviruses to cling to the cells of their hosts' respiratory systems.[20] Eventually, dead cells broken up by the virus clog the lungs, and if your body can't clean up the damage fast enough, you can suffer from respiratory distress and even suffocate to death. Thankfully, these coronaviruses usually are not lethal, Oldstone tells me. The common cold is probably due to a coronavirus, but so are the original SARS and MERS, both of which are much deadlier. And, he cautions, even less deadly viruses can be terribly destructive if they transmit effectively.

This wouldn't be much of a concern, except they are saying now that the virus has been with us for a while. The amount of genetic change shown between the original samples of the virus and more recent ones reveals to virologists like Andrew Rambaut at the University of Edinburgh that this new coronavirus has been circulating for about *two months*.[21] Trump promises that Xi's government is on top of it. But the worry in the scientific and medical community is the virus has a high transmission rate and has already traveled much farther than our government is admitting.

MONDAY, JANUARY 27, 2020

The basketball legend Kobe Bryant died in a tragic helicopter accident yesterday. Some corners of the internet say he was assassinated. But this is a hoax—a conspiracy theory pushed by one self-described psychologist.[22] There is an epidemic of false information, hoaxes, and conspiracies like this one on nearly any topic on any given day.

Take the hoaxes surrounding the new virus, for instance. Though many Americans learned about this novel coronavirus only a few days ago, one conspiracy theory—that Bill and Melinda Gates took out a patent on a coronavirus vaccine in 2015—has been retweeted at least fifteen thousand times.[23] A YouTube video promoting this hoax has over 2.6 million views.

Many conspiracy theories are openly partisan, insisting that members of the so-called Deep State are colluding with Democratic politicians. Others traffic in racism and xenophobia. One story claimed that 2.8 million people in China are infected and 112,000 have died, while the Chinese government manipulates WHO and the international news media to promulgate a lower count.[24] These numbers are preposterous, unlikely to happen in a country with modern healthcare. Hoaxers attach images of rioting people on the streets of Beijing to their posts, reinforcing barbaric stereotypes. These right-wing conspiracy theorists neglect to mention that, at least for now, Trump's message is that China has this new coronavirus under control.

In the past, news funneled through print media, radio, television, and film. Much of it, funded by big corporations or governments, was subject to some editorial oversight. Now, "the truth" has become a commodity whose manufacture is determined by the market. Any person can post an idea or a video that can go "viral"—absolutely no pun intended—regardless of its veracity. Now more than ever, market-driven "truth," hacked together on the internet, drives the news that major broadcasters tell. A massive 2018 study showed that false news spreads much more rapidly than truth in our social media-saturated society.[25] And some of it, via Fox News, reaches the president, who repeats, amplifies, and legitimizes the falsehoods.

WEDNESDAY, JANUARY 29, 2020

In his timeless book, *A Journal of the Plague Year*, Daniel Defoe recounts the fear that struck people before the pestilence spread through London in 1665. Frightened Londoners "thronged out of the town . . . Indeed, nothing was to be seen but wagons and carts, with goods, women, servants, children . . . all hurrying away."[26] Today, like so many times before in human history, people are running from plague.

Two hundred and ten worried US foreign service workers and their families left Wuhan and landed this morning in California.[27] The National Center for Emerging and Zoonotic Infectious Diseases, a division of the CDC, screened them—although this screening can't have been very telling, since it takes days for tests from the CDC in Atlanta to come back with results. Workers with the Administration for Children and Families (ACF), a division of Health and Human Services (HHS), will help them settle into the base today. From there, they can decide whether to remain in quarantine for three days or to travel to their homes across the country, where they will self-monitor for an additional fourteen days. Compared to the reportedly strict lockdown of Wuhan and the Hubei region, it is a modest intervention.

Meanwhile, Mike Ryan, executive director of the WHO Health Emergencies Programme, takes the podium at a hurried press conference in Geneva. Fifteen countries now have infected citizens. "They have to stop transmission," he says emphatically. He believes "chains of transmission can still be interrupted," but there is worry in his voice.[28] Coronavirus is spreading fast.

There is a lot we know. Right now, WHO reports 6,065 cases and around 250 deaths globally. Only a handful of infected people reside in the United States. We know it is another viral respiratory disease caused by a SARS coronavirus. Its most obvious symptoms include fever and a dry, persistent cough. We also know who it endangers the most. An article published in the *Journal of Medical Virology* charts the first seventeen deaths from Wuhan.[29] More males died from this disease than females—average age, seventy-five. Most people in this group lived only fourteen days from the time they reported their first symptoms. Two weeks from coughing to dead. Eleven showed comorbidities like diabetes, heart disease, cirrhosis of the liver, and hypertension.

Most of these comorbidities are associated with modern, stereotypically Western lifestyles. That's another reason for those of us in Europe and North America to hope the fifteen countries where the virus has been detected are able to contain it.

THURSDAY, JANUARY 30, 2020

Some health officials argue that yesterday's evacuations from China are an overreaction. "It doesn't make sense," protests Paul Offit, a prominent pediatrician and flu vaccine promotor at the Perelman School of Medicine at University of Pennsylvania, during a CDC telebriefing.[30] Influenza kills thirty thousand Americans a year, he says, yet we don't put an entire plane full of passengers into quarantine in California for that. We have detained people in the March Air Reserve Base, and there are *zero* Americans dead, Offit complains. He echoes the president, who again insists everything is okay, that the Chinese government has the virus under control.

Nevertheless, today, Trump asks HHS to launch the White House Coronavirus Task Force (CTF). Alex Azar Jr., the Trump-appointed head of HHS, will lead it. Azar signals HHS will soon declare this a public health emergency and confirms the suspicions first aired last Friday that Chinese scientists uncovered direct person-to-person spread.[31]

Creating a vaccine will be the only real solution. Companies like Johnson & Johnson have already started working on such a vaccine for the Chinese market. Vaccines for viruses are difficult to develop, though. We take them for granted now, but each vaccine represents many years, often decades, of research. Funding is often a problem in vaccine development. Back in 2016, researchers at the Center for Vaccine Development in Texas reported being unable to attract investors to finance work on the first SARS coronavirus.[32] Vaccine developers must avoid antibody-dependent enhancement, which occurs when a vaccine makes it *easier* for an infection to invade the host cell.[33] Even when safe and effective vaccines have been readily available for decades, increasing numbers of anti-vaxxers are encouraging completely unnecessary deaths. A shocking 142,000 *preventable* measles deaths occurred globally just last year.[34]

Until a vaccine is developed, personal protective equipment (PPE), including face masks, face shields, and gloves, will be the best way to protect against this new 2019-nCoV. Today, the Chinese government appeals to other countries to sell PPE to them, a move that raises eyebrows, given that Chinese manufacturers produce most of the masks on the planet.[35] There may soon be a strain on the world's PPE supply.

Even after a week of disconcerting news from China, Americans seem not to have noticed. Posts online continue to mourn Kobe Bryant, celebrate Joaquin Phoenix's Oscar nomination for *Joker*, gossip over Meghan Markle's impending departure from Buckingham Palace, and fret over Valentine's Day, which is just around the corner.

One exception is Laurie Garrett, a science journalist who won a Pulitzer Prize in 1996 for her work tracking Ebola. Garrett is sounding an alarm for anyone who will listen. Screening for this coronavirus won't work, she says, because it can spread without showing symptoms. Screening temperatures at airports only sets up a "false sense of defense," a kind of health theater. She, too, is concerned there is no vaccine for *any* coronavirus to date, especially because antibodies to coronaviruses do not persist—even if you have them, you don't stay immune for long.[36] It is surprising to hear someone of Garrett's prominence yelling so loudly while someone like Paul Offit claims that we are *over*reacting. Is Laurie Garrett a Chicken Little or a prophetic Cassandra?

While some are figuring out the science of the virus, others are already assigning blame. A French newspaper calls the virus the Yellow Peril, a racist phrase from the nineteenth century. It gets picked up in the US. Westerners blame the coronavirus on what they imagine are the Chinese habits of consuming bats and other exotic animals. Sinophobia has been a staple of American nativist rhetoric for two centuries. Americans blamed East Asians in the 1800s for the spread of smallpox, syphilis, and the plague partly as a justification for the US colonial project in the nineteenth century.[37] That stigmatization was one of the reasons for the passing of the Chinese Exclusion Act in 1882, which barred immigration based solely on race and was repealed only because the United States needed Chinese air bases to fight the Japanese in World War II.[38]

This attitude feeds into the low point of the day, when Commerce secretary Wilbur Ross claims that all the death and disruption in China has a silver lining. "I don't want to take a victory lap over a very unfortunate, malignant disease," he says, just before taking a victory lap over a disease, "but if the Chinese are too sick to handle the work, healthy Americans will step in and expand their businesses."[39] He does not seem to consider how easily the tables could turn if the coronavirus spreads here.

FRIDAY, JANUARY 31, 2020

Americans are now paying attention to the new coronavirus. It's a noticeable shift since just yesterday—probably because the Trump administration imposed a travel ban on the whole country of China.

I decide to examine internet search trends for the month of January to track the level of concern among Americans over this virus compared to the flu. My search reveals that people became much more interested in the term "corona*" (the asterisk captures any use of the term, regardless of syntax) on January 20, coinciding with reporting on the first case in Washington State. Simple enough.

It gets more interesting when I examine searches for "flu," looking at the past two years of flu seasons, from September 2017 through January 2020. Searches for "flu" were very high in the winter of 2018 and slightly lower in 2019. They are beginning to rise again in 2020. The year 2018 was a particularly bad one for the flu; CDC estimates were 79,400 deaths—a 0.16 percent mortality rate. In 2019, 42.9 million got influenza, with 61,200 deaths—a slightly lower 0.14 percent mortality rate. We are well into this year's flu season. Perhaps what we see at the end of this month just reflects the usual cycle of flu cases escalating.

And yet, three weeks ago, the NIAID's Anthony Fauci noted that flu levels in the second week of the year looked more like the levels on the fifth or sixth week of a typical year, when they tend to be worse. I worry when seeing these search trends that Fauci is only partly right—flu itself may have peaked early and already started to fade away. What if increases in searches this week are not really for the *flu*? According to Google Trends, there are a lot of people going online trying to figure out what to do about their flu *symptoms*. Could they have the novel coronavirus and not realize it?

Evidence is growing that coronavirus spreads even when the infected person is not showing symptoms—a point Chinese health officials made last week, and Laurie Garrett underscored yesterday. Today, physicians report in the *New England Journal of Medicine* (*NEJM*) that a businesswoman from China traveling in Germany spread the virus during a business meeting, though she wasn't obviously sick.[40] Add that to what we know about the original US patient in Seattle who was moving around for several days without symptoms only two weeks ago. It appears people could go days without seeming sick at all, all while actively spreading coronavirus.

Travel from China to the United States is banned, but what about the rest of the world? Across the political spectrum no one has interest in shutting down international travel. Banning travel only from China seems like an ineffectual smoke screen, a bit of "security theater," like we saw after 9/11, when entire populations were required to go through the motions of heightened security, which was ultimately shown to be ineffective.[41] All the while, individuals are not prevented from leaving China to go West, potentially spreading the virus before crossing the Atlantic via London or Frankfurt.

SUNDAY, FEBRUARY 2, 2020

Jerome Adams ✓
@JeromeAdamsMD

> Roses are red
> Violets are blue
> Risk is low for **#coronavirus**
> But high for the **#flu**
> So get your **#FLUSHOT!** 🙏

7:38 AM—Feb 1, 2020

Surgeon General Jerome Adams tweeted this Valentine's-themed poem yesterday. Save your real worry for the flu, he says. Physicians and politicians retweet it throughout the day. This assurance again ripples through national media: don't be frightened. Even if the virus does come in a real way to our shores, the *New York Times* assures us, the US, like other wealthy countries, will detect and contain it. It's countries with fragile healthcare systems, like India, the Philippines, and rural Russia, that will suffer.[1] The Sunday newspapers have spoken as a single chorus, from the largest national outlets, like *USA Today*, to smaller markets in the interior of the country.[2] Epidemiologists repeat it on their Twitter feeds. Even in Seattle, which has active coronavirus cases, the mantra is the same: the flu "is a much bigger threat than the new coronavirus."[3]

Media representing both sides of the political aisle seem to be welcoming this message. Left-leaning *BuzzFeed News* and *Vox* confidently proclaim this virus does not have the makings of a pandemic. This offers a chance to stop stigmatizing the Chinese. Right-wing media also welcomes the focus on the flu. Here is the opportunity to tamp down on what they have, from the beginning, seen as over-coverage of the coronavirus.[4] Any time an event looks as if it might challenge President Trump's leadership, it is critical they minimize that threat.

Trump himself hasn't tweeted or spoken about the coronavirus in three days. When he speaks to Fox News personality Sean Hannity today, he focuses on the upcoming election. "African American poverty numbers are the best they've ever had," he says. "So, I don't know how anybody could possibly beat me with that vote."[5]

What attention was being paid to this virus has slowed significantly in just forty-eight hours. Granted, there is still the online maelstrom of hyperbolic myths, conspiracy theories, and hoaxes. But so many other things have leapt up: LeBron James's LA Lakers are honoring the late Kobe Bryant at tonight's game, and there's Super Bowl LIV between the Chiefs and the 49ers. Maybe the journalists and advertisers who drive the news feel the need to move on to something more . . . entertaining?

MONDAY, FEBRUARY 3, 2020

The new coronavirus death toll is now over 360 in Hubei Province, higher than the original SARS in the 2002–03 outbreak.[6]

Chinese citizens are upset with their government's handling of the outbreak. Last Friday, ophthalmologist Li Wenliang died of the virus after trying to warn people that something terrible was happening. The Chinese government censored him in late 2019. Then, after he signed an official apology for "rumormongering," he contracted the virus. Today, on the popular Chinese online social network, the Wuhan Central Hospital mourns, "all-out efforts to save him failed." The outpouring of emotion from the Chinese people is overwhelming. One Weibo post says, "The only thing is not to forget."

That's right, of course. "The struggle of man against power is the struggle of memory against forgetting," penned Czech author Milan Kundera fifty years ago.[7] The tragedy of Dr. Li reminds us all that under the weight of a powerful and callous government, one can be made to apologize for one's own death. But one cannot be forced to forget. When the Chinese people agree not to forget Dr. Li, they refuse to relinquish to the regime the power that real History confers. They fight quietly to remember things as they were, as opposed to remembering a past that the powerful construct for them.

TUESDAY, FEBRUARY 4, 2020

WHO pronounces SARS2 not a pandemic, only an epidemic: a disease widespread but contained to a single region or population. To be called a pandemic, the disease must be uncontrolled in multiple countries and, though there are infected individuals in Asia, Europe, and North America, WHO doesn't consider it uncontained. News agencies broadcast this information with some amount of relief. Apparently, it's not critical that a cruise ship, the *Diamond Princess*, with ten cases, is now quarantining off the coast of Japan. The media likewise doesn't appear to be concerned that the US Food and Drug Administration (FDA) just authorized the broader production of coronavirus tests. Most of us are confident that the "people in the know" are handling it.

America's attention has shifted palpably away from this new virus. Perhaps all the "flu is worse" coverage makes it seem like China's lockdown of Wuhan and halting of travel for millions during Chunyun was overkill. We are instead caught up in other serious stories, like trying to understand what happened at the Iowa Democratic presidential caucus last night. (Two voting apps evidently crashed. No one yet knows whether Bernie Sanders or Pete Buttigieg won. This will certainly serve as proof to some that Democrats are too incompetent to defeat even an impeached president). The news is reporting that Greenland's ice sheet, which alone holds enough water to raise global sea levels by a staggering 24 feet, is melting seven times faster than it was in 1992.[8] And the trial of Harvey Weinstein, the film producer, continues, with more women coming forward to accuse him of sexual assault. Weinstein and hundreds of other perpetrators are finally being brought to a reckoning.

THURSDAY, FEBRUARY 6, 2020

Today's events highlighted a worrisome phenomenon that has been on the rise in scientific publishing for some years. It turns out the *NEJM* article released last week about the businesswoman from China who spread the new coronavirus in Germany before she started to show symptoms made an error. Evidently, the doctors who wrote the original article never interviewed this woman; she did have mild symptoms when she traveled to Germany, which seems to upend the claim that the virus can be passed by asymptomatic people.[9]

The *NEJM* released the article to the public as a preprint; it was posted to the internet before it was peer-reviewed. Since the 1800s, the process of peer review has been pretty much the same. Scientists and scholars conduct research, write up their results, and submit their work to an academic journal for consideration. The editor sends the article to several peer specialists in the same field who review the article and send their feedback on its merits back to the editor, who forwards the needed revisions, or the rejection, to the authors. Once the authors revise their article, it goes back to the peer reviewers again. The cycle might repeat four or five times. This model is ubiquitous; it is the hallmark of quality research in all fields.

There are problems with peer review, however, not least of which is that it can take *years* to get published. An alternative is to share research online, with peer review happening after the fact. Scientists post these "preprints" in central repositories like arXiv.org, viXra.org, bioRxiv, chemRxiv, and medRxiv.[10] Nearly all print journals have joined the rXiv trend and have some version of this preprint system running.

"Preprinting" gets information out quickly, but it has problems, too. The general public doesn't necessarily understand the difference between a preprint and a peer-reviewed article. Sometimes preprint articles that would not pass peer review are read by science journalists and bloggers who then report on them as though they were verified science. Those articles then get reposted hundreds and thousands of times, creating immense confusion. These days "eyeballs," "clicks," and "downloads" often matter more, even professionally, than careful peer review.[11]

In the wake of this most recent problem with the *NEJM* preprint regarding asymptomatic spread, WHO releases an equivocal report: "Transmission from asymptomatic cases is likely not a major driver of transmission. Persons who are symptomatic will spread the virus more readily."[12] So, we should be aware of people coughing and sneezing, but not worry so much that asymptomatic cases are floating around everywhere we go.

While that news is mildly comforting, this isn't: the first American citizen has died of coronavirus in a Wuhan hospital.[13]

Lastly today, something that should be historic and shocking yet feels anything but: the Senate voted not to convict the president. We knew that antagonistic partisanship determined this outcome weeks ago. The only noteworthy moment occurred when Mitt Romney (R-UT) became the first senator to vote his conscience for the removal of a president of his own party. Romney's moving speech reminds us of just how far this president will go to accumulate and retain power.[14] "It was a flagrant assault on our electoral rights, our national security interests, and our fundamental values," Romney intones. If Romney is right, then we have cause to worry that Trump might even be willing to withhold information about the dangers of this coronavirus from the American public, if it would serve his interests.

TUESDAY, FEBRUARY 11, 2020

At the suggestion of the International Committee on Taxonomy of Viruses, the coronavirus name was changed from 2019-nCOV to "SARS-CoV-2." No easier to say or spell, perhaps, but it links it clearly to SARS and MERS. The disease caused by this coronavirus is now called COVID-19, short for *co*rona*v*irus *d*isease 20*19*. Popularly, many call it "Rona," as in, "wash your hands, cough into your elbow, don't catch the Rona."

Even if the United States has dodged a bullet this time, our luck won't last forever. Our healthcare technology may be advanced enough to fight many diseases, but some experts warn that we are not prepared for an actual pandemic. David Himmelstein, a specialist in internal medicine at New York's Albert Einstein College of Medicine and a lecturer at Harvard Medical School, calls America's healthcare a "brittle, just-in-time" system. "It's a byproduct of being competitive rather than cooperative," Himmelstein emphasizes to me. "We don't think about what the community needs; we think about our position in the market." Even hospitals think this way.

That mentality emerged decades ago, Himmelstein says. It began in the late-1960s, with the tug-of-war between healthcare providers, insurance companies, and the federal government over Medicare. A key moment came in the mid-1970s, when Robert B. Fetter and John D. Thompson at

Yale formulated the diagnosis-related group (DRG) system. "The DRG system folded hospital capital into operating costs," Himmelstein explains. While this "managed care" slowed down the increase in healthcare expenses passed on through Medicare to the federal government, it created two unintended consequences. "Hospitals did not used to be operated like businesses—financially or 'spiritually,' for lack of a better term." But since these DRG reforms took off, hospitals understood they would have to generate not only enough revenue to keep the doors open but to build capital for facility improvement. "Your future then depends on surplus," clarifies Himmelstein. Since surplus couldn't be created from Medicare patients, the goal of hospitals shifted to attracting privately insured patients and submitting them to every reasonable billable treatment. "Clinical behaviors went out of control," as Himmelstein puts it. And the tension between healthcare providers, the government, and health insurers ratcheted up.

Now, even people *with* private health insurance can't afford the care they receive.[15] In just the last decade or so, health insurance premiums rose 55 percent, even though our earnings have only increased 26 percent. Deductibles have risen 200 percent.[16] So when you need to go to the doctor, you know you might have to pay a huge bill even if you're covered by an expensive health insurance policy.[17] Private equity (PE) firms—basically rich people acquiring and flipping companies for a profit—have been on a buying spree of healthcare facilities such as elder care homes in the last two decades. They slash staff and raise prices in order to increase revenue before selling them. Motivated only by short-term profit, these PE-owned firms make healthcare even more unaffordable, all while sacrificing quality of care.

The Affordable Care Act, also known as Obamacare, was supposed to help more people get insurance. And it did. Yet that didn't control costs. Moreover, the GOP has been trying to repeal or hobble it for the last decade. They talk of the "sanctity of choice" and the danger of "socialized medicine." They argue that if we were to enshrine every American's inalienable right to healthcare (as we protect the right to carry firearms), we would end up in some hellscape where overworked, communist doctors stage "death panels" to decide who gets to live or die.[18] It's ridiculous hyperbole. And, in any case, the notion that, even with insurance, we currently choose our healthcare is a joke. It's like asking me if I want to buy a Bugatti or a Ferrari. My answer is, well, I can't afford any of it, and so I will stay home and die.

As professor of sociology and public affairs Paul Starr and healthcare journalist Elisabeth Rosenthal have been pointing out for years, American healthcare has become a profitmaking juggernaut only tangentially connected to the job of helping the sick.[19] The motto is: "More treatment is always better; always default to the most expensive option," says Rosenthal.[20] It's so bad that when new doctors come out of medical school with massive debt, they feel they can't *afford* to become general practitioners or primary care physicians because they would do fewer procedures and, therefore, make much less money. Gastric sleeves and angioplasties—that's where the bank is. In our acute-care-based, fee-for-service model, physicians are disincentivized to consider cost to the consumer or quality of life if it means refraining from ordering another test.[21]

Prevention does not make the profit that procedures do, confirms Edward Hoffer, cardiologist and researcher in medical informatics at Massachusetts General Hospital.[22] Even if it is far better to help a diabetic manage their blood sugar through regular checkups that could keep them alive for ten more good years, it's more profitable to the organization—it "generates more surplus," to use Himmelstein's term—to amputate a foot when a patient comes in after years of little to no preventative care, all so they can live for five more painful months. No decent doctor would ever choose this course of action for a patient simply for profit. Yet it's worth emphasizing that all of us, from patient to physician, remain at the mercy of a healthcare payment system that currently places less value on preventative care than the bottom line.

THURSDAY, FEBRUARY 13, 2020

Historian of medicine Robert P. Hudson notes that infectious diseases are "dynamic social constructions that have biographies of their own."[23] Many of the most memorable ones—the 1918 flu, AIDS in the 1980s, Ebola just this past decade—craft dramatic narrative arcs to go with lots of carnage. I hope that is not true of this coronavirus.

Especially as I find myself flying across the country today.

In the Charlotte airport, I see on a TV that scientists in China recalibrated their infection count. Previously, Chinese physicians only counted a patient as having the novel coronavirus if they had a confirmation from their RNA-based test. Doctors can now use computerized

Timeline of Coronavirus Onset

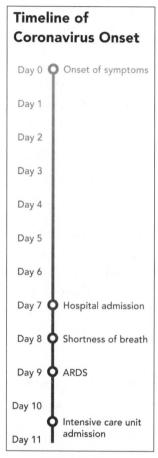

Day 0 ○ Onset of symptoms

Day 1

Day 2

Day 3

Day 4

Day 5

Day 6

Day 7 ○ Hospital admission

Day 8 ○ Shortness of breath

Day 9 ○ ARDS

Day 10

Day 11 ○ Intensive care unit admission

How the virus progresses from contraction to the intensive care. Data from C. Huang et al., "Clinical Features of Patients Infected with 2019 Novel Coronavirus in Wuhan, China," *Lancet*, Feb. 15, 2020. Image credit: Elsevier.

tomography (CT) scans to make diagnoses from patients' lungs. As soon as that criteria change took place, the number of COVID-19 cases shot up: around 15,000 new cases and at least 242 deaths reported *in one day*.[24] By comparison, about 8,000 people came down with the first SARS in *total* in 2003.[25] Without those other diagnostics, if China's physicians measured only when the RNA tests revealed coronavirus, the cases would have risen by only 1,508.[26] This means that their previous diagnoses were potentially off by a factor of *ten*. Does this mean *global* cases are far higher, too? Our new SARS is declaratively more menacing than its 2003 predecessor.

The TV blaring above me switches to the Democratic presidential primaries. Lots of people are "feeling the Bern" for Bernie Sanders in Iowa and New Hampshire, while poor Joe Biden is getting crushed. Meanwhile, I see *no one* being screened at any point in *any* airport, even people who are obviously, openly coughing. Maybe it wouldn't matter anyway; the CDC admits something went wrong in the first batch of tests they sent to state health officials over the last couple of weeks.[27] Judging by the news blasting in the airport, the media is too invested in the Democratic horse race to notice this mishap.

SATURDAY, FEBRUARY 22, 2020

News about the *Diamond Princess* feels like the Chernobyl meltdown mixed with a bit of *Gilligan's Island*—bad choices, none of which by themselves are too terrible, that cumulatively spell disaster. On January 17, an eighty-year-old man from Hong Kong flew to Tokyo to meet his family for a cruise. He hadn't visited any wet markets, but he had spent a day in Shenzhen, China, more than two weeks earlier. The *Diamond Princess* was scheduled to leave from the Yokohama port in Tokyo on January 20 with 2,666 passengers and 1,045 crew members for a fourteen-day tour of Kagoshima, Hong Kong, swinging around Vietnam, then Keelung in Taiwan, and back to Japan.[28] The day before departure, he developed a cough but boarded the *Diamond Princess* anyway.

Five days into the trip, he felt sick enough to get off the boat in Hong Kong. At Princess Margaret Hospital, physicians CT-scanned his lungs and saw signs of infection.[29] But only when his RNA test results arrived seven days later did the Hong Kong government officially announce he had coronavirus.

On February 2, the final night of the cruise, the *Diamond Princess* captain informed passengers about the ship's case of coronavirus. No one seem fazed. They went to shows, played games, and took dance lessons. To their surprise, the next day, instead of disembarking in Yokohama, Japan, they stopped at a spot off the Daikoku Pier, with no word of when they might dock. Two days later, on February 5, officials ordered a lockdown of the ship, and the news finally broke that no one would be leaving for two weeks.[30]

Passengers with fevers waited for days to be tested while sick staff wandered the ship serving others. On February 17, the US chartered *Diamond Princess* passengers back to the very same naval base where the American diplomats from China arrived just a couple of weeks ago. Even today, 1,300 passengers and crew remain onboard.

All of this seems worryingly *ad hoc.* The Japan Ministry of Health says that from the first day of the quarantine, February 5, to February 22, active cases swelled from 10 to 634.[31] How can we be sure that the people who left the boat weren't sick? If we now know people can spread coronavirus without obvious symptoms, then have these actions by multiple governments just facilitated viral dispersal around the world?

SUNDAY, FEBRUARY 23, 2020

There's dire news out of Italy and Iran. Social media videos show body bags stacked in closets and mass graves. Consequently, Americans are paying attention to the virus again.

Looking back on American internet searches, I can see that that our initial interest lasted through January 31. But then Americans stopped searching for information on coronavirus until just this weekend. Why this lull through February?

My first suspicion is that television media went quiet in its coverage of the virus, diverting attention to politics and celebrity. To test this hypothesis, I ask two research assistants to track and chart as much media coverage as possible of the coronavirus since January. They go off to comb the major networks: CNN, MSNBC, ABC, CBS, NBC, and Fox News. More on that later. I also wonder if Americans' declining interest in coronavirus could have been related to the widespread message that the flu is worse. Or, perhaps, Americans believed Trump's assertion that Premier Xi had it under control.

Either way, we are paying attention now. Two people dead in Qom, Iran, and they have shut down the schools. Italy, which had ten cases ten days ago, has 152 today. These cases are not all connected to the Italian man who originally contracted the virus in China. This means that there is community spread in Italy now. Milan, Venice, and other towns in Italy have closed opera houses, postponed the carnival, and scrubbed soccer matches. Giorgio Armani was forced to show his new collection for Fashion Week solely online.[32] In response, Austria is halting all trains coming from Italy at the Brenner Pass, where Mussolini and Hitler met to celebrate their Pact of Steel in 1940. Italian officials swear that none of these people have been to China.[33] Similar news comes from South Korea, which has leapt from 28 cases nine days ago to 763 today. Clearly, the second SARS coronavirus is moving quickly through Europe and the Middle East. It was not contained, as Trump assured the world.

MONDAY, FEBRUARY 24, 2020

I'm in a waiting room at the doctor's office. Rush Limbaugh's televised recording of his radio show is playing on the TV, mounted high in the corner of the room. I often ask to turn off blaring televisions in doctors' offices, but I don't think the tight-lipped receptionist is giving up the remote control. She stares intently at the screen.

As a scholar who works on the history of propaganda, I acknowledge Limbaugh's mastery of tried-and-true agitprop techniques. He repeats specific adjectives and phrases when referring to opposition groups, describing Democrats as overly emotional, uninformed dupes, or mentally ill. "Crazy Bernie" is his nickname for Bernie Sanders, who looks on track to be the next Democratic presidential candidate. Female Democrats he calls "feminazis." The press he labels "corrupt." Black and brown people he insinuates are dangerous in some way—he infamously dubbed the NBA the "Thug Basketball Association."[34] Limbaugh slots people into archetypes, offering a simple and predictable worldview to his devotees, one filled with heroes and villains, paladins and thieves. It is a classic approach, intended to unify one's target audience in opposition to a shared, monstrous enemy.

In addition to name-calling and stereotyping, Limbaugh mobilizes the techniques of classic agitprop as he shapes each of his broadcasts around one critical argument, repeated during each segment. Today, it's "this coronavirus thing." Like any propagandist, he chisels his argument from the bedrock beliefs of his audience. Step One: disprove and dismiss the standard narrative—the lies told by "elitists" controlling the media. On the video broadcast, you see him sit up, almost bouncing, in his seat. He takes off his glasses and puts them on his desk, then leans toward his gold-plated microphone. "Now I want to tell you the truth about the coronavirus." He raises both arms up beside him like he's trying to hold a pregnancy ball. "The coronavirus is the common cold, folks! The drive-by media hype of this thing"—he draws out that last word, "thingggg"—"as a pandemic, as the Andromeda Strainnn, as OH MY GOD if you get it you're dead!" You can see and hear the scorn in his voice as his arms flap up and down. He stumbles looking for the right word, "the survival rate is 98 percent?!?" Any media reporting on the dangers of the virus, he suggests, must conceal a hidden agenda.

A few seconds later, he moves into Step Two: identify additional enemies. "It probably is a ChiCom [short for "Chinese communists"] laboratory experiment that is in the process of being weaponized," he says. "All superpower nations weaponize bioweapons. They experiment with them. The Russians, for example, have weaponized fentanyl." Never mind that Trump has defended Xi from criticism over his handling of the outbreak. Limbaugh's message resonates because it feeds into his listeners' established suspicion of Chinese perfidy. A good lie always has some truth to it. It begins by reminding the audience that the Chinese state steals intellectual property—a phenomenon that has been known to happen. Using this verified piece of information, Limbaugh can argue to susceptible audiences that myriad Chinese crimes are in the works. It is not a big leap to believe that they could also design and release a terrible bioweapon in order to give themselves a global trade advantage.

Step Three: establish a "real" truth that makes it possible for the people in the group to believe that they are able to see reality while everyone else remains in the dark. This truth reaffirms what the audience already believes. After a tangent about the relative harmlessness of fentanyl when taken in small doses (!), he points out to his listeners that the stock market has collapsed by nine hundred points in the wake of this coronavirus scare. He pauses and sighs, letting his exasperation sit in the silence. He raises his left hand in a shooing, dismissive gesture, like a scientist responding to a claim that the sun revolves around the earth. He repeats that only 2 percent of people with the virus die, far less than the flu. He goes on to claim that the whole story is just media hype meant to generate audience interest. He mentions again the idea that the Chinese have weaponized the virus, and then he closes, "By virtue of the media, I think this is an effort to bring down Trump. And one of the ways is to scare investors."

Limbaugh's performance presents a series of fragmented realities that create a whole world in which even the deceiver is deceived. It generates a sense of unity, founded on delusion, that demands we ignore its contradictions. For instance, if the Chinese have weaponized a lethal virus, they mustn't have done a very good job since Limbaugh is also arguing that the virus is no more of a threat than the common cold. He speaks of the virus only killing 2 percent of the population. Yet, if everyone on the planet contracted this virus, and the virus has a 2 percent mortality rate, *152 million people* would die. Upwards of *3 million* Americans would die. That's one whole city of Chicago, two Philadelphias, four Washington, DCs, or nine New Orleanses, wiped out. Limbaugh is arguing that the press of the entire world cares so much about us Americans that they concocted this apocalyptic scenario to scare our investors—all just to hurt Trump. What hubris and ego are required to believe that the press of the world spends this much time thinking about us?

An estimated thirty-five million listeners, including the other people in this doctor's office, hear Limbaugh say that this virus is a political ploy engineered by communists and the liberal global press to tear down their president. Limbaugh has not just politicized the virus; he has transformed it into a moment of identity building. His audience will be expected to perform in a certain way in order to reaffirm this message and assert their identity as conservatives. He has made dismissing the coronavirus part of the larger performance of being "in the know," "owning the libs," and "melting the snowflakes." By invalidating the realities of this virus, he makes *his reality* real for his listeners.

This performance wields tremendous power. "The spectacle is the bad dream of a modern society in chains," philosopher Guy Debord wrote.[35] "If we've been bamboozled long enough," warned scientist Carl Sagan, ". . . we're no longer interested in finding out the truth. The bamboozle has captured us."[36] Now that Limbaugh's audience has seen the spectacle, possibly been captured by the bamboozle, they will repeat it on social media, at the bar, before the meeting, around the dinner table. If we reach a moment when the nation must come together to fight this virus, this spectacle could do incalculable harm.

TUESDAY, FEBRUARY 25, 2020

In 2018, the Trump administration actively signaled it did not take the possibility of a pandemic seriously by scrapping the country's major response capability, including the National Safety Council's entire global health security unit. They removed $15 billion in health spending, cut the operational budgets of the CDC, DHS, and HHS, and even eliminated the Complex Crises Fund.[37] This was part of the GOP's scaling back of government services they deemed necessary in order to grant tax breaks, mostly for the wealthy.[38]

This trend continues today when Secretary Azar—Trump's man in charge of the White House Coronavirus Task Force (CTF)—asks for $2.5 billion from the Senate Appropriations Committee, only half of which will fight the coronavirus, and simultaneously, maintains that the virus is well under control. Even Senator Richard Shelby (R-AL) raises an eyebrow and asks Azar if he's sure they need so little. "If you low-ball something like this, you'll pay for it later," Shelby warns.[39]

The messaging on the virus is not consistent, and it is unclear whether or not we should worry. At one point today, Dr. Messonnier, director of the

CDC's NCIRD, warns it's not a matter of "if" this virus will hit the United States, but "when."[40] At the same time, the director of the US Economic Council says on cable news that there is nothing to worry about. It is not clear what—or who—to believe.

One thing is clear: American businesses are taking a hit.[41] United Airlines, for instance, is seeing its numbers of passengers decline by at least 5 percent.[42] The oil industry's prices are dropping. Apple says production of its iPhone will be seriously disrupted.[43] Sales of new cars in China have fallen by a staggering 92 percent.[44] In the last twenty-four hours, stocks across the globe plummet.[45] All the gains of the last two months on the US stock market have vanished in just the last forty-eight hours.

Our country has been fortunate: only fifty-seven cases so far, forty of which were from cruise ships. Limbaugh's histrionics notwithstanding, this virus is not a conspiracy to bring down Trump. However, it is potentially more widespread, harder to control, and trickier to manage than anything we have seen before. We could very well be standing on the brink of something monstrous.

WEDNESDAY, FEBRUARY 26, 2020

News of the virus is steady now. It generates a low hum of worry that accompanies me as I prepare lessons and meet with students. In the office, my colleagues and I wonder how we could possibly teach during a pandemic. For now, we put it out of our minds and go back to work. In the meantime, in the nation's capital, the Democrats push to give four times more funding than Azar's request—$8.5 billion—to stave off an emergency.[46]

In the afternoon, the president comes to the Coronavirus Task Force press conference. Other officials, white, older, and almost all male, stand around, smiling nervously. In disjointed comments, Trump repeats even now that "Xi has it under control." He goes on:

> We had a great talk. He's working very hard, I have to say. He's working very, very hard. And if you can count on the reports coming out of China, that spread has gone down quite a bit. . . . As opposed to getting larger, it's actually gotten smaller. In one instance where we think we can be—it's somewhat reliable, it seems to have gotten quite a bit smaller.

He then pivots to a soon-to-be-available vaccine:

> The vaccine is coming along well. And in speaking to the doctors, we think this is something that we can develop fairly rapidly, a vaccine for the future, and coordinate with the support of our partners.[47]

Trump shrugs and agrees to take whatever amount of coronavirus money Congress offers. Then he invokes his own version of a flu mortality statistic that appeared in the media earlier this month: "25,000 to 69,000 people a year" die of the flu. He claims we'll be down to a handful of infected people soon. He mentions a Johns Hopkins University report that the US is the "most prepared in the world" for a pandemic.

Then, oddly, the president places Vice President Pence in charge of the CTF, though Azar is still there, still *also* the head of the CTF, still saying that the risk to everyone is low, that the containment policies are working. The CDC's Anne Schuchat, one of the few women in the room, also seems to be saying that our quarantining of the individuals from Wuhan and the *Diamond Princess* worked. But then she makes a little warning that businesses and schools should get their "pandemic preparedness plans" together. Why would we need to prepare for a pandemic if there isn't one, if the quarantining worked? Also, *are* there pandemic preparedness plans? Who has these? I'm pretty sure my kid's school doesn't have these. Nor does my work.

Fauci then gets up and says that it is going to take a year to a year and a half to create and test a vaccine. This is not surprising, but given how quickly this second SARS appears to be spreading, it is a little disconcerting to hear that timeline stated so bluntly. A year to a year and a half is a long time.

THURSDAY, FEBRUARY 27, 2020

About a month ago, a dozen workers from the HHS's Administration for Children and Families (ACF) greeted hundreds of evacuees from Wuhan, China, at the March Air Reserve Base near Riverside, California, with its open expanse and palm trees lining the road. Another dozen met with more evacuees at Travis Air Force Base in Solano County, California. Some HHS workers wore full hazmat gear; a significant number of the ACF workers had little to no protective equipment, though they were interacting with potentially infected people.

Earlier this month, a whistleblower inside ACF complained about the oversight. In her complaint, she added that ACF workers left quarantine after these unprotected interactions with evacuees from Wuhan, even traveling on commercial flights to other parts of the United States.[48] If coronavirus spreads through people without symptoms, as several agencies have reported, then our own government employees may have inadvertently seeded the country. Azar's HHS office responded by assigning the whistleblower to a different job; she was told she would be fired if she didn't accept the reassignment.

Today, it looks like coronavirus has emerged in none other than Solano County, California. This new case signals open community spread of coronavirus, like in China, Spain, and Italy. Northern California might be headed toward a Wuhan-style lockdown. The infected woman in Solano County—like the Seattle man returning from Wuhan back in January—met dozens of people before seeking medical attention. Ten contact tracing specialists from HHS are on their way to California to help ensure that those to whom she may have spread the virus also quarantine.[49]

Why are we relying on whistleblowers to bring this to our attention? Have members of the executive branch lost their sense of whole-community obligation? Has the horse officially bolted from the stable?

FRIDAY, FEBRUARY 28, 2020

This morning, self-proclaimed "Rush baby" (what Limbaugh fans call themselves) Mick Mulvaney, Trump's acting White House chief of staff, affirms the narrative that people are overreacting to coronavirus at the Conservative Political Action Conference (CPAC). Like Limbaugh, he claims it's a conspiracy to bring down Trump.

By the evening, the idea of coronavirus as a hoax has had a chance to settle in the president's mind. He confirms it first to a CNN reporter who asks about Mulvaney's comments. Later, at a rally in Charleston, Trump grabs the podium, swaying under the lights. "Now the Democrats are politicizing the coronavirus," he tells the crowd. "They have no clue; they don't have any clue. . . . And this is their new hoax. But you know we did something that's been pretty amazing. We have 15 people in this massive country," he says, referring to the number of reported COVID-19 cases from earlier in the week, now inaccurate. He then turns to his flu numbers, "So a number that nobody heard of that I heard of recently . . . 35,000 people on average die each year from the flu. . . . It could go to a 100,000 . . . and so far we have lost nobody to coronavirus in the United States."[50] Though he inflates the flu numbers again, he is right, technically: None of the dozens in this country with the novel coronavirus has died.

It feels like a crack has emerged in our society's understanding of this virus. Some believe it's a hoax. Others believe that it presents imminent danger. It is not clear if this rift started with Limbaugh, but you can see it break open just this week—a widening crack that could very well bring the whole house down.

Despite the hoax rhetoric from the right wing, the financial markets have sensed something is wrong. This week has been the worst for Wall Street since the Great Recession of 2008–09. The Dow Jones index saw the worst drop in its *history* today—a sell-off that mirrored what has already happened from Asia through Europe.[51] Clorox and 3M, manufacturers of products useful for a viral pandemic, successfully rode out the slide. Insurance companies have been hit hard, presumably because investors know coronavirus is *not* a hoax.[52] Actual people will be headed to actual hospitals and filing actual claims. Also hit are the major airlines and hotel chains. Even within Europe, travel to Italy is dropping dramatically after the Italians declared two hundred new cases. Some cancel cruises, not because they're afraid of coronavirus, per se, but because they do not want to risk being quarantined on board, à la the *Diamond Princess*.[53]

It is true that we only have a small number of cases here. But two additional cases reported today have no clear link to China or any other place that is currently experiencing an outbreak. This means "community spread"—that they got it from somewhere here in America, many times removed from the original host.[54] The president assures us that the very best people are working hard and that his travel ban against China stopped it. But what happens if it is coming not just from China but Europe or western Asia as well? Trump's ban will have been of little use. Also, many of the tests issued by the CDC either did not work properly or were not administered correctly, which means we have *no idea* how pervasive this virus really is.[55]

SATURDAY, FEBRUARY 29, 2020

As I feared, yesterday's report of two new coronavirus cases, thought to be instances of community spread, turned out to be wildly optimistic. Today, we learn that we have closer to *one hundred cases*. Seventeen cases were evacuees and travelers from China or members of their families from January. Forty-two coronavirus cases came from the *Diamond Princess* and were quarantined at military bases after disembarking. The past two days revealed new cases not connected to the previous fifty-nine: A school worker in Lake Oswego, Oregon. Two people from Santa Clara County, California. A high school student in Everett, Washington, the town where the original patient from Wuhan appeared in January. None of these individuals have recently traveled overseas. None have had any contact with a traveler or any person known to be infected.

This morning, Governor Jay Inslee of Washington State declares a state of emergency when a man in his fifties dies from COVID-19 at Evergreen Hospital in Kirkland, becoming the first American to die inside the continental United States. The original coronavirus carrier lived in Snohomish, Washington, about twenty miles away, and no one has established a connection between them.[56] There is a suspected outbreak at a long-term facility in Kirkland, but the man who died has no connection to that place, either. Surely all of these individuals could not have gotten the virus from people traveling out of China. The CDC affirms the source of this spreading illness is unknown. Coronavirus is loose in the Pacific Northwest and perhaps across the entire West Coast.

I'm not sure we will be able to recontain it. In the meantime, the story that the virus is not real continues. Thrumming across social media and comments to news articles is the growing crescendo of that spectacle unleashed this week: It's a hoax, the Democrats have politicized it, Bill Gates is profiting from it, it's a Chinese weapon. Now on the list of symptoms of the illness that could doom us is our propensity to stitch every crisis, even a pathogen, into our partisan identities.

MONDAY, MARCH 2, 2020

Pediatrician and vaccine expert Paul Offit is again appearing on the national stage, this time on Christiane Amanpour's global affairs show on

CNN. At the CDC briefing on January 30, he said the flu is worse than coronavirus. He is again insisting people are making too big a deal of it. "I would be really surprised if this virus were able to catch up to the devastation that influenza virus causes," he reassures viewers. Between eighteen thousand and forty thousand Americans (a number quite a bit lower than Trump's) have died of the flu during this season alone. Coronavirus has killed two. What worries Offit is not this "outbreak," but that Americans will panic and "overwhelm the healthcare system" by demanding assessment of phantom symptoms. "It's really fear that we have to combat more than the virus itself," Offit opines, conjuring FDR's claim that "the only thing we have to fear is fear itself."[1] This is not the really serious kind of pandemic, he reassures, with a slight sardonic smile. If you have respiratory symptoms, you should "do what you ordinarily do with coughs and colds."

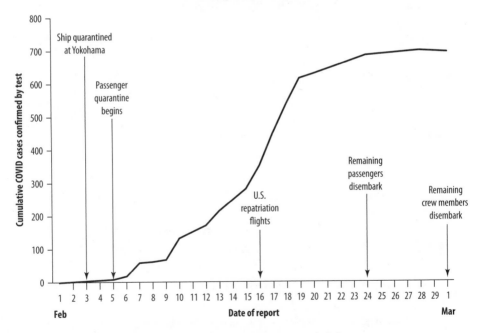

Timeline of the *Diamond Princess* Combined with Growing COVID Case Rates

Cases from passengers on the *Diamond Princess* have exploded even as passengers have disembarked. This does not bode well. (CDC, Statista)

At work, we talk occasionally about the virus, wondering if the schools will shut down. We shake our heads and hope for the best. We cannot begin to fathom how we would finish the semester or get our kids through the rest of the school year. Some people have begun to hoard emergency items like household cleaners, disposable gloves, hand sanitizer, and masks. It started last weekend in most of Europe and now seems to have spread to the US. Germans call this behavior *Hamsterkauf*—panic-hoarding, much like hamsters filling their cheeks with food.[2] Videos on YouTube suddenly show empty store shelves, runs on masks at hardware stores, and, hilariously, instructions on how to make hand sanitizer using vodka.

FRIDAY, MARCH 6, 2020

It seems like the nation is beginning to suffer from some cognitive dissonance in the face of the growing threat of coronavirus. Since the 1950s, social psychologists have identified "cognitive consistency" as one of our core human traits—we want to think of ourselves as thinking and acting in ways that line up with our stated identities.[3] This means when we act in ways that do not line up with who we consider ourselves to be, we become uncomfortable and willing to do almost anything to alleviate the dissonance.

In 2015, research psychologists Michael R. Ent at Towson University and Mary A. Gerend at Florida State University told participants in a study they would be taking an unpleasant test for a virus. But it was important because the virus was known to spread among their demographic. Interestingly, Ent and Gerend named the fictitious malady Human Respiratory Virus-27 (HRV-27). The test required the insertion of a very long cotton swab up the nose to the back of the throat. They even had the demonstrator, dressed in scrubs, lay out "latex gloves, hand sanitizer, multiple swabs, and a medical specimen bag on a table." Indeed, this sounds like the procedure being used globally right now for the SARS-CoV-2 tests. Ent and Gerend broke the subjects into two groups: The first group was told that they did not meet the required health criteria to receive the viral screening. The second group was told they *were* in fact eligible to be swabbed.

Ent and Gerend hypothesized that those who were told they were good candidates for the tests would complain that they didn't actually need it.[4] This is exactly what happened: Participants who were told they were eligible came up with excuses for why they didn't need it—all while holding to the idea that they were not the sort who would turn down a medically beneficial test just because it would be unpleasant. The psychologists concluded that if a beneficial decision also costs us somehow—in dollars or discomfort—we look for any excuse to get out of it rather than recognize our own personal unwillingness to absorb those costs.

It makes one wonder about the United States in 2020. We all think of ourselves as people who care about the public good, but no one really wants to wear a medical face mask or deal with the inconvenience of society shutting down like in China. Instead of acknowledging that we, in fact, are unwilling to put the public good ahead of our personal comfort, we will look for excuses that allow us to have our comforts without facing the implications of our decision. Limbaugh, and increasingly the president himself, are providing easy-to-follow mental paths out of cognitive dissonance—you can dismiss the virus and ignore the health experts, and it doesn't mean that you're a bad person. What will happen if officials here do close down large gatherings, like sporting events? Americans might easily contrive justifications for refusing to comply; that would save us from having to admit that we are prioritizing personal entertainment over public health.

In this week's *Atlantic*, two journalists wrote about how many coronavirus tests the United States has done.[5] I assumed the answer was "thousands." The FDA said earlier in the week we'd be able to do a *million* tests soon, and just two days ago, Vice President Pence concurred. That number makes sense: we've known about the virus and how dangerous it is for two months. American scientists have had the genetic sequence of SARS2 in their hands for six weeks. But after surveying health departments in all fifty states and in DC, the authors of the *Atlantic* article could verify that only 1,895 tests have been conducted. Just as frighteningly, it turns out, contact tracing and airport screening led to no testing.

Unfortunately, tests are not the only problem. Many of the world's face masks, especially the N95 one, which filters out viruses, are made in China. A supply line staunched for the moment and panic-buying this week has healthcare facilities fearing a shortage of masks.[6]

This week, Trevor Bedford, a computational biologist at the University of Washington, published his analysis of the likely spread of coronavirus in Seattle. He argues there are more cases than we've tested for; given the testing shortage, this seems a certainty. Bedford's model shows Seattle is where Wuhan was on January 1. In other words, Seattle, and perhaps the rest of Washington, if not the country, is at a crossroads. To curtail the spread of the virus, the city could put in place what he calls "large-scale non-pharmaceutical interventions to create social distancing"—ending mass gatherings, fastidiously disinfecting surfaces that could carry coronavirus, washing hands like crazy, and working from home when possible. "China averted many millions of infections," Bedford points out, but it took the Chinese government three weeks and a severe lockdown. If Seattle really clamps down, they might stop the spread and avoid a more aggressive lockdown. But it would certainly cause discomfort; many would denigrate the seriousness of the coronavirus and pressure officials to keep things up and running in order to deal with their cognitive dissonance.[7]

This is surely why Chinese officials were slow to recognize the threat in December, choosing to intimidate Dr. Li and the other whistleblowing physicians instead. The State and the people who run it are no less susceptible to the vagaries of cognitive dissonance.

SUNDAY, MARCH 8, 2020

This weekend, the internet is awash with claims that Black people cannot die from coronavirus. It started when Kem Senou Pavel Daryl, a twenty-one-year-old Cameroonian student living in Jingzhou, China, contracted the disease and then began to recover.[8] On February 14, before Senou was released from the hospital, an anonymous post sent through the Nigerian portal of Opera News Hub—an open content, fee-per-article platform—claimed Senou, "remained alive because he has black skin, the antibodies of a black [sic] are three times stronger, powerful and resistant compare [sic] to that of white."[9] Posts appeared claiming that Chinese scientists had confirmed "Africanness"—having "African" DNA or blood—confers resistance to coronavirus. Other claims were made about protective qualities of melanin.

"Believe it or not, this claim is a holdover from *nineteenth century* scientific racism on twenty-first century social media," physical anthropologist Jim Bindon says. Bindon, who specializes in the impact of race on medicine, has seen these misconceptions about race reemerge when crucial health decisions are on the line for a half century. "Nearly all genetic diversity in the world already exists in African populations," Bindon asserts. And since all humans are descended from African ancestors, our genetics are shared. "There is no specific 'Africanness' found in genes or blood." Obviously, the biochemical melanin found in the skin cannot protect from infectious disease, whether it is malaria or coronavirus.

Today, Jennifer Caudle, a Rowan University professor, attacked the pernicious myth that people of African descent, including African Americans, cannot contract coronavirus or, if they contract it, will be protected by melanin: "I'm Black. You might be Black. There is no evidence to say that Black people cannot get Coronavirus. THIS IS A MYTH, okay?! Anyone can get coronavirus. Now we know it mostly affects older people more seriously. It seems like younger people are spared or have milder disease. But guys! In terms of races, Black people can get coronaviruses."[10] The myth she's debunking reflects, tragically, old race science that justified keeping Black slaves in the fields harvesting sugar and cotton while tropical diseases crept from the Caribbean to Boston.

Though white folks don't often acknowledge it, this legacy of scientific racism continues to impact the daily practice of American healthcare. In 2016, researchers found that a sizable number of white laypeople, medical students, and medical residents believed that African Americans didn't feel pain as acutely as white people did. This, in turn, impacted how they treated pain and the kinds of interventions they recommended for a Black patient.[11] According to Bindon, this same racism allows white doctors to disregard the pain that Black women feel during pregnancy.[12] These biases are dangerous in a medical setting, especially because, historically, minorities suffer disproportionately *more* during episodes of infectious disease spread, not less.[13] Viruses may not discriminate, but humans so often do.

TUESDAY, MARCH 10, 2020

Michael Osterholm, an expert in public health and infectious disease at the University of Minnesota, is today's guest on the wildly popular podcast *The Joe Rogan Experience*.[14] Rogan asks Osterholm right off the bat if we should fear this novel coronavirus. Unlike Paul Offit, Osterholm says we absolutely should. This coronavirus spreads easily through the air, you can infect others before you show symptoms, and most importantly, because it is new, it could be *ten to fifteen times* worse than the worst seasonal flu outbreaks. His research group estimates *over 480,000 deaths* over the course of 2020 if America takes no precautions. Honestly, it's refreshing to hear someone speak so clearly, given the noise in February and now into March that the flu is so much worse. But it must be an overestimation. I cannot imagine half a million people dying in this country, even with its problems.

Osterholm describes the brittleness of the US pharmaceutical supply chain, how it hampers our ability to fight many diseases, coronavirus among them. We are surprisingly reliant on China for our supply of medications for chronic illnesses, such as heart disease and diabetes. Coronavirus has disrupted pharmaceutical manufacturing and distribution in China. Almost seven hundred thousand Americans have end-stage renal disease, for instance, and the major drugs to treat it come from China.

Rogan presses him, Aren't there treatments [for COVID-19] to keep people safe? Not really, shrugs Osterholm. "What about probiotics," Rogan wonders. No, those won't do anything, replies Osterholm, with an eye roll. Social distancing, persistently washing hands, and protecting the most vulnerable through more aggressive non-pharmaceutical interventions will slow the spread. Probably some shutting down of schools will be necessary, not because kids are getting sick but because they will take the virus home with them. The American public needs to be ready. He says we absolutely must pass along the knowledge that this is coming, just like the National Weather Service warns of hurricanes. We're going to be hit; we have to prepare. The worst possible thing is to assure people the risk is low.

But the message of low risk is precisely what much of the country's leadership is sending. Osterholm confirms what science journalist Laurie Garrett was saying back on January 30. No vaccine has yet been developed to fight the deadly SARS1 or MERS because we lose interest once a crisis passes. We are a nation that prioritizes acute care, Osterholm laments.

David Himmelstein agrees: "We have a tendency to neglect public health." As he sees it, part of our neglect is because we're overly focused on the dramatic events that almost certainly won't happen. We spend billions of dollars preparing for improbable military attacks and very little stockpiling masks or developing plans for how hospitals, schools, towns, and workplaces can defend themselves against more probable infectious diseases.

"Why this massive discrepancy?" I press Himmelstein.

"Deterioration of public health has been part and parcel of our shift to a capitalistic model in medicine that prioritizes revenue over a healthy populace," is his response. Capitalism, rooted in generating revenue, does not see an easy route to profit-making through the stockpiling of masks.

Warehouses of ventilators and Metformin do not create increasing markets, and they do not provide spin-off opportunities for money making. They may defend the nation from the possible complications of a pandemic, but they are boring compared to the production of F/A-18 jets. Those are a part of a multibillion-dollar industry. They help the military recruit. And the Blue Angels fly them at air shows while singer Lee Greenwood reminds us how proud we should be to be American.

In a strange echo of what Daniel Defoe chronicled in *A Journal of the Plague Year* three hundred years ago, charlatans offering quick solutions to the crisis are finding a receptive audience. Jim Bakker, the white televangelist best known for his meteoric fall from the religion-entertainment complex in the 1980s, has been caught promoting colloidal silver as a cure to coronavirus. This particular quack medicine is known to cause argyria, a chronic condition that turns your skin literally blue-gray. New York attorney general Letitia James ordered Bakker, who has already done jail time for embezzlement, to stop promoting it.[15] This week, the FDA and the Federal Trade Commission went after him, and now Missouri attorney general Eric Schmidt filed a restraining order against Bakker and his church, Morningside USA, for taking advantage of poor white evangelicals.[16] The problem is that some people *prefer* quack treatments to inconvenient interventions mandated by experts. Defoe noted this in 1722, also. Quack treatments tend to be easier to take and promise magical results. People are hearing misinformation directly from their most respected leaders.

While coronavirus continues to spread, the stock market falls, and toilet paper is disappearing, Trump repeats his mantra about the flu being far more dangerous, to encourage spending in restaurants, bars, and stores and to protect the stock market. We are collectively witnessing a hurricane develop, and he tells us to go swimming.

WEDNESDAY, MARCH 11, 2020

It is 9 p.m. EST, and the president is behind the Resolute desk. Televised Oval Office addresses were regular enough during earlier administrations but a rarity for the present occupant of the White House. He scoots up to the desk, folds his hands on his unopened folder, squints at the teleprompter, and starts: "My fellow Americans, tonight I want to speak with

you about our nation's unprecedented response to the coronavirus outbreak that started in China and is now spreading throughout the world. . . .
This is the most aggressive and comprehensive effort to confront a foreign virus in modern history. . . . From the beginning of time, nations and
people have faced unforeseen challenges, including large-scale and very
dangerous health threats. This is the way it always was and always will be."
He goes on to indict the European Union for "fail[ing] to take the same
precautions [as the United States] and restrict travel from China and other
hotspots."

Aside from the fact that one should never use the phrase "from the beginning of time" in a speech, the president's reference to the virus as "foreign" is a jarring reversal of his earlier praise for Chinese and European
handling of the outbreak. It is what Limbaugh did two weeks ago, linking
disease and foreignness as dangers to the collective "us."[17] Even blocking
travel from continental Europe, but not the UK, which the president announces tonight, rings of, in the words of Edward Said, orientalist "posi-
tional superiority," in which America and Britain enjoy the "upper hand" in
the world. In no way can this ban be effective as an actual bulwark against
the disease, clearly already here.[18] It may, nonetheless, fulfill other purposes as it rallies Trump's followers behind familiar causes and enemies.[19]

We know there is nothing uniquely Chinese about the coronavirus, just
as there was nothing uniquely French or Italian about syphilis when it appeared in Europe in the 1500s.[20] Pandemics have frequently carried foreign
names. The 1918 "Spanish flu" had nothing to do with Spain; it only got
that title because Spain's uncensored press did not suppress the story as the
French did, who called it the *maladie onze*, or "disease eleven."[21] Doctors
named Ebola and Zika after places in Africa, even though those diseases
spread far beyond any particular people or region. For this reason, in 2015,
WHO adopted new naming conventions for novel diseases to avoid animals, since the etiology of disease is often unclear, and stopping the practice of naming diseases after places and populations. And yet, here in 2020,
Trump is labeling the virus "Chinese," after defending China for months.

"This is not a financial crisis," he continues, "this is just a temporary
moment . . . we will overcome together as a nation and as a world. . . . No
nation is more prepared or more resilient than the United States. We have
the best economy, the most advanced healthcare, and the most talented doctors, scientists, and researchers anywhere in the world."[22] These are com-

forting words. Yet, we appear not to have set ourselves up to "significantly impede the transmission of the virus," as Trump says we have. True, as of today, "only" 1,248 Americans have tested positive for coronavirus, though 38 have died. If we look back to America's last major pandemic, a century ago, it seems we stand at an important point right now. Have we learned any lessons from history to make us "prepared," "advanced," and "resilient"?

On September 11, 1918, the city of Pittsburgh recorded its first death from the "Spanish," though it likely originated in Kansas, influenza. Two weeks later, the death count was increasing quickly. City administrators met but waited to ban large gatherings or close schools until October 3. By then, there were 20,000 cases in the city. By October 16, six weeks after its first death, Pittsburgh recorded a mortality rate of 0.8 percent.[23] In the end, of the half million people living in Pittsburgh, 4,748 died of influenza.[24] Barely *three weeks* elapsed from the first death until city leaders finally decided to implement lockdown orders. If Pittsburgh had hit the 2 percent rate that Limbaugh belittled a couple of weeks ago, and that the president now repeats with abandon, around 12,000 denizens of the Steel City would have been laid in the ground from the worst flu outbreak in recent American history.

The clock is ticking for us in 2020. The first death from community spread was on February 29—that's twelve days ago.[25] Though a small number of mayors have issued restrictions, no one to date has gone as far as they did in Pittsburgh in 1918 by banning public gatherings or closing schools.

Why haven't we moved so quickly this time?

Perhaps it is because American interest in coronavirus palpably decreased in February. Last month, I asked my researchers to catalogue the news stories on the coronavirus by the major television networks. After examining over two thousand television news stories about coronavirus broadcast over the first nine weeks of the year, we are forced to conclude that the television media was *not* the culprit for the February lull in public attention on the virus. In fact, ABC, CBS, NBC, MSNBC, CNN, and Fox News consistently covered coronavirus as it unfolded around the world. In fact, *Time* magazine criticized the media for *over*-sensationalizing the virus on February 7.[26]

So why did American interest in coronavirus decrease across the board in February, if media stories themselves did not decrease? Perhaps, as

Adam Smith suggested long ago, the majority of us thought of it as an "over there" problem, as exclusive to China. Perhaps we also believed what was actually reported by many of those two thousand news stories: that the CDC and HHS and WHO experts were handling the problem.

In any case, America seems to be jolted to awareness now. Tom Hanks and Rita Wilson are sick with coronavirus in Australia. Just before the president's address, the NBA stopped a game between the Oklahoma City Thunder and the Utah Jazz after Utah's Rudy Gobert tested positive for COVID. Before Trump finishes speaking, the NBA reports that it has shut down its entire season.[27] The NHL soon follows. Athletics calling a halt to its seasons feels like more of a turning point in this coronavirus story than the president's address.

But why did it take *entertainment* to wake America up? Seventeen days ago, Limbaugh was telling his disciples that coronavirus was a liberal hoax. Two weeks ago, the president of the United States echoed him. Now the country appears entrenched along typical partisan lines. Can we draw that lesson from Pittsburgh a century ago that we need aggressive, politically unified, nonpartisan government intervention before it is too late?

THURSDAY, MARCH 12, 2020

Businesses are locking their doors. "Will we be furloughed or just let go?" immediately becomes the question around proverbial water coolers. And it makes sense: throughout the day, the stock market plunges to the worst daily drop since the stock market crash of 1987. Perhaps the president triggered this when he claimed incorrectly in his address last night that travel and cargo from twenty-six European nations has been halted.[28]

The news comes at a breathless rate all day. In the wake of the NBA announcement last night, most professional sports pause their seasons. College basketball eliminates tournaments. Then school systems educating millions in Virginia, Ohio, New York, New Mexico, Tennessee, Washington State, Kentucky, San Francisco, and Connecticut announce long-term closures. Universities move courses online. The Disney and Universal Studios theme parks close, as do the Smithsonian Museums, the Metropolitan Museum of Art, and the National Zoo. The lights go out on Broadway.[29] New York City mayor Bill DeBlasio announces that gatherings of more than five hundred are prohibited. Mayors in other major cities follow with even more restrictive policies. Television shows agree to stop in-studio recording. Movie studios put films on hold mid-production. Theaters won't be showing many anyway, now. Domino after domino is falling.

FRIDAY, MARCH 13, 2020

Masks are nowhere to be found. There is no toilet paper, soap, ramen noodles, mac 'n' cheese, soup, flour, yeast, beans, frozen French fries, popcorn, bananas, eggs, tomato juice, peroxide, bleach, Lysol, rubbing alcohol, rubber gloves, baby wipes, Advil, Tylenol, cough drops, heartburn medicine, thermometers, paper products, or, weirdly, tofu.[30] I admit, in my nightmares of future plagues, a run on Charmin and Clamato juice just did not figure in.

Apparently, the Transportation Security Administration (TSA) and Customs and Border Protection (CBP) couldn't thoroughly screen the people flying from countries covered by the various travel bans, both because they are short-staffed and because so many with coronavirus do not show obvious symptoms. People who are now reporting being sick, likely catching the illness in Europe, were not screened at all before entering the United States.[31] All the touting of America's superior preparedness looks to have been wishful thinking.

People turn to the president for answers. He quickly conjures an old favorite culprit. In numerous tweets and calls into Fox shows, Trump claims Obama did not handle "his pandemic" well when the 2009–10 H1N1 influenza outbreak during the first year of his administration killed an estimated 12,469 Americans.

I decide to figure out if this is the case. The first diagnosed case of H1N1 appeared in the United States on April 12, 2009.[32] HHS declared a public health emergency on April 26, 2009, when twenty cases of H1N1 were in the United States.[33] Two days later, Obama's administration requested, and Congress approved, research and vaccine funding for $7.65 billion—a stark contrast to the $1.25 billion request made by Azar's HHS last month.[34] Six months later, Obama declared a national emergency. Vaccine discovery came quickly, but the rollout was slow.[35]

Trump declared an emergency on January 31, 2020, then banned most Chinese nationals from traveling to the country. Today, they invoked the Stafford Act, promising $50 billion in unspecified COVID aid, and the National Emergencies Act (like Obama passed in October 2009). On the

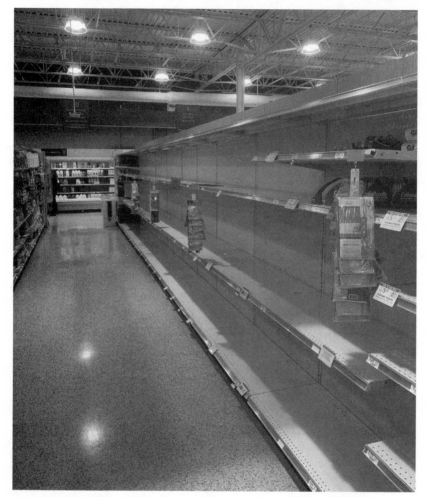

Empty grocery-store shelves during the first panic of the lockdowns. (Erik Peterson)

surface, it looks like Trump's response is not far afield from Obama's. Criti-
cally, however, the scale of response that the coronavirus demands seems to
be many degrees greater than with H1N1. H1N1's fatality rate was .02 %;
the novel coronavirus looks to be ten times worse.

The real contrast is in other realms of leadership. Trump won't admit
that we are in trouble. Imagine how powerful his message would be if he
compared this virus to the attacks on 9/11 and Pearl Harbor. Get in front of
the nation with an American flag waving behind you! Tell everyone that this

is a moment of crisis and then give clear instructions on what each American needs to do to fulfill their patriotic obligations to the nation. Call upon the American population to rally against this terrifying foe like George W. Bush and FDR did. Stop saying that there is nothing to worry about.

MONDAY, MARCH 16, 2020

Fifth day after shutdowns began—4,300 cases of COVID-19 (unless otherwise indicated, COVID case and death numbers refer only to the United States)

Each morning, I forget for just a moment that the world is in flux, that reality right now might be fundamentally shifted by the time I return to bed at night. I don't know how my kids are going to finish school now that they have been sent home. I don't know how I'm going to do my job. I don't even know how to find flour and toilet paper, and I have this strange compulsion to sew and bake bread.

A blaring warning siren comes in the economic news. The Federal Reserve announces it will cut interest rates down to a range of 0 to 0.25 percent.[36] The hope is that people will start borrowing money to spend it, which will help the companies that sell what they spend it on stay in business, which will help people to keep their jobs, so they can make money and . . . keep spending it. This is the Keynesian cycle inscribed on the life of every American. The Federal Reserve also starts buying billions of dollars in bonds, something they do when they want to put more cash in the economy so people will make and spend more. The Fed did the same during the 2008–09 financial crisis. These moves are meant to stabilize the economy and stop the slide that led to the Great Recession.

Despite these efforts, today, the futures market collapses. High-risk traders don't feel confident enough in the economy. Artificial "circuit breakers" kick in this morning and temporarily stop the selling when prices start to plummet. Once Wall Street starts trading, however, the true crash begins. The Standard & Poor's 500 Index, the Dow Jones Industrial Average, and the NASDAQ Composite lose 12 to 13 percent of their value in a single day. It's the largest loss in history.[37] While this news could impact our job security, most of us won't see much immediate change in our daily lives. The majority of Americans don't own much of the actual value that is wrapped up in the stock market. The newspapers and broadcasters "do the numbers" every morning, telling us whether stocks are "up" or "down," but one third of all Americans have less than $5,000 in savings and do not feel they can save much, if anything, for retirement.[38]

The economic shutdown will hurt all of us, however, and it is pervasive. Venues that support everyday life are shutting their doors and laying off workers. McDonald's and Chick-fil-A close their seating areas, though you still can't walk up to the drive-through. Washington governor Jay Inslee closes the dining areas of all restaurants in the whole state, followed by bars, gyms, movie theaters, and other social gathering spots. Sadly, these establishments are staffed by some of the country's most vulnerable workers, paid hourly without health benefits.

Closures are happening faster now because lots of people are suddenly starting to die. Thirty-five elderly residents in the Life Care Center near Seattle have passed away. Today, King County Public Health officials announced 488 cases and 43 fatalities, an infection rate of 53 cases per 100,000 people. New York City posts similar reports, with over 2,100 cases, an unexpected leap of 1,000 from yesterday. *One thousand* cases in one day—such an overwhelming number, like we saw in China two months ago. Minnesota, like Washington, closes its bars and restaurants. Santa Clara County, California, is going even further, ordering its seven million residents, including the entire city of San Francisco and much of Silicon Valley, to "shelter in place."

On top of this, voting in the presidential primary elections still has to happen. Ohio governor Mike DeWine, a Republican, petitions to delay state primaries, scheduled for tomorrow. For most states, though, deciding whether or not to delay because of the virus has turned into a partisan fight. Republicans, taking cues from the president who continues to minimize the danger of the virus, say delays are unnecessary. Democrats feel strongly about avoiding the spread of the virus, as no one is sure how to bring that many people together safely to vote. The president called Governor DeWine's request to delay the voting "unnecessary"; the election will go forward as planned. Ohio voters, understandably confused by the back and forth, will appear at the polls tomorrow or find themselves excluded from the electoral process.[39]

In the meantime, at a CTF press briefing tonight, President Trump rates himself a "ten out of ten" for his response to the pandemic.[40] Dr. Fauci and Dr. Deborah Birx, White House coronavirus response coordinator, talk about the importance of social distancing. If we stand six feet apart, they say, we should be safe. The president brags that closing "our borders to China" is what saved the United States from being in a "very bad position, much worse than what's happening now." Perhaps there was no way that we could have stopped the virus from coming here. We are a globalized society, after all. The real test is how we manage it. Already over four thousand Americans have tested positive for COVID-19, and I read that Phase 1 trials of a coronavirus vaccine just began. No matter what the president says in front of the cameras, it *feels* as if we're about to be in a "very bad position, much worse than what's happening now."

WEDNESDAY, MARCH 18, 2020

8,000 cases

Today, Congressman Michael McCaul of Texas, the top Republican on the House Foreign Affairs Committee, claims China committed "one of the worst cover-ups in human history."[41] It is not clear whether this claim is valid. Chinese scientists sequenced and publicly released the genetic data of the virus in early January. The Chinese government alerted its citizens and put them on severe restrictions during Chunyun—the equivalent of our government suspending travel through Chicago O'Hare at Thanksgiving. Obviously, these were clear signals from China that this coronavirus was not to be taken lightly. In December 2019, China brought WHO, though not the CDC, into the reporting process, allowing Western journalists in to follow its quarantine and death toll. All of these were actions China did *not* take during the SARS1 outbreak in 2003. The Chinese government now admits that they made some mistakes—something they refused to do during the original SARS epidemic seventeen years ago—including sharing that they missed the earliest cases back in mid-November 2019.[42]

Nonetheless, for the Trump administration, China has been a blank slate for any meaning deemed expedient at the moment. Initially, Trump defended Communist leader Xi, emphasizing the resumption of Chinese factories' operations as an indication that the pandemic was waning globally, even though no medical organizations supported that claim.[43] Now, he is reinscribing China with the bigoted tropes of its people as cunning, dirty, dangerous backstabbers, and continues to use the term "Chinese virus." As always, most Republican politicians scramble to genuflect, change their positions, and delete old tweets to match Trump's current stance. It seems to me our government has more in common with the "Chi-com" behavior, as Limbaugh calls it, than any of them would care to admit.

But why the switch to anti-Chinese language? The American media broke the Dr. Li story and the distrust of China by its people almost two months ago—at the same moment the Trump administration was loudly telling the American public to calm down because the Chinese government had the outbreak under control.[44] Back then, the narrative was that flu was worse than coronavirus.[45] Now, the stock market has tanked, and the Play-Place at McDonald's is closed.

FRIDAY, MARCH 20, 2020

We learn today that our institution, its 45,000 students, faculty, and staff, will be going fully online for the rest of the term. We have five days to reconfigure the next six weeks of lectures, discussions, readings, papers, tests, and exams. Students are being told to go home immediately, without packing up their dorms. Every educational institution is experiencing the same mass upheaval, from kindergarten through graduate school. For the moment, learning will take a backseat to safety.

The whole of New York City seems to be shutting down. New York State processed 10,000 additional coronavirus tests in just the last twenty-four hours, which pushed the count up to nearly 8,000 coronavirus cases—a number *ten times* higher than earlier in the week. New York City alone accounts for 5,600 of them.[46]

The same thing is happening in Chicago, Los Angeles, Philadelphia, Boston, and Washington, DC. All have issued stay-at-home orders for those who do not qualify as essential workers. Ohio, Virginia, North Carolina, and others have called up their national guards to help distribute medical supplies.[47] Even places that resisted the first lockdown orders last week are giving in, turning off, and locking up. Starting Monday and continuing through the week, states and major cities limited restaurants to delivery and takeout orders and closed bars and nightclubs until at least the end of the month.[48]

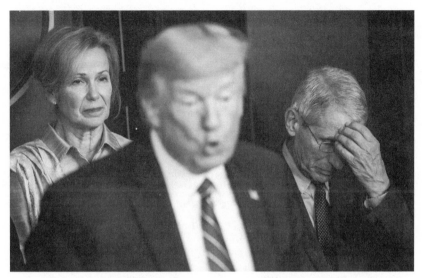

The facepalm that was heard around the world. Drs. Fauci and Birx attempt to remain stoic at a CTF press conference on March 20, 2020. (Jabin Botsford, Getty Images)

Congress passes the Families First Coronavirus Response Act after a week of debate. In this second piece of coronavirus legislation, the government will provide paid leave, free coronavirus testing, and expanded food assistance as well as additional money to states to manage the pandemic.[49] Unemployed folks, and there seem to be more every day, are supposed to receive an additional $600 a week on top of state unemployment to encourage them to not go out to look for work right now.

SATURDAY, MARCH 21, 2020

Day 10 after quarantines began. 23,700 cases.

Hopefully that $600 per week is enough, because the Department of Labor reports a new "epidemic": first-time unemployment insurance claims, which rose this week from 240,000 to 3.28 *million*. The previous record—695,000—was set in October 1982, during the Reagan recession. It is so bad that in order to visualize the data, the Department of Labor has to change the scale of its charts.

Travel, retail, transportation—anything that relies on physical work done outside the house and close to strangers—felt the pinch weeks ago.

Any business that relies on public service—bars, restaurants, theaters, clubs, salons—is obviously hard-hit, but so are businesses that service other businesses, like advertising and head-hunting firms. How do you advertise to a market that is not there? Our progressive new "gig" economy, full of service workers and computer programmers doing piecemeal work with an almost nonexistent economic safety net, proves not so progressive after all.[50]

"This is the 9/11 for the restaurant business," Larry, a restaurant owner in Destin, Florida, tells me.[51] In anticipation of spring breakers, he just spent hundreds of thousands of dollars buying perishable foods, hiring staff, and training them. He's not happy about the sudden shutdown order in the face of very few coronavirus cases; it brings into stark relief the difficult situation business owners are in. They want to protect public health but also themselves against financial ruin. His staff will be scrambling to build up his take-out business while he pays his employees for as long as he can. He's also worried employees might quit because the new federal $600 per month in addition to state unemployment benefits is better than what he's paying them.

Not surprisingly, elite management seems to have a buffer. Some are making noble gestures, like Marriott's Arne Sorenson, who, sick with cancer, has suspended his own pay. Two days ago, Sorenson recorded a video message to his employees:

> COVID-19 is like nothing we've ever seen before. . . . But here are the facts. . . . COVID-19 is having a more severe and sudden financial impact on our business than 9/11 and the 2009 financial crisis combined. . . . The restrictions on travel, gatherings of people, and required social distancing is having an immediate impact by depressing demand for our hotels. . . .
>
> Given these circumstances, we have been forced to take proactive steps . . . We have stopped all hotel initiatives for 2020 and have gone dark on our brand, marketing, and advertising during this period. Both Mr. Marriott and I will not be taking any salary for the balance of 2020 . . . Above property around the world, we are moving to shorten work weeks. . . .
>
> At the property level, contingency plans . . . for open hotels include closing food and beverage outlets, reducing staff, and closing floors of hotels.[52]

The video has gone viral. Today, *Forbes* hails it as "a lesson in authentic leadership." That may be the case, but given that his salary was $13 million in 2018—over *four hundred times* the salary of the average Marriott front desk associate—he's probably not collecting food stamps just yet. Meanwhile, his hotel staff find themselves "reduced" as Marriott furloughs two-thirds of its payroll.[53]

For many Americans right now, there exists a deep tension between going to work to pay the bills and staying home to, as we're told, "flatten the curve." On March 11, Trump called us a resilient nation. But it's more accurate to say we are a fragile society where few of us can stay home for the public good and still pay for those homes. Many of us are now caught in an unavoidable dilemma.

MONDAY, MARCH 23, 2020

42,700 cases—ten times as many as last week

Much is closed now. The freeways are clear. No school buses. Hardly any planes. America sits at home, holding its breath.

Trump tweeted in all caps last night, and then again this morning: "WE CANNOT LET THE CURE BE WORSE THAN THE PROBLEM ITSELF."[54] He undoubtedly does not want to be at the helm if the nation experiences a cataclysmic economic collapse. From an actuarial standpoint, it might be possible to weigh the thousands of lives that have been, and will be, lost to this pandemic against the impact that a nationwide shutdown has on the lives of Americans. But it feels profoundly cold and calculating to argue that we should be willing to sacrifice human lives in exchange for economic solvency.

Andrew Cuomo, governor of New York, Joe Biden (now almost assured of becoming the Democratic nominee for president—what a difference a month makes!), Dr. Birx, and Dr. Fauci, who have both been appearing in the White House CTF briefings, collectively fill the president's leadership vacuum. In public appearances, they try to offer data-driven advice, empathy, and thoughtful guidance. Even they are desperately unclear at times in their messaging. For his part, Surgeon General Jerome Adams walks a tightrope between giving accurate information and not angering the president. On NBC's *Today*, Dr. Adams admits, "it's going to get bad."

Collectively, we have got to "flatten the curve," he says—there's that term again. Adams at least explains it: we must restrict our own movement. Otherwise, so many will be infected that we will clog hospitals and bring down the level of care for everyone. The real determinant of our ability to handle this outbreak is the availability of hospital beds. It seems clear the virus will spread; our only intervention is to manage its speed. We cannot afford to all get sick at the same time.[55]

This new reality has come on shockingly fast. In the last two weeks, we have leapt from six hundred cases to over forty thousand, with five hundred deaths. The comparison to Pittsburgh in 1918 I made a month ago seems uncomfortably on point. What's scarier is that these numbers cannot possibly be accurate. The Association of Public Health Laboratories admits that American testing, already woefully delayed, continues to lag.[56] We can be certain that more people have COVID than we know.

Craig Spencer, director of Global Health in Emergency Medicine at New York Presbyterian Hospital, recounts his experiences in the COVID ward.[57] He allows me to print this record of his daily life here.

Wake up at 6:30am. Priority is making a big pot of coffee for the whole day, because the place by the hospital is closed. . . .

Walk in for your 8am shift: . . . There is a cacophony of coughing. You stop. Mask up. Walk in.

You take signout from the previous team, but nearly every patient is the same, young & old: Cough, shortness of breath, fever. They are really worried about one patient. Very short of breath, on the maximum amount of oxygen we can give, but still breathing fast.

You immediately assess this patient. It's clear what this is, and what needs to happen. You have a long and honest discussion with the patient and family over the phone. It's best to put her on life support now, before things get much worse. You're getting set up for that, but . . .

You're notified of another really sick patient coming in. You rush over. They're also extremely sick, vomiting. They need to be put on life support as well. . . . Two patients, in rooms right next to each other, both getting a breathing tube. It's not even 10am yet.

For the rest of your shift, nearly every hour, you get paged: Stat notification: Very sick patient, short of breath, fever. Oxygen 88%. Stat notification: Low blood pressure, short of breath, low oxygen. Stat notification: Low oxygen, can't breathe. Fever. All day . . .

Sometime in the afternoon you recognize you haven't drunk any water. You're afraid to take off the mask. It's the only thing that protects you. Surely you can last a little longer . . . One more patient . . .

When your shift ends, you sign out to the oncoming team. It's all #COVID-19. . . . low oxygen, lymphopenia, elevated D-dimer. . . .

Before you leave, you wipe EVERYTHING down. Your phone. Your badge. Your wallet. Your coffee mug. All of it. Drown it in bleach. Everything in a bag. Take no chances. Sure you got it all??? Wipe it down again. Can't be too careful. . . .

You reflect on the fact that it's really hard to understand how bad this is—and how bad it's going to be—if all you see are empty streets. Hospitals are nearing capacity. We are running out of ventilators. Ambulance sirens don't stop.

Everyone we see today was infected a week ago, or more. . . .

We were too late to stop this virus. Full stop. But we can slow its spread. The virus can't infect those it never meets. Stay inside. Social distancing is the only thing that will save us now. I don't care as much about the economic impact as I do about our ability to save lives.

You might hear people saying it isn't real. It is. You might hear people saying it isn't bad. It is. You might hear people saying it can't take you down. It can. I survived Ebola. I fear COVID-19. Do your part. Stay home. Stay safe. And every day I'll come to work for you.

TUESDAY, MARCH 24, 2020

52,600 cases

Almost all schools in America have closed. Idaho was a holdout. Texas, Colorado, and Missouri waited until yesterday. The closures put working parents, especially single ones, in a terrible bind. Teachers and parents scramble to figure out what education at a distance looks like.[58] Apparently, we are all moving to an online video chat tool called Zoom. Overnight, it becomes the connective tissue of American education, business, and social interaction. By unspoken consensus, it is the platform for get-togethers, work meetings, birthday parties, keeping tabs on elderly parents in nursing homes, and even court hearings.[59]

Philosopher Martin Heidegger argued that technology is dangerous because it controls how we experience the world.[60] The medium defines the message, creating distances and technologically reliant relationships that inhibit real human contact. It is hard to deny that tools like Zoom will control our reality in millions of incalculable ways. As long as we are interacting online, we will be defined to some extent by this technological framework. Heidegger couldn't imagine Zoom, WhatsApp, Marco Polo, Voxer, Parler, or any of the other internet-based technologies that hold this current world together.

At the same time, there is some undoubtable good to tools like Zoom. They are making the continuation of life through this pandemic possible. Kids can stay in school at a distance; some of their parents, at least, can keep their jobs. People can see a doctor, order groceries, and connect with friends and family, and not be so alone.

Zoom, like the computerized turn of the last forty years, also reveals the fault lines of wealth and poverty in this nation. To participate in this online world, you must have a computer, an internet connection, and a space to work. The ubiquity of expensive smartphones has muted the conversation about this divide. Nevertheless, students in public schools, colleges, and universities across the country have been sent home to finish a whole semester online, which is nearly impossible to do on a phone with only cellular connectivity. It's a line of demarcation between the haves and the have-nots. Students and teachers alike teach or complete assignments on their phones. Many of my own students are the first in their families to attend college. Internet is not available in some of their towns, or if it is, only at the public libraries, now closed. I have students who are paper-mailing assignments to me. We may be heading into an era in which internet access becomes something that the nation has to provide, much like electricity and telephone in the 1930s and '40s.

Even with internet access, online education sculpts learning, because it changes the calculus of *attention*. In my class with hundreds of introductory students, I can record and post a powerful lecture on the lessons that the Holocaust has to teach, but I've already discovered that most of my students will not watch it. We read Svetlana Alexievich's *Zinky Boys*, but our Zoom discussion of the Soviet invasion of Afghanistan, and the scars these brutal wars left, grows thin. These discussions matter. They teach the importance of empathy, of the fragility of life. But, despite my scolding, students keep their phone notifications on. They are distracted and disconnected. I can't imagine what it must be like to teach younger kids over Zoom. Having to engage a session full of third graders seems terrifying. Teachers will have to be careful about correcting their students, given that parents are watching just offscreen.

We have been living in a digitally mediated reality for decades, and perhaps this moment is merely the culmination of a process that began a hundred years ago, when Heidegger first made his observations. Actual learning requires undivided attention. Social media, texts, video games, streaming— they are designed to distract. And when you're already locked on a screen for school, there's no escape, no way to hone the practice of what Georgetown University computer scientist Cal Newport calls "deep work."[61] I fear what will become of education if this state of affairs lasts too long.

WEDNESDAY, MARCH 25, 2020

900 deaths from COVID-19

In a Fox News interview yesterday, the president claimed: "You're going to lose a number of people to the flu, but you're going to lose more people by putting a country into a massive recession or depression. You're gonna lose people. You're gonna have suicides by the thousands."[62]

This is Trump's fifth major argument against taking collective action to stop the coronavirus. First, it was that the virus was far away in distant China. Then came the argument that it was a hoax manufactured by the left to scare investors and undermine his presidency. Third, he claimed that the flu is worse than the coronavirus, so we should do nothing to confront the growing pandemic. Fourth was his warning not to let the "cure," that is, stay-at-home orders, be worse than the "problem," meaning, as far as anyone can tell, that the stock market shouldn't be hurt trying to halt the deaths of citizens. Unbelievably, other right-wing personalities express this even more sharply, suggesting that older folks should be made expendable to keep the economy running.[63]

Now we are being told that shutting down will cause us to kill ourselves. Perhaps Trump is imagining the old canard that during the stock market crash of 1929, deeply indebted people took their own lives. This was proved a myth—an intentional bit of "fake news," made up by *New York Times* columnist Will Rogers.[64]

The sad truth is that we don't need an economic crash for suicides to happen. The National Center for Health Statistics report that the national suicide rate has risen by about 35 percent over the last twenty years, even more sharply since 2006, when times were good. By 2019, suicide leapt into the top-ten causes of death for Americans.[65]

According to the Substance Abuse and Mental Health Services Association, mental illness (always a risk factor for suicide) is statistically linked to how much access to care people have, their exposure to social media and smart phones, and their relative levels of isolation.[66] As Émile Durkheim in the nineteenth century and Johann Hari in the twenty-first century argued, mental illness and suicide are terrible byproducts of our always-connected-yet-always-lonely modernity. No stock crash necessary.

If coronavirus deaths stay below 45,000, and suicide rates remain on their current pace, then suicide numbers will indeed outpace this pandemic's casualties by year's end. Unfortunately, last week's projection by Imperial College London (ICL) suggests we're in for a greater COVID death count than 45,000, unless the US is very serious about this shutdown strategy. The ICL study suggests we need strict non-pharmaceutical social interventions for as long as a year until reliable vaccines are made available.[67] The White House, however, seems completely unwilling to let shutdowns go past early April, let alone until there's a vaccine.

If we give President Trump the benefit of the doubt that he is truly worried about suicides due to loss of income, then he will certainly celebrate the Senate's passing of a *$2 trillion* stimulus bill tonight. Several notable items in what they are calling the CARES Act: $500 billion for municipalities and corporations, expanded $600 per week unemployment insurance through the end of July, and most encouragingly, a direct payment of $1,200 to each adult and an additional $500 per child for parents. It includes $100 billion to hospitals, $1 billion to the Indian Health Service, and billions for expanding health equipment capacity.[68] Also, the Trumps are specifically blocked from getting any of this money—a restriction unnecessary for any prior presidential family.[69]

THURSDAY, MARCH 26, 2020

Stay-at-home orders started two weeks ago—82,000 cases

With more COVID-19 cases over the last two weeks than China had during its entire outbreak, the United States is the center of the pandemic.[70] Elmhurst Hospital Center in Queens reports a line outside of people with symptoms waiting for tests. Even if they're admitted, they are not guaranteed a bed. Nurses, lacking personal protective equipment (PPE), wear trash bags. A refrigerated truck becomes an overflow morgue. A federal hospital ship is on the way but won't be useable for weeks.[71] All the while, leaders are offering platitudes about America being the most advanced nation in the world.

South Korea and Japan, which learned they had infected citizens at the same time as the United States, managed to "flatten the curve" with aggressive contact tracing, lots of public service announcements, and widespread testing.[72] Singapore worked so hard at tracing and quarantining that they were able to reopen schools within two months. By contrast, our contact tracing has been negligible. We are seeing mysterious outbreaks popping up in places like Albany, Georgia, far away from major cities, with no known connection to travelers from Asia or Europe.[73]

Why are we so *unprepared*—now an object lesson for the rest of the world? Scholars, epidemiologists, and politicians will study this question for decades to come, but I am convinced here, at the end of March, these failures do not just belong to the Trump administration. It is true the president and his supporters have put personal agendas before the lives of other citizens by not promoting a unified public health message. But even the political left missed the chance to create effective messaging. Medical experts failed on basic issues like whether we should all wear masks; it's clear we should. Our media so often courts controversy and spectacle over harder, slower science, giving voice to nonexperts who pontificate without actual knowledge. And, as the historian Tom Engelhardt notes about the toxic legacy of American "victory culture," when we believe in that story of national exceptionalism—pride in our ability to ignore rules and beat the odds as atomized *individuals*—it makes us incapable of humility or sacrifice for the common good.[74]

MONDAY, MARCH 30, 2020

160,000 cases—quadrupled since last week

How much authority should the central government hold versus the state governments? In theory, the Tenth Amendment protects the rights of states to control the spread of dangerous diseases within their jurisdictions. The Supreme Court reinforced this in *Gibbons v. Ogden* (1824), a unanimous ruling that states have the right to impose quarantines. More cases like it have followed, meaning quarantines and business restrictions must happen at the state level.[75] Today, the issue is that, with some governors refusing to implement or extend stay-at-home measures, coronavirus will spread more. If New Mexico shuts down, for instance, but Texas does not, how can New Mexicans avoid infection from Texas?

Because there is no federal management of resources, states are now competing among themselves for medical equipment and PPE. Louisiana, a poorer state than New York and Washington, has emerged as an epicenter in the national outbreak. But it will lose a bidding war for ventilators to richer states and their hospital corporations.[76]

In the meantime, in our "advanced," "exceptional" nation, desperate people, myself included, have formed socially distanced mask-sewing groups, coordinated over the internet, donating masks to hospitals and nursing homes. Others 3-D-print parts for hospital equipment like ventilators.[77] They are wonderful gestures, similar to French taxi drivers carrying soldiers to the front in WWI, but they aren't sustainable at scale, and they reveal a serious failure in infrastructure. Providing masks and ventilators to hospitals is, arguably, something the federal government should be doing. The system is overwhelmed, doctors are saying. If the central government were ever to step up and glue the states together, this is the time. Is this not a perfect example of how our competitive, privatized, just-in-time medical system is inefficient and—dare we say—inhumane?

FRIDAY, APRIL 3, 2020

All but seven governors have now issued stay-at-home or shelter-in-place orders—the governors of Alabama and Missouri are waiting until today to decide. Florida closed down on Wednesday and only, according to Governor Ron DeSantis, because New Yorkers have fled there.[1] The Axios/Ipsos Coronavirus Index shows fully half of Americans quarantining this week.[2]

There is some ambiguity about what the orders mean. People should stay in their homes, except for runs to the grocery store or doctor appointments. "Essential" work continues, however, and therein lies the ambiguity. Who, or what, is essential? Physicians and nurses, certainly. What about bankers? Liquor store workers? Walmart, Target, and Home Depot employees? Are any of these "essential" workers going to receive PPE to protect themselves?

The seven states still holding out against the shut-down orders—Arkansas, Iowa, Nebraska, North Dakota, South Dakota, Utah, and Wyoming—are largely rural. Most refused the Medicare expansion promised by the Affordable Care Act, known as Obamacare, over a decade ago. Several of these states perennially invest the least in healthcare per capita of any state.[3] More concerning is that these are the states with citizens who rank among the highest in risk factors associated with COVID-19, including diabetes, obesity, and heart disease. In just the last few weeks, health professionals in these states observed higher death rates among younger patients than they have seen before.[4] Because there are no COVID checks at state borders and interstate travel is still allowed, these states become sieves for infection spread.

Right now, however, the eyes of the nation are fixated on New York City, where the situation grows ever more dire. Some of the most essential workers are Rikers Island prisoners. For six dollars an hour, they bury the COVID dead in a mass grave on Hart Island, east of the Bronx, in Long Island Sound.[5] They wake up in the small hours, under the blue morning light, and are taken to this gloomy gravesite, with the ruins of an old mental asylum teetering around them. There, they unload grandmothers, grandfathers, sisters, brothers, mothers, fathers, daughters, and sons—none of whom had a funeral, all of whom, because of COVID-19, died alone—into the ground. Someone sits inside the cage of a bulldozer, steadily moving dirt over the pine coffins, stacked neatly in a massive pit, like shipping containers at the docks nearby.

A month ago, we saw similar images via satellite of mass graves in Qom, Iran.[6] It would be nice to believe the urban United States is medically and economically advanced enough to avoid the same fate as Iran.

And yet, seven thousand people have already died, about double the casualties from 9/11.

New projections from the University of Washington suggest over 80,000 Americans could die of COVID-19 by July.[7] The CDC warns between 100,000 and 240,000 might die during the entire pandemic.[8] Such numbers seemed unreasonably pessimistic only about a week or so ago, when there were just over 1,500 deaths.

I find myself desperately seeking out friends and family on Zoom. In the two weeks of this quarantine, I have spoken to old roommates and former students I had lost touch with long ago. We all seem to have this need to see each other, to hear each other's voices, to talk about where we are and how we are coping, and to make sure that we are all still alive. It is reassuring in ways that are hard to articulate.

And yet, even then, I hear the persistent whisper of two famous refrains: Langston Hughes, "O, let America be America again—The land that never has been yet—And yet must be . . ." And the other, T. S. Eliot, "April is the cruelest month . . ."[9]

SUNDAY, APRIL 5, 2020

Almost 10,000 dead

I wake up, fumble for my glasses, and check my phone. I do this every morning now. There is a kind of dread that settles over the first thirty seconds of every day. I know I will see dozens of emails from coworkers and students who need answers to questions I never imagined they would ask. This low-level panic scaffolds our "new normal."

One student writes that she is now living in her car without a computer for her classes. She charges her phone at a gas station and has a circuit of churches she goes to for food each day. She is worried she won't be able to complete the semester without access to the library. When I ask her about going home, she—a trans woman—says this is not an option. It is not safe; I don't press her. I think the university has funds to help students in an emergency. I start scrambling to find her housing.

"Here's who to contact to find a dorm room," I tell her later over Zoom, "and here are the mental health counseling phone numbers." She laughs. The counseling offices are closed, she reminds me. And even when they were open, it was a six-month wait for an appointment. She says this in a bright tone, not at all suited to her predicament. I wonder if she will be able to navigate all this by herself. I offer her a room at my house, but she politely declines. It's Sunday, so she will be in her car for at least tonight. I schedule to meet her at the gas station near campus. I am sure I have an old computer in my closet that she can use.

As I grab my things, I see another email from a student whose father in New Jersey has been admitted to the hospital with COVID. She needs extensions on her assignments. Below that is a message from a graduate student, unable to keep up with his work because he has had to move his sick father and "awful stepmother" into his one-bedroom apartment.

And they're just the tip of one iceberg. I've read social media posts from families powerless to intervene, saying goodbye online to loved ones in New York and Detroit and Seattle and New Orleans. The news on TV shows hospitals so overwhelmed that they are rationing care.[10] Even when I turn to my friends on Zoom for comfort, the pain and fear and confusion can't be avoided. I hear from a friend stuck living with her estranged husband, despite their recent divorce. An artist with a career-shaping gallery showing in New York canceled. A worried friend about to have a baby in the potentially virus-laden hospital. Another friend who needs a mastectomy and will have to go alone to the hospital for the surgery. Some have lost jobs; they can't get through to the unemployment office and won't be able to make rent. Any of these situations would be scary in ordinary life, but now, no one knows how to even begin to handle them.

This coronavirus pandemic isn't one trauma; it is many, all the time, and it is happening to nearly everyone. By the end of the day, I run to the kitchen for a glass of wine. Then two. Then three. It takes a lot to shut down these days.

MONDAY, APRIL 6, 2020

360,000 cases—double last week

Back in late February, while the rest of the Trump administration was promoting the "coronavirus is a hoax cooked up by Democrats" message, Secretary Alex Azar requested that relatively small funding increase to fight coronavirus. The Democratically controlled House eventually granted them much more funding than they asked for, with the proviso that they should use it to fight the coming outbreak.

This last week, HHS conducted phone surveys of 323 hospitals across forty-six states plus Puerto Rico about how things are going and how the HHS money is being spent.[11] The anecdotes included in the report sound like they come from local clinics in some banana republic instead of the touted American healthcare system. One administrator writes that the supplies the hospital received "won't even last a day." One health system reported receiving one thousand masks, five hundred of which were for children, unusable for adult staff. One hospital reported receiving 2,300 N95 masks that were so old the elastic bands had dry-rotted. Another hospital reported its last two shipments from a federal agency contained PPE that had expired in 2010.[12]

Hospitals are spending their own money to make up for the lack of government supplies. Unfortunately, the prices of basic supplies have skyrocketed. Masks that used to cost fifty cents now cost six dollars apiece. It's true that around 100 of the 323 hospitals surveyed are located in rural areas or small towns, so maybe it makes more sense that supplies might not be on hand. However, 34 of those surveyed were either major teaching hospitals associated with the nation's top universities or centers specializing in treating infectious disease. The report suggests that even these hospitals are understaffed, under-resourced, and generally not at the level they should be to face a pandemic. New York governor Cuomo puts the need succinctly:

Andrew Cuomo ✅
@NYGovCuomo

Our single greatest challenge is ventilators.
We need 30,000 ventilators.
We have 11,000.

11:49 AM—Mar 25, 2020

Strangely, Cuomo's pleas triggered the president to lash out at the cited shortage. Trump's deal with auto manufacturer General Motors to produce ventilators has fallen through, and he refuses to use the Defense Production Act to force manufacturers into producing the needed supplies.[13] Having failed to secure more ventilators, Trump attacks the whole notion of

New York needing ventilators.[14] In one of the nightly CTF briefings, and again on Fox News, the president claims they don't need so many ventilators.[15] And, to top it off, he dubs a reporter's question about the lack of federal response "threatening."[16]

Dustups between the president and the press distract from two other important issues. First, ventilators *used to be there*, stockpiled, gathering dust, but the cost of storing ventilators for a future pandemic became too expensive. Economic shortfalls, some of which were caused by the lack of federal preparedness funds, led to New York selling its stock of emergency ventilators.[17] This is another example of what happens when you have a just-in-time healthcare system. The second issue is even more harrowing. In 2018, in remembrance of the one-hundredth anniversary of the 1918 H1N1 influenza pandemic, NYC Health + Hospitals ran an executive-level pandemic-response workshop. Administrators and healthcare providers found massive holes, resulting in recommendations about data sharing, training, communication, and payment systems.[18] Apparently, none of these pandemic suggestions were implemented.

WEDNESDAY, APRIL 8, 2020

14,600 deaths—fourth week of quarantine

Good news arrives today: the city of Wuhan has reopened. After ten weeks of lockdown in a metropolis of eleven million, it appears they've beaten the first wave of the virus.[19] Trump says nothing about this, even though he praised Xi all through January and February for his handling of the outbreak.

The nation's perception of time has become warped over the last month. "Blursday," people call it. Anthropologists say the feeling is tied to the loss of "temporal agency," or the sense that we no longer have the ability to control and structure how we use our time.[20] Our lives through most of history were shaped by the agricultural seasons. During the Industrial Revolution, our time, a measure of our value as workers, was even less ours to control. Life revolved around the clock, waking for a work shift at an hour designated by a boss, spending set times at our studies (if we were lucky enough to get to study), following schedules for entertainment and leisure.[21] The most extreme example of having no control over one's time was the experience of enslaved people (although even they found ways to carve moments for themselves). The point is that we desire temporal agency—a belief that we can control our time—even if we don't really have it. One way we give ourselves this sense of agency is by "tricking time," by planning for a future we think we can predict.

The problem arises when we lose our tether to this sense of a controllable future—when we become locked in what anthropologists call "enforced presentism."[22] All we know is now; we cannot know tomorrow, and it is not a good feeling. Maybe this explains why I keep needing to connect with my friends and family, why I have this desire to establish a set hour each morning for exercise and another for lunch, why 6 p.m. is universal glass-of-wine time, and why, despite all these efforts, the days still feel like a blur, still uncontrollable. I need to be able to think about some point in the future as being different from today. But there is no vacation to plan, no family reunion at the park, no Friday afternoon at the bar.

Space has also been altered by the pandemic. The rooms of the house take on new uses; the den is school/gym. The kitchen doubles as office/school. It's crowded. Adults working from home, kids "learning" from home. Truth be told, by now "school" has devolved into an hour of Zoom in which teachers give out reading assignments, musical instrument practice, exercise routines, and math problems that never quite get explained in the allotted time.[23] In suburbia, parents try to keep kids learning by creating science experiments, allowing them to take apart that old clock, signing them up for online sewing classes. We are afraid to send our kids outside. I am half-worker, half-parent, half-teacher. I feel like I am doing a half-assed job at all of it.

Young professionals move whole offices to their apartments and set alarms to remind themselves to stop working at 7 p.m. Families buy work-out equipment, video game consoles, and screen projectors for at-home movie nights. I see details around the house I never noticed before, like the water stain on the ceiling where the roof must be leaking. I run my hands along my worn furniture and throw out a broken lamp I've inexplicably kept since college.

And we are the lucky ones, with stable jobs and money and family and friends and older kids. My friends with younger children don't seem to be able to work at all, or are bankrupting themselves paying for babysitters who, justifiably, expect hazard pay to work masked up during a pandemic.

And so many millions have to move in with parents or take whatever work they can find or collect their extra unemployment insurance and try not to lose their homes.

Our computer and phone screens are somehow even more central in our lives than they were before. We "doomscroll" the terrible news or amuse ourselves with cooking shows and memes. At first, everyone around me seemed to be carried along by an apocalyptic mentality: worry over the actual virus combines with a *frisson* at the idea of living through such a historic time. There was a manic, frenetic energy to those first weeks, like holding tight to the bars of a roller coaster as you careen toward the earth. But it's hard to stay panicked indefinitely. Now televisions, streaming services, and internet ads fill with commercials that start with soft music and the phrase, "In these challenging times . . . ," followed by an expression of solidarity by the company with their loyal market. The apocalypse has become quotidian.

People are looking for good news, I suppose. Sunday's *Today* started this week by featuring good deeds by regular folks. There's Sue from West Islip, New York, who cheerfully hands out hand sanitizer at the local grocery store. John Krasinski's *SGN* (Some Good News) YouTube channel reminds us we can still find kindness in the world. My favorite piece of happy news is also quite practical: the segment on the morning news show on Fox 8 in Cleveland, Ohio, called "What Day Is It? With Todd Meany." He literally just tells you what day it is. I need that. And apparently, so does everyone else.

FRIDAY, APRIL 10, 2020

Twenty-nine days since shutdowns began

US Surgeon General Jerome Adams just pulled out a red asthma inhaler in the White House briefing room. "I've been carrying around an inhaler for forty years," he says. With this dramatic gesture, Adams is hoping to emphasize some of the first data to emerge from this pandemic's progress through the United States. And it's not good. COVID-19 is tracing the racial fissures in the landscape of America.

African Americans die from respiratory illnesses at a much higher rate than other groups. Maybe two to three times higher. Part of this relates to lower amounts of health insurance coverage, part has to do with physicians occasionally prescribing cheaper, less effective medications for African American patients.[24] While journalists continue to report that disease does not "discriminate" by race, historians of epidemics have long known that's misleading. And now we have data to show this coronavirus is killing African Americans at much higher rates than whites.[25] From Milwaukee, Detroit, Chicago, and New Orleans, the numbers look bleak. Chicago is about one-third African American, but over two-thirds of its COVID-19 deaths are in the Black community. Louisiana and Michigan report the same disproportionate numbers. Milwaukee is even worse.[26]

It would be easy to attribute such data to some innate difference tied to "Africanness"—the negative image of the myth refuted just a month ago that skin color made one immune to coronavirus. Surgeon General Adams thankfully moves on quickly; no genetic predisposition to dying of COVID-19 exists.

At the same time, Adams chooses not to address the real causes of disproportionate deaths. The factors killing minorities are socioeconomic, not biological. Take "essential workers," for instance, which we often think means physicians and firefighters. Right now, the term also encompasses cashiers, bus drivers, meat packers, mail and food deliverers, and sanitation workers.[27] During lockdowns, these essential workers still do their jobs, often for low wages. They receive few, if any, paid sick days. They often have no PPE. They cannot work from home.[28] They have to return to work even if exposed, as long as their symptoms aren't bad. They rarely have adequate health insurance. Often, these vulnerable workers are racial minorities.[29] They are still transporting, cleaning, keeping the grocery and hardware stores running. They are delivering increasing amounts of stuff to the folks sheltering at home. So, one explanation for why racial minorities in the largest American cities are dying disproportionately during this pandemic is because of occupational segregation—so many workers from minority groups are on the "front lines," unable to hide from the virus at home.[30] Surgeon General Adams dodges this fact entirely.

Instead, in what can only be described as cringe-worthy TV, Surgeon General Adams launches into a lecture about behaviors that will help out nonwhite communities: "Avoid alcohol, tobacco and drugs. . . . Do it for your Abuela, do it for your Grandaddy, do it for your Big Mama, do it for your Pop-Pop. . . . We need you to step up and stop the spread." He defends his language in the Q&A afterward, saying these are terms used in his family. But it sounds suspiciously like blaming the victim. Where were these comments about behavior modification when politicians were urging white people to stay at home?

What makes this tone especially egregious is that government in this country seems *nakedly disinterested* in helping African Americans protect themselves from the virus. There's the problem of "masking-while-Black"— Black men reporting run-ins with police simply because they're wearing medical masks in public.[31] Yesterday, an officer inside an Illinois Walmart followed two African American men through the store and told them they "cannot wear masks."[32] Today, a Miami-Dade officer handcuffed an African American physician for passing out masks.[33] It looks like you can either wear a mask to stay safer from the coronavirus or not wear a mask to stay safer from white cops.

Wisconsin's presidential primary election on Tuesday provides another example. Had government at any level been truly interested in protecting minorities in, say, Milwaukee, where we know coronavirus is hitting the Black community especially hard, mail-in balloting or delayed voting would have prevailed. Instead, Republican justices ruled elections had to continue as normal. "Normal" meant few polls open in Black areas and, consequently, long lines of people, not all of whom had masks or felt safe to wear them even if they wanted to "do it for . . . Big Mama."[34]

SUNDAY, APRIL 12, 2020

Easter Sunday. 550,000 cases—the day Trump originally said the country was going to "open"

Some churches hold Easter services in person today, despite it being illegal basically everywhere. At Maryville Baptist Church near Louisville, Kentucky, parishioners toss nails and tacks in front of the church driveway to keep police vehicles out.[35] Perhaps these parishioners believe themselves to be immune from the coronavirus and justified in dismissing the laws. Maybe they simply put their need to be in person above the law or public health.

On the other end of the Christian spectrum, Pope Francis writes an Easter message stressing that this pandemic could be the right time to consider "a universal basic wage." Such provisions would make it possible for people to stay home and pay their bills. It might help stop the virus. The idea seems to fall on deaf ears here in America.

Meanwhile, "essential" workers are being laid off. The Smithfield Foods pork processing plant in Sioux Falls, South Dakota, one of the largest in the world, is closing "indefinitely."[36] In its announcement, Smithfield doesn't mention any COVID-positive employees, only that coronavirus is in all kinds of production facilities all over the country. But two hundred of the Smithfield Sioux Falls plant employees have tested positive, bringing its per capita case rate higher than that of Seattle or Chicago. Yesterday, South Dakota governor Kristi Noem, a staunch Trump supporter, and Sioux Falls mayor Paul TenHaken requested the plant close for cleaning and employee quarantining for just fourteen days—not "indefinitely."[37] In response, the Smithfield CEO basically threatened the state and the nation: Either we stay open and make pork, or you go hungry and have lots of extra pigs running around. Nowhere does the company say what it's doing for its employees. This behavior is not surprising. Smithfield waged a fifteen-year long fight against workers unionizing. The company's labor is largely comprised of low-wage, vulnerable immigrants from around the world. In the past, workers have accused Smithfield of calling immigration raids on them to disrupt the ability of labor to organize.[38]

Holding the other end of the retail-food supply chain are grocery store employees. Last week, the largest food workers' union, the United Food and Commercial Workers International Union (UFCW), pushed the CDC to issue new guidelines for how grocery stores should operate. They seem straightforward: stores should mandate social distancing of six feet or more, allow employees time to wash their hands every thirty minutes or so, sanitize the heck out of anything touched, place barriers between customers and cashiers, supply PPE and mandate that employees wear it, and make sure shoppers are also wearing masks. UFCW also argued that meatpacking plants like Smithfield must be held to the same standards.[39] We're one month into shutdowns from this pandemic and this demand by the union is only now being lodged. At least forty-one grocery workers have died of coronavirus so far.[40]

Also, there were well over *one hundred* tornadoes this Easter weekend, killing dozens and injuring hundreds. That kind of natural disaster used to make the front pages.

WEDNESDAY, APRIL 15, 2020

One month and three days after shutdowns began—around 28,000 deaths

Ordinarily, today is Tax Day. This year, it's been moved to June or July; I'm not sure. Again, as with the tornadoes, what would be major news becomes a footnote.

Instead, the news follows the right-wing groups, many from rural Michigan, that have been staging anti-lockdown protests at the statehouse in Lansing. Today, they have implemented Operation Gridlock—their plan to shut down the city's main thoroughfares with their cars, trucks, and RVs. They are complaining about Governor Gretchen Whitmer's stay-at-home order extension, which bars travel back and forth from vacation homes on the lake. She also removed more businesses from the "essential" list, including landscaping and gun stores, so they'll have to close. Operation Gridlock blocks ambulances from getting to the nearby hospital on a day when Michigan is recording 28,000 cases and over 1,900 deaths.[41] The Michigan Nurses Association label the protest as "irresponsible."[42]

A handful of white, anti-lockdown protesters step out of their trucks with rifles and walk purposefully through the city streets. Dozens of others assemble in front of the statehouse, their "Trump 2020" and "Don't Tread on Me" Gadsden flags waving. No police interfere.

SUNDAY, APRIL 19, 2020

Erin Bromage specializes in infectious diseases at University of Massachusetts-Dartmouth.[43] He offers a synopsis of what we know about this virus at the moment.

On the question of where the virus came from, Bromage declares that it was definitely *not* intentionally engineered, as some still speculate; it's not a Chinese weapon. That said, scientists cannot rule out at this time that the virus escaped accidentally from a lab.[44] Most likely, however, this was a bat-to-human zoonotic event, perhaps with a scaly pangolin host in between—the standard story for over a month.[45]

On the question of whether or not COVID-19 was in global circulation early last year, Bromage declares that it was not. The first major crossover event occurred in November in or near Wuhan, but not necessarily at the seafood market.[46] The United States had a few cases but contained them and shut down travel from China by the end of January.[47] Most cases in the United States, according to Bromage, likely came from Europe and ran through the East Coast, *not* from China and the West Coast. Still, recent news suggests the so-called China travel ban let in a staggering 430,000 people, many of whom were not screened. American airports proved porous barriers.[48]

Right now, the RT-rPCR test is the most common tool for assessing if someone has COVID-19. It involves jamming a cotton swab on the end of a long stick up your nose until it feels like it hits your brain. They spin out your cells, use reagents to boost it, and *Violá*, you can read if there's coronavirus RNA floating around in your mucus membranes. A positive result is very accurate; it means there is actual SARS-CoV-2 ribonucleic acid in your body, even if you're not sick from it yet.

Unfortunately, false negatives with this RT-rPCR test appear with worrisome frequency, because either the swab was taken incorrectly or the patient has insufficient "viral load" for the RNA to show up.[49] This almost certainly led to China's methodological shift away from lab-based diagnostic measures toward clinical ones like chest X-rays. This also led to China's upward revision of cases and deaths—headlined as a "surge" instead of a change in diagnostic practice—in February.[50] I woke up in a cold sweat last night, wondering if we have thousands of people in this country who have received false negatives and are unwittingly spreading the disease.

WEDNESDAY, APRIL 22, 2020

Globally, car and airplane traffic has almost completely stopped. Water and air pollution has shrunk dramatically.[51] Residents of Jalandhar, India, can see the snowcapped Himalayas from their homes for the first time in decades. Noise pollution, too, is down—much appreciated by whales, birds, and the scientists who study them.[52]

While humans have been confined to their homes, animals are on the move. Goats stroll down village streets in Wales. Lions lie on empty safari park roads in Kenya. Leatherback sea turtle hatchlings in Oregon travel from their nests on the beach into the ocean to start their lives without being disrupted by nosy people.[53] Ibex lope down Israeli streets. A very large alligator crawls toward a strip mall in South Carolina. Many read this as a redemptive narrative—this idea that something good has come of the virus as the earth "heals itself." Online, eco-activists declare that "we are the virus."

It is nice to see the natural world getting a break. But who knows how long it will last? We're still extracting and combusting to make our electricity. The Antarctic and Greenland ice sheets haven't slowed their melting. Massive floral and faunal die-offs continue unabated.[54] Long-term trends have not budged much. Given how hard it's been to come together as a nation to address a pressing pandemic, it's easy to worry about our ability to address long-term threats like climate change, even if we vote a new leader into office come November.

THURSDAY, APRIL 23, 2020

Six weeks since stay-at-home orders began—44,000 deaths

Today, at a CTF briefing, the president says to Bill Bryan, acting undersecretary of the Science and Technology Directorate at DHS: "So, supposing we hit the body with a tremendous—whether it's ultraviolet or just very powerful light. . . . supposing you brought the light *inside* the body, which you can do either through the skin or in some other way, and I think you said you're going to test that too. . . . and then I see the disinfectant, where it knocks it out in a minute. One minute. And is there a way we can do something like that, by injection inside or almost a cleaning. . . . you're going to have to use medical doctors. . . . But it sounds . . . interesting to me."[55]

In other words, President Trump, in front of cameras, in his official capacity as an authority speaking to the country, speculated that a bright light could be shined into the body or some disinfectants put "inside" the body to heal coronavirus. The makers of Lysol disinfectant release a public service announcement immediately, warning people, "under no circumstance should our disinfectant products be administered into the human body (through injection, ingestion or any other route)."[56]

Lysol has reason to worry. Surveys show more than three-quarters of American voters show intense emotional connections to their chosen political party's leaders. They *are* their party. Emory University psychologist Drew Westen argues even when it is irrefutably clear that a leader in your party has committed a serious ethical violation, people will work,

"Houdini-like," to escape from those facts in order to retain an emotional connection to their party.[57] Cognitive dissonance resolved. It will be tough reconciling this one.

In the same briefing as his "bleach speech" (as the press quickly labels it), Trump touts an "awe-inspiring" economic recovery already underway.[58] No evidence supports this claim. Yet, there is a huge population who will choose to believe him because to do otherwise invites discomfort and dissonance.

MONDAY, APRIL 27, 2020

980,000 cases—ten times the number one month ago

Only rarely does the *New York Times* print a story about the suicide of a noncelebrity. But the death yesterday of Lorna M. Breen, the medical director of the emergency department at New York-Presbyterian/Columbia University Allen Hospital in northern Manhattan, symbolizes something profound. Before she died, Dr. Breen described patient after patient being pulled out of ambulances, already lifeless. In less than a month, close to sixty people died in her hospital alone. She contracted COVID herself, then returned to work after only ten days of convalescence. Dr. Breen hadn't fully recovered, and the hospital put her on leave again. She died at her parents' home in Virginia only two weeks later. Friends and family blame her dramatically altered behavior on longer-term effects of the virus.[59] These facts, of course, neither plumb the depths of Breen's pain nor explain her death. And it's worth noting that hers is not the kind of suicide the president warned about on March 25.

It looks like COVID is killing people in unexpected ways. Younger people with no known comorbidities are dying of stroke, apparently tied to COVID.[60] In the first major analysis since this outbreak began, Yale School of Public Health researchers found *far* more deaths in March and April than usual, even accounting for those coded as COVID. The actual death count in New York City, for instance, is 6,300 higher than normal for this time in the year (*not* including deaths marked as COVID).[61] Surely, not all of these excess deaths have been due to coronavirus. But the number does raise concerns that either we are undercounting the number of deaths from COVID or people are dying from other disorders at an escalated rate, perhaps because of poor medical attention due to the overwhelming number of coronavirus cases flooding hospitals and clinics.

Equally frustrating is the insistence coming from the right-wing media that physicians exaggerate fatality numbers to profit hospitals unjustly. On Laura Ingraham's Fox News show, Senator Scott Jensen (R-MN), who is also a physician, hinted that the federal government payout to hospitals incentivizes them (and, by extension, their physicians) to exaggerate COVID claims.[62] Ingraham played a clip of the April 8 White House CTF in which a reporter raised the notion "that the number of COVID-19 deaths are being padded." At that meeting, Dr. Fauci responded that these conspiracy theories are "nothing but distractions." Ingraham then invited Jensen to respond to Fauci's claim. This pandemic, Jenson replied, is indeed making hospitals and doctors rich. And Fauci, he implied, is wrong.

Jensen seems to have gotten his evidence for this claim from a *Kaiser Health News* article that, ironically, draws a contradictory conclusion. The initial $30 billion government payout to hospitals went to facilities based on their "historical share of revenue from the Medicare program for seniors—not according to their coronavirus burden."[63] So, hospitals in largely rural, largely Republican areas that are not suffering much from this pandemic (including those represented by Jensen in Minnesota) are ending up with *more* money being doled out to them through government welfare than some hard-hit New York City hospitals. Zero evidence exists for the claim that physicians are participating in system-gaming in New York City or Detroit or Seattle or Chicago or Miami—the coronavirus hot spots. (To be fair, even Jensen later admitted this.) If anything, it's hospital *corporations* protected by their big donations to GOP insiders gaming the system, though through Medicare mis-billings, not COVID-19 payouts, as Jensen insinuates.[64]

TUESDAY, APRIL 28, 2020

Over the last month, the president has spouted several contradictory messages. When people asked him to shut down the country last month, he claimed that he did not have the authority to tell governors what to do. Now he says repeatedly that states must reopen and that his "authority is total." On April 16, his administration released reopening guidelines. As the Michigan militia has been taking to the statehouse these last two weeks, he called on his supporters to "LIBERATE MICHIGAN!" Confusingly, he *opposed* Georgia's planned reopening just last week. He also recently moved to block green cards for most immigrants on the pretext that coronavirus *wasn't* under control in the US.[65] Two days from now, the initial federal stay-at-home guidelines are set to expire, which should cede further decisions to the states. On April 6, the country had around ten thousand COVID deaths. Three weeks later, on April 24, we had *fifty thousand*. No curve has been flattened. And our tests are barely more reliable—or available—than they were over a month ago.[66]

Making matters worse, the debate that began in *February* over whether the flu is worse than COVID, continues. The logic from those protesting stay-at-home orders is that, if the seasonal flu doesn't trigger lockdowns, why should this coronavirus?

So, let's settle this. Is the novel coronavirus pandemic just like a bad flu year?

To find out, I investigate the much longer history of the CDC's influenza statistics. The CDC's estimates of how many people die from seasonal influenza each year do look scary, with upwards of fifty thousand deaths per year. The tragic 2017–18 season saw eighty thousand people die from flu.[67] This statistic puts the ordinary flu up with some of the most tragic killers in the United States *every* year: accidents, suicides, and so on.

But the CDC's system of counting flu deaths is *not* the same as its method for counting coronavirus deaths. The CDC counts a COVID-19 death when "COVID-19" is listed as the cause of death on the death certificate.[68] In contrast, they do not count a flu death based on "flu" being written on the death certificate. Instead, they use models and projections of how many deaths *could* have been caused by flu—not how many actually died of it. Before 1950, states, cities, and individual physicians used their own subjective discretion in reporting whether someone died of "flu." WHO and the CDC realized this sort of monitoring was deeply flawed and started mathematically modeling excess deaths due to influenza combined with pneumonia by using sample groups to predict flu deaths, hopefully catching another viral outbreak before it happened.

Over the years, the CDC updated its modeling. Each time, it updated the model *upward*, arguing that increasing numbers of people were getting sick and dying from the flu. They did this ostensibly to encourage increased funding for public health and because the flu often goes undiagnosed. Current models estimate that for every influenza related hospitalization, "between 11 and 365 more" cases occur—an enormous margin.[69] Importantly, the flu mortality rate is also based on this sort of overcount.[70] The point is that flu deaths are likely lower than the models suggest. One ER physician, in response to the "flu is worse than coronavirus" argument, recently claimed he had seen only *one* death by influenza over his career, in contrast to the many deaths he has seen from COVID-19.[71]

Rumors presently circulating on social media fixate on an *overcount* of coronavirus deaths at fifty thousand, though an *undercount* is more likely.[72] A heart attack or stroke triggered by the infection was likely to have been missed. Counting excess deaths rather than actual COVID-labeled death certificates—the same technique we use with the flu, in other words—will likely show many more deaths above the ordinary this year.

WEDNESDAY, APRIL 29, 2020

Over 55,000 deaths

I am aware that I am drinking more than usual. It is both dismaying and comforting to read in the news that I'm not alone, and that alcohol consumption has tripled in the last two months.[73] Sometimes, I struggle just to get out of bed. Sometimes, the worry and uncertainty register as physical pain, running from behind my eyes to my swollen hands to my chest. I realize I'm forgetting to breathe.

Chrystos, the renowned Menominee two-spirit poet, writes me. "Thinking of covid & death . . . trapped in a sprawling city with not enough land around us for protection . . . Rain has come falling softly on the thirsty earth . . . Stupified with grief.—me today. (sic)"

"Thank you," I write back. "I am glad to know that I am not alone."

Historically speaking, all this drinking is perfectly appropriate. Generals have known for centuries that drink lifts confidence and suppresses fear. In 1940, Lord Woolton, British minister of food, declared that beer was essential for keeping up public morale during World War II. Soviet soldiers received rationed portions of vodka in their MREs in Stalingrad in 1943. British soldiers got rum, Americans, whiskey. Alcohol manages stress. It also blurs reality.

An old friend emails me about joining AA in March. What a time to decide to get sober.

In early March, on my forty-sixth birthday, I polished off a bottle of Jameson and a bottle of Jägermeister in four hours. When I woke up the next morning, I was leveled by this overwhelming depression and anxiety. For the first time, I had real thoughts of suicide. I hated myself and all that I had become, all that I had lost. I realized that I was standing on the edge of a knife, facing a life-or-death choice, maybe the last choice I had to make. . . .

What I have learned since then is that AA is really a course on how to live a manageable life and how to go to bed at night with a sense of integrity that comes from being honest and humble . . . Drinking made my ego huge. . . .

Deciding to get sober during a pandemic was a blessing and a curse. . . . When the virus hit, the bars all closed, which meant that I was buying liquor by the bottle and drinking it at home. I drank three times as much in those two weeks. It seems like everyone started drinking more heavily after the shutdown. . . .

The virus also made getting help harder. After my birthday, when I decided that I had to do something, all the meetings were over Zoom. I got on the computer and tried one meeting. It was absolutely ridiculous. There I am, staring at a screen with thirty-five other people and I'm trying to have that first, really hard conversation. I knew instantly that if I was going to succeed at this, it wasn't going to be on the internet. I told a friend in the program. . . . She texted me, "We are going to be at the park tomorrow at 7:30 in the morning. Just show up." When I got there, there were nine other people there, and I knew six of them.

I have gone every day since. It is against the law to meet in person, but I wouldn't be alive without it. We meet in the park every morning. Twice the cops have approached us, but they let us continue when they find out why we are there. All I know now is that there are three things I need to do every day: don't have a drink, go to a meeting, and talk to my sponsor. I am willing to risk this virus and the police to make those things happen.

THURSDAY, APRIL 30, 2020

Seven weeks since stay-at-home orders began, most expire today

Today, in Lansing, Michigan, grown men—all white—brandish assault rifles inside the state capitol, hollering insults, looking down on the state senators from the second-floor balcony, as you would fish in a barrel. Senator Dayna Polehanki tells me that everyone was terrified.

It's worth dwelling on these images for a minute. True, flashing weapons in the statehouse chamber is not illegal. But it's not illegal to hold a toy gun in a park either. Nevertheless, in 2014, it took Cleveland police less than two seconds to kill Tamir Rice, an African American twelve-year-old who was merely holding a toy gun. Here are grown men, with fingers on triggers, threatening elected officials, and cops stand by motionless. This is the third or fourth such "reopening" protest there this month. Gone are people holding signs begging to be able to go to their lake houses. These guys are here to send Governor Whitmer a more threatening message.

Outside, another spectacle: a crowd on the steps of the courthouse flies the Confederate battle flag—a flag that, a century and a half ago, thousands of men from this state bled to defeat. Two girls dance. One wears a Trump mask, the other an artificially darkened Barack Obama mask—literally, in blackface. A truck parked nearby bears a gallows with a noose. "Tyrants get the rope," reads its sign.[74]

Only blocks away on Michigan Avenue, healthcare workers at Sparrow Hospital, many of whom are African American women, wage a different sort of battle. They call on the hospital corporation and the government to enforce the stay-at-home rules and to provide more help and protective equipment.

Both of these groups insist the needs of a community must be protected. But *which* community and by what means? Each group questions governmental legitimacy, though one side sees the political leadership as too invasive, the other, not invasive enough.

The militants at the state house hear the president declare that, even without a vaccine, the virus is just "gonna go. It's gonna leave."[75] They believe there's no pandemic, that they are strong enough to withstand any illness, or, fatalistically, that if this doesn't kill them, something else will anyway. They ignore the danger they represent to the grocery store clerk with diabetes, the elderly parent, or the healthcare worker to whom they become a mobile viral time bomb.

April is over. It was indeed a cruel month. Despite my concern in February that we weren't taking it seriously enough, I never imagined *over 1 million cases* or *57,000 deaths*. How is that possible, given our "advanced" medicine and economy? I know people are clamoring for the country to go back to "normal." Agreed: I don't want this Zoom-mediated, alcohol-medicated life either. I want the kids to go back to school, businesses to open, to hug my elderly mother. But if we don't do something as a community now, will it not just get worse?

Senator Dayna Polehanki ✅
@SenPolehanki

> Directly above me, men with rifles yelling at us. Some of
> my colleagues who own bullet proof vests are wearing
> them. I have never appreciated our Sergeants-at-Arms
> more than today. #mileg

11:38 AM—Apr 30, 2020 from Lansing, MI

FRIDAY, MAY 1, 2020

Fifty-one days since lockdown—over one million cases

Today is May Day, or International Workers' Day. The US has seen over one hundred labor actions so far in this pandemic, a number higher than all of 2019.[1] Workers at Amazon demand extra pay or extra equipment. Meat-packers' strikes continue as Smithfield and other corporate shills blame their largely immigrant labor force for outbreaks.[2] Autoworkers successfully lobby GM, Chrysler, and Ford to delay opening until assembly lines can be made safe.[3] Workers in nursing homes have threatened to walk out if management refuses to help keep them safe and provide hazard pay.[4] Even employees at the LSL Healthcare, a PPE manufacturing plant in the western suburbs of Chicago, are presenting demands, after learning one of their own was ill with COVID and management knew but kept it from workers.[5]

Workers in jobs deemed essential, many of whom are people of color and immigrants, have continued to stand in the firing lines against this virus for almost two months. They are joined now by contractors, landscapers, manufacturers, and retail assistants who have been ordered back to work amidst the "reopening," whether or not it is safe. If school boards decide to open schools in August, teachers will be added to this list of essential workers.

"May Day" can mean advocating for laborers. But it's also the urgent call of a pilot whose plane is going down.

TUESDAY, MAY 5, 2020

1.19 million cases

A week or so ago, Shelley Luther, hairdresser and owner of Salon a la Mode, in Dallas, Texas, defied the lockdown order and opened her business. She received a reprimand and decided to ignore it, ripping it up in public. Today, a Dallas County judge sentenced her to a week of jail and a $7,000 fine.

Many people see Luther as a defender of individual rights against encroaching state control. They are the same people who believe the state should be *more* intrusive in other ways, such as preventing a woman from getting an abortion. They seek to ban abortion because they value life, they say. Yet, they will not agree to stay home, which would stop the spread of the coronavirus—and save lives. Luther and her supporters argue the financial cost of closing their businesses is too high. But they seem not to consider the financial cost to the public—the cost of caring for the people they will infect by keeping their businesses open. They say they are defenders of "law and order," but they seem to want that law and order only when it protects their own financial interests.

Allen West, a highly decorated retired Army officer, an African American running for the chair of the Texas Republican Party, compares Shelley Luther to civil rights icon Rosa Parks. This is galling. Parks risked everything, defying seventy years of Jim Crow laws relegating African Americans to permanent second-class status. Shelley Luther defied a forty-five-day law temporarily restricting the work of hairdressers during a global pandemic that has already taken the lives of around seventy thousand Americans. Parks put her life on the line to fight for equal rights. Luther opened up her shop one week earlier than all the other business owners who chose to follow the law.

Before the judge today, Luther mobilizes the politics of childhood and maternity to justify her actions: "I have to disagree with you, sir, when you say I am selfish, because feeding my kids is not selfish. I have hair stylists who are going hungry because they'd rather feed their kids. So, sir, if you think the law is more important than kids getting fed, then please go ahead with your decision, but I am not going to shut the salon."[6] Luther conjures the age-old image—a cliché, really—of a desperate parent breaking the law to feed their children. To some, she now joins the ranks of Eisenstein's mother in *Battleship Potemkin* and Jean Valjean in *Les Misérables*. Few images are more potent than the hungry, dirty, and orphaned child to motivate a population to rage and revulsion.[7] People have used the image of the threatened innocent child to justify every action under the sun. Giving a prohibited wash and trim to the quarantine can now be added to the list.

Meanwhile, healthcare workers all over the country make hard sacrifices. A North Carolina ICU nurse named Kate tells me how she sits in a chair at the foot of her basement stairs to talk to her family at the top of the stairs for a little bit each night. She misses them but knows it's safer this way. Karl, an ER physician, comes home to an isolated room. Sometimes he plays board games with his children through a window, pushing the pieces with a broom handle. Kate, Karl, and countless other medical professionals sit alone at night, hoping more people will take shelter-in-place orders more seriously, so they can hold their kids soon.

Further challenging Luther's hard-luck story is the account of Isabel Castro-Garcia and Brenda Stephanie Mata, arrested in Laredo, Texas, for running a salon out of their homes. Undercover officers ran a sting operation to catch the two Latina women violating the same Emergency Management Plan that Luther openly flouted in Dallas. Will the "Resistance" branding breaking out on Twitter for Luther extend to Castro-Garcia and Mata—and their children, who are suffering actual economic anxiety while their mothers await jail time?[8] Being poor and nonwhite in 2020 means you can be arrested for the exact same activity that valorizes a white woman.

And it's not just a double standard. There's actual danger. Today, a video appears online from events back in February. Two white men gun down a Black man named Ahmaud Arbery in the middle of the day on a residential street in the seaside town of Satilla Shores, Georgia.[9] The video shows Arbery jogging on the left side of a road. A white pickup truck with the Confederate battle flag prominently displayed stops in the right lane. A white man with a handgun is standing in the truck bed. Another white man gets out of the driver's seat with a shotgun. While the camera shakes, the two men collectively fire three shots into Arbery, who struggles to knock the shotgun away from the driver. Arbery then tries to run away and makes it five steps, stumbles to the ground, and stops moving, his life snuffed out.

Why did it take until today for Ahmaud Arbery's extrajudicial killing to go public? One of the shooters, Gregory McMichael, is a retired police officer; he has also worked as an investigator with the local district attorney's office. He was the one standing in the truck bed. His son, Travis, drove the truck and fired the shotgun. Local law enforcement and the broader justice system in southeast Georgia appear to have buried evidence and slowed the investigation for two months. Right now, the McMichaels remain free men.

Other unbelievable events took place today but went largely unnoticed. A former US Green Beret along with his two former special forces buddies thought it would be a good idea to lead three hundred Venezuelan militia out of the South American jungle and try to overthrow Venezuelan president Nicolás Maduro.[10] The plan failed, to put it mildly. Two US citizens, both former Green Berets, are now in Venezuelan custody. Alleged ties connect this coup attempt to close associates of Trump.[11] In the "before time," this would be a scandalous story akin to the Bay of Pigs disaster. In 2020, we just call it Tuesday.

WEDNESDAY, MAY 6, 2020

It's like standing in front of an open fire hydrant.

For the first time in American history, the Supreme Court hears oral arguments over an audio stream today (the highlight is the "flush heard 'round the world," when someone uses the loo in the middle of arguments).[12]

Yesterday, scientists published evidence that the virus circulated the globe much earlier than previously believed. After examining the viral RNA of over 7,500 samples, researchers in London suggest the new coronavirus crossed from its animal host into a human sometime in September or October 2019. The coronavirus mutated several times as it traveled through Asia, Europe, and North America, even crisscrossing its own path. At present, the virus found inside each country reflects the mutation paths of SARS-CoV-2 around the world. This means each region had *multiple* introductions, *multiple* networks of transmission. We aren't going to find a "patient zero" for each country. Every nation is full of carriers of multiple strains, with multiple pockets of infection.[13] And the virus will continue to change.

But rather than paying attention to this new and pertinent scientific information, millions of people are watching a "Plandemic" conspiracy-theory video on the internet. It is the third-most popular internet search term and the accompanying book, a bestseller. Dr. Fauci, as the theory goes, is an evil genius in cahoots with international scientists and businessmen who orchestrated the outbreak for personal profit. Ominously, "Plandemic" misinformation has leapt from the internet onto real signs at real protests calling for pandemic restrictions to be dropped, coast to coast.

THURSDAY, MAY 7, 2020

Today, Texas governor Greg Abbott sets free the hairdresser-turned-Rosa Parks hero of American consumer liberties, Shelley Luther. The popular morning show *Fox & Friends* has invited Texas Republican congressman Dan Crenshaw to talk about Luther's role in fighting the good fight.

> Yeah, these so-called leaders and these so-called judges across the country arresting moms and dads . . . , they need to take a civics lesson. These laws will not be respected if they are not respectable laws. People are not dumb. They can understand and they can assess whether a law makes sense, whether it's based on data and public health. . . . It's because they're drunk on power. They're drunk on power. They think we're stupid . . . And this is why you're seeing people rise up. Americans are sick of it. . . . [14]

Dan Crenshaw, himself a powerful member of the federal government, rails against the drunk-on-power "they." But who is this "they," exactly? Democrats? Advocates for public health? Or is Crenshaw angry with anyone who tells him and his supporters they can't have exactly what they want right this second (because "liberty" is defined by customer desires)?

"Othering"—creating a "them" in order to create an "us"—is a vital part of modern political culture, according to historian Edward Said.[15] "They" serve as a useful enemy, defined not by a static meaning, but by the need to justify a group's beliefs and retain societal power. At present, "they" includes the judge, whose sentence has been overturned, and anyone else who would advocate for more rigorous non-pharmaceutical interventions.

Why is this debate over public health versus individual freedoms so loud during this pandemic? This debate, while not exclusively American, is a critical part of our national identity. From our inception, the founders established the nation's commitment to defending freedom and the pursuit of happiness—for a particular group of propertied white men. The freedoms and rights, even the *lives*, of others had to be secondary. Posed against that is the common welfare; literally the common*wealth* as John Adams framed it back in 1780, and as Kentucky, Virginia, Massachusetts, and Pennsylvania continue to insist.[16] Adams argued that *everyone's* liberties are worth representing and defending by elected officials, even if it means limiting the actions of the few. Adams recognized this does not have to be a zero-sum proposition, though this is how it's being constructed today.

It is hard to ignore that Crenshaw's "they" often aren't white. The Dallas judge who fined Luther is Harvard-trained Eric Moyé. He is African American. For Crenshaw, Luther, and their supporters, "law and order" seems great when applied to the "others." In Ohio, for instance, Black people are being arrested for violating social distancing at a vastly disproportionate level compared to white people.[17] Dallas city councilmember Omar Narvaez, who is Latino, best sums up the hypocrisy he sees—how law and order is essential when it applies to minorities but is labeled "socialism" when applied to white people like Shelley Luther:

> All I know is that [minorities] are always told to fall in line because "we are a nation of laws." . . . Everyone watches us with a microscope for when we make a sudden move. Black men are literally slain on running trails or arrested trying to get into their own homes. . . . What makes [Luther] different? She has child support, a very nice home, nice cars, beautiful furniture and was the recipient of a fully funded small business loan through the CARES Act . . . Her difference is her privilege of being a well-to-do ultra conservative white woman. If she cared so much about her kids all she had to do was apologize and she'd have been home with those same kids she was so worried about feeding and preparing to open her salon on Friday like all the other folks that all followed the law and were waiting.

FRIDAY, MAY 8, 2020

Back in April, the Cheyenne River Sioux and Ogala Sioux erected check-points on South Dakota roads entering their reservations. The Bureau of Indian Affairs issued a memorandum saying that tribes could only restrict access to tribal lands after they had "consulted and reached an agreement" with the state.[18] The Sioux didn't budge. South Dakota's governor, Kristi Noem, had refused to mandate business closure and stay-at-home orders. On April 17, at least 634 workers at the Smithfield Foods facility in Sioux Falls tested positive for COVID. Workers reported that they were not given any protective gear or hand sanitizer. There was no social distancing, with lunchrooms holding five hundred workers at a time.[19] That afternoon, Noem launched the only state-run hydroxychloroquine trial.

Today, Governor Noem writes letters to the Oglala Sioux Tribe and the Cheyenne River Sioux Tribe, demanding that they close their checkpoints. "The State of South Dakota objects to tribal checkpoints on US and State Highways regardless of whether those checkpoints take into consideration the safety measures recommended by the South Dakota Department of Transportation." She threatens the tribes with legal action.[20] Later, Cheyenne River Sioux tribal chairman Harold Frazier responds: "We will not apologize for being an island of safety in a sea of uncertainty and death." He cites the Fort Laramie Treaty of 1868, reminding the governor that no white people can be permitted to occupy or pass through their lands without the "consent of the Indians first."[21]

Noem perhaps has forgotten that Native American communities have long-standing reasons not to trust white leaders. Their tribes were destroyed in the seventeenth century by viruses that Europeans brought into their communities.[22] Native American populations suffer from high levels of diabetes and heart disease, which put them at increased risk of death from COVID. Their access to healthcare is precarious. The Indian Health Service provides $4,078 per capita in healthcare spending, less than half what is spent on federal prisoners.[23] The one hospital on the Cheyenne River Sioux Reservation has no ICU. In the Navajo Nation, 4,253 cases and 146 deaths have been reported, with a case rate of 22 percent.[24] They don't even have an accurate understanding of how bad their case rates are; the CDC did not start reporting race and ethnicity in its COVID outcomes until April, and even then, it slotted Native Americans into the "other" category.[25] As Kerry Hawk Lessard, executive director of Native American LifeLines, notes, the lack of reliable data means that resources can't be allocated. Reservations lack ventilators and PPE; hospitals run out of medical gowns.[26] In the meantime, case rates in Native American communities continue to grow, and the Cheyenne River Sioux, understandably, man the ramparts.

SUNDAY, MAY 10, 2020

Mother's Day

I make turkey sandwiches and celery sticks, all wrapped individually in wax paper, to meet my mom and her roommate at the park. We wave at each other from opposite sides of the pavilion, my kids lined up awkwardly on one side of a picnic bench so that their grandmother can see them. She is too far away for real conversation. We eat our sandwiches and watch the big tugboats move down the Black Warrior River to the Gulf of Mexico.

My mom moved to a retirement facility two years ago and has been locked inside since the pandemic began. I try not to worry too much about her. She was a nurse her whole life and has a relatively stoic view of her role in this pandemic. "When people like me die, it might be a heart attack or cancer or a virus that gets you, but really, you're just dying of old age," she says.

"The quality of your death matters, mom. You know that," I reply. She looks away and nods. "Sometimes you don't get to choose that."

She looks like a little old lady now, but she was a nurse in Quang Ngai, Vietnam, during the Tet Offensive in 1968. She has pulled shrapnel out of babies. It might not matter to her how she dies, but it does to me. COVID-19 is taking her generation right out from underneath our noses, while we are stuck in Zoom meetings. If they enter the hospital, we might not even get to say goodbye.

Meanwhile, our leaders dither over mask ordinances and how hard to come down on the Shelley Luthers of the nation. All I can think as I bite into my sandwich is how so many people have had to die alone. If only we had acted sooner, maybe we could have saved some of them.

MONDAY, MAY 11, 2020

Two months since the NBA shutdown

"No moral code or ethical principle, no piece of scripture or holy teaching, can be summoned to defend what we have allowed our country to become," Matthew Desmond says in his transformative book, *Evicted*.[27] Six million Americans are out of a job. Many are surely losing healthcare, unable to pay the rent, have children going hungry. But this situation has been happening to the poor in our major cities long before the pandemic. This helps explain why the latest Gallup poll measuring the percentage of American adults who consider themselves to be "thriving" has dropped ten points. That represents about twenty-five million people, worse than 2008 recession levels.[28]

Today, Trump claims "Obamagate" is to blame for . . . something. When asked point-blank what the current president is accusing President Obama of doing, he has no answer.[29] In Trump's Twitter tirade yesterday, it was clear that he hopes the word "corrupt" sticks to Obama and Biden like "crooked" stuck to Hillary Clinton.[30]

More information about the shooting of Ahmaud Arbery comes to light today. The men who shot him planned the attack and received institutional support in the cover-up. This news underscores how we remain two Americas, with two histories and two realities. One America believes in law and order as a protection provided to all. The other America views law and order as a tool for supporting a white, wealthy, nativist status quo. It allows certain people to shoot a man three times and walk away free.[31] In the words of Trevor Noah, host of *The Daily Show*, "It's funny how in America if you break the law and look a certain way, you're a criminal. But if you break the law and look a *different* way, then you're a freedom-loving American exercising your rights." Arbery literally ran into that second America, where white men assumed they could do what they pleased. Arbery must have thought, or at least hoped, that law and order would protect him, too.

WEDNESDAY, MAY 13, 2020

According to marketing analysts at *Forbes*, we have entered the "Escapism + Optimism" phase of our virus experience. *Forbes* tells marketers how best to profit off the moment. They have been tracking, and can evidently predict, our consumer behavior, even during a pandemic. Evidently, in the early days of the shutdown, Americans searched for how to make a home office and how to cut our own hair. The following month, people searched for what to send in a care package and what to wear while they worked from home. Now, these marketers claim, we are in the third phase. A VP at marketing analytics firm VaynerMedia says Americans are now interested in spending their money on positive and hopeful plans that project their "utopian view of a post-COVID world."[32] Searches for "virtual sleepover" jumped 800 percent, as have those for "free virtual field trips" and "kids virtual birthday party." People are looking for apartments they might move to and wedding venues in which to someday celebrate. Many are already planning for the wonderful summer they expect will come after states relax health restrictions, which is already happening. This desire for temporal agency creates profit-making opportunities, they say. For marketers, utopias are the perfect commodity, pitched as something people can access through their own consumer activism.[33]

All of this marketing data is critical to firms looking to expand. In spite of antimonopoly laws designed to protect capitalist interests, we are witnessing mergers that would have been blocked before the pandemic. Many companies are using the "failing firm" argument, claiming to be in danger of folding under the pressure of the lockdowns and arguing only a merger with a former competitor can save them.[34] It used to be very difficult to get government approval based on this argument because it eliminated competition. But antitrust regulators are increasingly allowing it, which means the companies that come out of this pandemic are likely to be larger, more powerful, and face less competition.[35]

Companies are also using a different "failing firm" argument to declare that they must reopen, regardless of the danger to employees or customers. Tesla Motors CEO, Elon Musk, decided to open his Fremont, California, factory and informed his employees. Flying in the face of California law to benefit his company, Musk says workers must come to work now if they want to keep their jobs.[36]

SUNDAY, MAY 17, 2020

"Imagine I'm a closeted lesbian that is back in a homophobic house because of COVID-19," Avery Smith, a podcaster and leader in the LGBTQ+ community, shares with me. Smith hosts a highly respected podcast *Blessed*

Are the Binary Breakers and writes the blog *Queerly Christian*, highlighting the struggles and triumphs of the LGBTQA+ and gender nonconforming community.[37] For too many younger LGBTQA+ and gender nonconforming people, these stay-at-home orders have become nightmarish. "Or say you're at college, living away from the people who are maybe even hostile toward you." Smith's voice drops, "There's a pandemic. You're sent home. You're stuck now—you're *stuck*. . . . You don't have your ordinary connections."

"I have a friend group . . . that consists almost completely of trans-plus-autistic and/or otherwise disabled young adults," continues Smith. "This group of friends meets every Sunday evening at the house four of them rent to make and eat a meal, play games, and just chat and have fun together. They have not been able to hold these weekly dinners since February. And for some of the group, that was the one time all week they could be themselves: wear the clothes they like to wear, talk about trans and autistic stuff with people who Get It, and/or not have to worry about getting misgendered nonstop. So, it really sucks that the dinners can't take place. A lot of my friends are experiencing some bad drops in mental health because of that loss of community."

And there are still more tangible difficulties now. "For instance, say a cishet person becomes homeless because of pandemic, and so does a transgender person. The cishet person might be able to find a homeless shelter to stay in; meanwhile, the transgender person may not be able to find a place that will take them in or that will guarantee their safety from transphobic violence. Another example: say a trans person ends up in the hospital for COVID. They may face transphobic remarks from hospital staff, misgendering, or even outright refusal to treat. I know of many trans persons (and other LGBT persons) who will not go to the hospital unless they're literally on death's door because they've been traumatized by health providers in the past. And it's a pandemic!"

WEDNESDAY, MAY 20, 2020

Over 1.5 million cases

I spend an hour this morning looking at my favorite paintings on the internet, trying to get collected for another day in the new normal. If you have ever stood in front of a Kandinsky or a Vrubel or a Glenn Ligon, you know that no image on a screen or on a page can begin to capture the awe-inspiring, lived experience of art. I suspect that, in order to truly emerge from the trauma of this year, we will need the shared-language-that-lives-before-language that art provides.

I speak with Zachary Levine, director of Archival and Curatorial Affairs at the United States Holocaust Memorial Museum. The world's museums and libraries closed back in early March, many permanently.[38] Well-known spaces with large endowments—the Met or the Smithsonian—will survive. Others have been working to move online. Historical archives, where people like me do our hardest work, are digitizing their materials to allow scholars and students (and now homeschooling parents) access. The role of the museum, Levine argues, was already starting to shift before the pandemic from being an authority delivering information to passive visitors to a convener of people around a particular subject. People want to participate and engage. With the pandemic, the successful programs will be those that include the visitor in an active dialogue, even if it is only online. Eventually, there will be an opportunity "for cultural organizations, museums, and art galleries to work very differently from what we've seen in the past." While lots of media attention is focused on the closure of sports and music venues, Levine reminds me that it's institutions like his that we'll need the most in the long run.

Study after study shows the economic benefits of cultural institutions to cities and neighborhoods; they bring many, many more dollars than they cost. Besides, Levine reminds me, "in the wake of all this death and loss caused by coronavirus and the lockdowns, the role of museums—of those that survive these few months, anyway—will become even more central." Museums help us work through tragedies precisely like the one we're experiencing now. Perversely, the museums are closing. "You know, there are estimates that 50 percent of museums could fold right now," Levine says.

THURSDAY, MAY 21, 2020

Debate still rages over the fatality rate of this virus. In a controversial and problematic Stanford study, the authors say they tested a large population of Santa Clara, California, for COVID-19 antibodies. They found the number of people with the antibodies (meaning they have been infected and recovered) was 85 times higher than anticipated. This implies most of the population has already had the virus and, in turn, the mortality rate was not 2 percent but closer to 0.12 percent—roughly the same mortality rate as the flu. Conservative groups pounce on the study as proof that the nation's response to COVID is overblown.

Within days, a whistleblower complaint emerges; the study was actually funded by the JetBlue CEO, who opposes the recent lockdown measures. John Ioannidis, a respected member of the social sciences, has attached his name to the study. Famous for exposing the bad scientific methods of others, Ioannidis is now linked to a study with slipshod statistics, unreliable tests, and a conflict of interest in its funding. And of course, the article was a preprint. That doesn't automatically invalidate the study, but it is fair to wonder if these scholars went looking for something that met a particular economic and political goal—and then found it.[39]

Perhaps the upending of good inductive science is helping to sink us. Or perhaps it is the clear rejection of science from the highest peaks of power that has hampered our nation's response. Just three days ago, the Florida Department of Health fired the manager of its COVID tracking website, Rebekah Jones, after she reported that Florida was purposely underreporting its numbers. The state had not met its own guidelines for relaxing restrictions. But Florida needs tourism, and the governor insisted they open. Jones refused to distort the numbers; she had to go.[40]

These seemingly small decisions to ignore or obfuscate data has had real-life implications. A Columbia University study suggests over 50 percent of deaths to date could have been prevented had we quarantined the country *one to two weeks* earlier—a lesson we could have learned from the development of the 1918 flu pandemic. Over *fifty-eight thousand* people might not have died. That's more than ten times the victims of the 9/11 attacks, which we spent trillions of dollars avenging.[41] The Columbia study goes on to project that if the country fails to issue stay-at-home orders again when cases tick upwards, as they surely will now that states are relaxing enforcement, we will have an even higher surge of cases than we did in March and April. If the country delays two weeks, we could see a daily peak of over 30,000 new cases and 32,379 additional deaths by July.[42]

The research group at Imperial College London (ICL) has been accurately tracking trends through this entire pandemic; it is also releasing a report showing likely case counts for states and regions in the US.[43] Like the unrelated Columbia University study, this one suggests that, in the middle of the country, things will get worse before they get better. More surprisingly, it reveals a negligible number of the American public has developed antibodies to this coronavirus. At the high end, 16 percent of New Yorkers show that they've been exposed. In other states, 1 percent or less of their populations show antibodies, the ICL report estimates. Absent more strict social distancing or extension of quarantine, we will see many more people get sick before we're out of a "first wave" of coronavirus.

It's been less than three months. We are already creeping up on one hundred thousand dead, nearly as many Americans lost as were killed in a full year of the bloody First World War.[44]

SATURDAY, MAY 23, 2020

Ten weeks since lockdowns began (the same duration that Wuhan experienced)

Harvard historian of medicine Charles Rosenberg made the argument years ago that epidemics play out dramaturgically, in three acts.[45]

In Act One, people deny an epidemic is happening. They cannot imagine it as a reality. Physicians may see it first, but they say too little because no one wants to incite panic, exactly what Wuhan authorities scolded Dr. Li for doing in January. The epidemic inevitably causes economic loss, the derailing of plans, and social upheaval. Only when the bodies start to accumulate do officials face up to what's happening.

During Act Two, according to Rosenberg, the community settles on an explanation for the epidemic. In the very old days, we blamed human sin or the capriciousness of the gods. Later, we looked to the movements of astronomical bodies, unbalanced humors, or bad air (*mal aria*) to understand the crisis. Only in the late nineteenth and early twentieth centuries did we learn to blame practically invisible viruses and bacteria. Yet, even in this age of science, we hang on to the old notion of sin: we Americans blame others for making choices that increase their risk of getting sick. Because of this, Act Two is the time when pandemics take on moral, social, and eventually political meaning. Blame rubs off on the poor, the foreign, and the darker skinned. When they die, the wealthier, lighter-skinned people in the community identify preconditions in those other people's lifestyles, customs, and environment to explain their deaths. Syphilis and cholera unleashed fear and hatred toward the poor in the nineteenth century, as did AIDS toward homosexual men in the 1980s.[46]

Finally, notes Rosenberg, the public cobbles together colloquial practices and more formal public health measures. This is Act Three. In Europe's plague years, beginning in the 1340s, this meant quarantining, burning tar to clean the air, fasting, and praying. We still have quarantining but with new rituals. We have embraced social distancing, based on an arbitrary six-foot rule dating back to the 1930s.[47] We wear masks, scour surfaces, follow one-way direction arrows in store aisles. We clip hand sanitizer bottles to key chains and backpacks, celebrate graduations and birthdays with "parades" in which everyone stays in their cars. We buy quack treatments like colloidal silver, deploy ultraviolet light-emitting robots to create sterile spaces, doomscroll until our phones fall out of our sleeping hands, stand on big Xs taped exactly six feet apart in lines at the DMV or pharmacy, and adopt virtual backgrounds for our never-ending Zoom meetings, parties, cocktail hours, and get-togethers. We still do a good bit of praying, although presumably not inside a church or temple or mosque. Perhaps most tellingly, we watch a *lot* more television during Act Three, our collective Blursday the thirtyteenth of Maprilay.[48]

"Epidemics," Rosenberg says, "ordinarily end with a whimper, not a bang."[49] On the one hand, it appears case numbers are dropping nationally. On the other hand, daily cases now climb in twenty-four states in the interior of the country.[50] Here is hoping we are on the back end of this nightmare. Stores are opening all across the United States this weekend. And, as I can smell out my window, much anticipated Memorial Day barbecues and pool parties are firing up.

SUNDAY, MAY 24, 2020

Lillie Lodge works as an RN in the cardiac catheterization lab at WakeMed in Raleigh, North Carolina. After almost all of the elective or nonemergent procedures were canceled in March, she was working only about twenty hours per week. So, she voluntarily moved to the COVID ICU, believing she would be there for only two weeks. She is still there many weeks later.

At the beginning of all the COVID craziness, the entire unit was designated to care for COVID patients. . . . I was assigned to take care of two patients in rooms next to each other. . . .

One of my patient's kidneys had failed. They were on continuous dialysis for days and days, but the machine had started clotting despite a heparin infusion . . . The ventilator settings are still so high and we are unable to wean them. They have what we call a watershed stroke, impacting areas of the brain. . . . They have sepsis, the white blood cell count climbs daily, even on multiple antibiotics. We are unsure where this is coming from. I removed the hemodialysis line, the only line that could be removed. . . . We will have to put another in tomorrow though, because they need dialysis. In the morning, there was concern that the patient had a pulmonary embolism. . . . Their lungs looked awful on the scan. The nurse practitioner said, "This is really, really concerning. It's like we have made no progress at all. And see this part? That's *dead* lung tissue."

The patient's family can't see them, can't understand the full impact. They want to continue. To do everything, full court press. They believe God is going to work a miracle. . . . God is not going to work a miracle. Yes, I know miracles do happen. But I have seen this story again and again in my ten years. Dying slowly. No matter what we do, what we try next, it will end in death. The timing will just depend on the family. Until they tell us to stop, we will prolong the process . . . continue, continue, continue.

My second patient has been in the hospital for thirty-one days [with] a tracheostomy to facilitate weaning the ventilator, which we have been trying to do for . . . I don't remember . . . at least ten days. . . . The issue is ICU delirium, withdrawal from all the medications they required for sedation when they were at the peak of infection. . . . Most likely, they will live in a nursing home for months after they are discharged from the hospital.

You can see when things take a turn for the worse. . . . [T]here is a fast downward spiral . . . and then you are gowning up, putting on your PPE helmet as fast as you can to run in the room and start chest compressions, calling for help . . . the drugs you need to be passed through the door because the crash cart is impossible to clean so meds are passed one by one instead of bringing the whole cart in. . . .

Administration wants to tighten up as much as possible because the hospital has lost money. . . . It's frustrating to be unable to deliver the kind of care you want to. It's frustrating to have to go from one room to the next without enough time to talk to your unintubated patient, who is already so isolated.

We are tired, exhausted. And we go on, knowing that we have to because there is no one else to do it.

MONDAY, MAY 25, 2020

Memorial Day. 91,000 deaths.

As I do nearly every day, I pull up the "COVID Cases by Population" map on Johns Hopkins University's COVID-19 website. Today looks different. There are the typical urban hot spots of the virus in Chicago, New York, and Detroit. Now noticeable, however, is an enormous red stripe showing a high density of COVID-19 cases slashing down from Virginia, through the Carolinas, south of Atlanta, and west to New Orleans. These are not cities. These are rural towns in the American South. I feel a tingling on the back of my neck, like I'm looking at a ghost. I have seen this map before.

I find it. Here is a map drawn after the 1860 US Census, which was the last census to show concentrations of enslaved people. These two maps—2020 and 1860—look shockingly similar (see insert). Both tell the stories of poverty, neglect, and want, of institutionalized grift—the untold history of the United States. Coronavirus may be slowing in New York City, but it is finding a new, more pernicious foothold in places with the fewest recourses, the farthest distances to a hospital, the worst experiences with healthcare. This map similarity is not a coincidence. "Christ-haunted" land is what Flannery O'Connor called these parts.[51] Coronavirus is settling now in counties where, 160 years ago, white plantation owners ran forced-labor camps for enslaved Black people, then practiced segregation and capital divestment ever after. The worst of this pandemic may be yet to come.

TUESDAY, MAY 26, 2020

I've always wondered what would happen if a truly cataclysmic threat appeared—another world war or an alien invasion. I once thought a pandemic would do the trick. It would be our "One for all; all for one" moment. Now, I'm not so sure.

The day started with a presidential tweet railing against mail-in ballots, claiming it will be a fraudulent election. Election Day is over five months away, and one can only wonder if Trump, who himself has voted with mail-in ballots for decades, is already making plans to salt the earth if he loses. Colorado, Hawaii, Oregon, Utah, and Washington already allow mail-in voting, with no evidence of fraud.[52]

The right-wing think tank Heritage Foundation created a very official-looking document, now displayed on the White House website with "1,071 Proven Instances of Voter Fraud" emblazoned on the front.[53] That's the total instances of voter fraud that are supposed to have occurred between 2000 and 2016. Assuming *all* of them are genuine fraud, which election experts strongly dispute, this balances out to roughly sixty-seven cases of voter fraud nationally a year.[54] Given the 1,116,808,339 ballots cast during that time, voter fraud occurs at a rate of 0.000096 percent (rounding up).[55] Plus, most of the examples are exclusively related to local, not presidential, elections. Nonetheless, it is a powerful reminder of the different ways alternative truths can be packaged: it always seems to be the narrative that nonwhite immigrants are out to destroy law and order.[56]

Twitter tags Trump's morning tweet with a little blue exclamation point. "Get the facts about mail-in ballots," it says, with a link to the data. It is the first time any social media company has done this. It's one small pushback from Twitter; one giant shot across the bow from the corporation that serves as Trump's official/unofficial connection to his "base." The press cheers, the president fumes. It's all very newsworthy.

Until about noon. Then America turns a corner.

The first piece of news is an update on Ahmaud Arbery's story. Three men are now indicted. The case languished for months behind the desk of Waycross Judicial Circuit district attorney George Barnhill apparently for personal reasons, including connections to the accused men. The news media is portraying the story as a tragic but typical instance of racism in a small town in the conservative Deep South.

Almost before the story wraps, a second one emerges, this one in "liberal" New York City. Yesterday, on Memorial Day, Christian Cooper, an avid bird-watcher, asked a woman to leash her dog, as required in that part of Central Park. Christian Cooper recorded the encounter on his phone. In the video, the woman, Amy Cooper (no relation), becomes livid, wrenches her dog violently by the collar, and approaches Christian. He asks her to back away. Then she yells, "I am going to tell [the police] that there's an *African American man* threatening my life." She looks straight at him to stress the point—she knows he knows what her threat means. She follows through on that threat, saying three times to the police that she is being threatened. Each time her voice grows more distressed, even though Christian Cooper has not moved or even spoken much. Amy's dog pulls hard, even flipping itself over and yelping while she yanks on the leash and weeps white woman's tears, eventually begging, pleading for the police to come, "an *African American man*" she stresses to the police. Amy is clearly assuming that her whiteness and femaleness will make the police take her side—perhaps even violently. Melody, Christian's sister, later posts the video and dubs Amy a "Karen"—a term that has been around for a while but by tonight is common parlance. This is the moniker we will now use to describe white women who deliberately weaponize their privilege to control a situation.

Melody Cooper ✓
@melodyMcooper

Oh, when Karens take a walk with their dogs off leash in the famous Bramble [sic] in NY's Central Park, where it is clearly posted on signs that dogs MUST be leashed at all times, and someone like my brother (an avid birder) politely asks her to put her dog on the leash.

12:03 PM—May 25, 2020

On the heels of Amy Cooper is another video, shot last evening and also posted to Facebook. The television media shows only short clips, always with a disclaimer that it is "disturbing." A tall Black man is chest-to-the-ground behind the right rear tire of a Minneapolis police vehicle with multiple police officers kneeling on his back. One white officer in his forties has his left knee buried into the man's neck. Over and over again, the man pleads, "I can't breathe."

It's the conclusion to the threat that Amy Cooper leveled earlier.

On a bystander's Facebook page, you can watch what happened after George Floyd, a forty-six-year-old security guard at a local bar, was arrested by police, handcuffed, and knocked to the ground. Darnella Frazier starts filming after Floyd is down. One of the officers claims, with an apologetic shrug to the crowd that is assembling, that they had been trying to get Floyd in the police car for several minutes, and that Floyd had been resisting. But what Frazier's video shows is officers kneeling on Floyd's legs, back, and neck while he uses what breath remains in his lungs to beg for his life. The bystanders call ever more frantically for the police to get off him. Clearly, if Floyd was resisting before, he cannot move now.

George Floyd calls for his mother, which is when I, and I imagine, everyone else watching this video, start to panic. He is about to die. The white officer on his neck remains motionless—his hands in his pockets, of all things. Either he doesn't believe there's anything wrong, or he does and *doesn't care*. Four minutes into the video—eight minutes and forty-six seconds after Officer Derek Chauvin put his knee into George Floyd's neck—Floyd is dead.

Here are the words George Floyd spoke in the last eight minutes and forty-six seconds of his life:

God
It's my face man
I didn't do nothing serious man
please
please
please I can't breathe
please man
please somebody
please man
I can't breathe
I can't breathe
please
(inaudible)
man can't breathe my face
just get up
I can't breathe
please (inaudible)
I can't breathe shit

I will
I can't move
mama
mama
I can't
my knee
my nuts
I'm through
I'm through
I'm claustrophobic
my stomach hurts
my neck hurts
everything hurts
some water or something
please
please
I can't breathe officer
don't kill me
they gon kill me man
come on man
I cannot breathe
I cannot breathe
they gon kill me
they gon kill me
I can't breathe
I can't breathe
please sir
please
please
please I can't breathe

These accounts of white-on-Black violence braid tightly together to-day. Ahmaud Arbery, Christian Cooper, now George Floyd. Police are the tip of the white weapon aimed at the head of Black Americans.

Millions have seen these videos today. Minneapolis seethes by the late afternoon. Hundreds gather outside Cup Foods on Chicago Avenue and

East Thirty-Eighth Street, where George Floyd was killed last night, to protest. At first there's just milling around. But then they start chanting "I Can't Breathe." This chant is not new. Black Lives Matter (BLM) marchers adopted it after NYPD killed Eric Garner in a chokehold in 2014.

News filters in that the four officers involved have been fired, and for a moment, the crowd celebrates. But we're smarter than we were after Trayvon Martin in 2012 or Michael Brown in 2014. Everyone knows all too well even an indictment doesn't mean justice is coming for killer cops. Around 6 p.m., the growing crowd marches off toward the Third Precinct police station on Minneapolis's South Side. A few angry young men break off from the main group, spray-paint a police car, and throw some rocks at the precinct building. The local news reports that it's not especially loud or violent. After dark, as soon as everything begins to calm down and people begin to go home, police launch tear gas and a flash grenade straight into the crowd.[57] All spring, we have watched white men carrying weapons into government buildings to protest state-ordered lockdowns with no push-back from police. Now, when a multiracial group gathers to protest unjustified police violence, noxious gas starts to flow.

I don't even know what today *was*. Everyone wants to relegate violent racism to the South or to rural areas. But what we saw today was in New York and Minneapolis. Is this a turning point or just another bout of America's deeper sickness?

WEDNESDAY, MAY 27, 2020

Day 2 of Black Lives Matter protests. Almost 94,000 deaths from COVID.

At some point in the next week, one hundred thousand Americans will be dead of this new pathogen. That's more Americans than were killed in the Vietnam War, Pearl Harbor, Hurricane Katrina, and September 11 combined. It happened in about three months. The *New York Times* published a breath-stopping front-page obituary of one thousand of the victims of COVID-19.[58] The number is both overwhelming and incomprehensible. And, as CDC numbers of excess deaths suggest, it's an *under*count.[59]

Historians fight over casualty numbers; nations use them as evidence of honorable sacrifice. But critics use milestones like these as proof of the nation's failure, especially when that nation's leader decides to mark it by golfing. Lest we forget for a moment, each of those numbers represents a person who sat at the center of their own life's drama, now cut short.

FRIDAY, MAY 29, 2020

Day 4 of BLM protests. 1.73 million cases.

The protests over police brutality symbolized by George Floyd's death have spread to more cities. Thousands of people march and shout. There are increasing reports of looting and property damage, though it is unclear who is committing it. Police are agitated, firing into crowds with tear gas and rubber bullets.

Protest protected by the First Amendment is complicated during a pandemic. Minnesota governor Tim Walz wants people to stay at home if they can't maintain proper six-feet distancing during a march. Yet, he recognizes the anger and frustration on the streets: "Right now, I know there's a lot of folks out there [saying], 'I'll believe [that the state is reforming] when I see it. . . . I'll believe it when equity actually means something. . . . I'll believe it when my child gets the same education as your child and that color didn't matter . . . We're asking an awful lot to be based on faith."[60]

The streets are exploding in part because Floyd's murder is both horrifying and *typical*. In March, just after lockdowns started, Louisville, Kentucky, police issued a no-knock warrant to raid the home of Kenneth Walker and Breonna Taylor at 1 a.m. Walker, believing it was a home invasion, shot back in self-defense, striking an officer in the leg. Eight officers then fired into their home twenty-two times, killing Taylor in her bed. Police claim the home was being used as a drug drop site, but searches found no evidence of that. Protests continue as police do nothing to address what is being called a "botched" raid.[61] Not one cop has been arrested or indicted for Breonna Taylor's murder. Last night, seven people at the ongoing Louisville protests were shot; police claim they were not involved. All across social media, a quote of Dr. King's reappears: ". . . a riot is the language of the unheard."[62]

Starting at around 7 p.m. (CDT), looters hit businesses in Minneapolis: a supermarket, a Wendy's, an AutoZone, the local Target. Police stand on top of the Third Precinct, occasionally firing flash grenades and tear gas into protesters on Lake Street, who are not looting, just chanting. At 9:30 p.m., a group of police come down off the building and form a cordon. Firefighters arrive at the AutoZone, which is ablaze now. A half hour later, police push what is left of the protesters and bystanders, many of whom appear to be very young, down the street. Meanwhile, another rioting group sets the Third Precinct ablaze. Police must have abandoned it sometime during the evening.[63]

You can see partisan battle lines being drawn online. Everyone acknowledges that the death of Floyd is horrendous. There are plenty of people seeking to excuse it, however. "The violence by protesters is equally bad," some say. "George Floyd was a criminal and probably deserved it," chime others. Floyd's death is a bellwether of a nation that was already in crisis, and now . . . ?

SATURDAY, MAY 30, 2020

Day 5 of protests

This morning, the president praises the Secret Service for coming down hard on protesters last night, threatening those who have taken to the streets with "vicious dogs" and "ominous weapons" (a reference perhaps to Birmingham's Bull Connor terrorizing civil rights activists in the 1960s) and criticizing Washington, DC, mayor Muriel Bowser for not calling in more police to manage protests near the Capitol.[64] He calls on his white supporters to make tonight a "MAGA night," all while he finalizes plans to spend the evening watching the first commercially manned flight launch from the Kennedy Space Center in Florida. A leader leaving the nation's capital to distract an angry populace is a classic move. It happened on the eve of the Russian Revolution in February 1917, too. This moment also feels eerily like Mussolini calling up his Blackshirts or Hitler goading his followers into *Kristallnacht*.

Videos of police violence from the last few nights accumulate on Twitter and the news. Like the broadcasts of Chicago in 1968, they show images of police shoving, beating, spraying, tackling, kicking, and punching seemingly peaceful protesters, often with their hands up through the beatings. Cops conceal their identities.[65] This is not new: in Chicago in 1968, police also removed badges and name tags before beating protesters. The anonymity makes these actions feel even more like we're witnessing the secret police of history's worst authoritarian regimes.

On social media, Representative John Lewis, who experienced this in the 1960s, tries to tamp down the rage of the protesters by emphasizing nonviolence. Predictably, the debates from fifty years ago rise again like phoenixes. *How long* must we wait? How patient must we be? Why must Black bodies remain placid and nonviolent while white police power wields whatever weapon is at hand?

A protester descibes what he is seeing in Miami. He was prepared to take the risk of protesting, both from the virus and the police. "To speak against police brutality and the killings of innocent black Americans like George Floyd and others. . . ." It was a chance to say their names, to chant, to march, to say "no more" to police violence. As night fell, police responded aggressively: "We were peacefully gathered in front of their precinct in downtown Miami when they began to throw teargas cannisters [in] to the crowd."[66] Police shot rubber bullets, and "chaos ensued," he says. The crowd retaliated, "lighting police cars on fire for about two hours, then the looting in Bayside Marketplace began."There may be some protesters destroying property, but there is no evidence of them attacking people. The same cannot be said of the cops.

We are in the middle of a pandemic that has already taken the lives of as many people who died in all American military engagements after World War II combined, and Minneapolis police just choked a Black man to death, remorselessly, on camera.[67] *That's* what's on the streets tonight: exhaustion, frustration at the apathy of our national leaders. Their response: more gas, more batons, more rubber bullets.

As images, stories, videos, and posts flood in, I keep thinking I'm witnessing Hungary in 1956, Prague in 1968, Tiananmen Square in 1989. Not the Land of the Free in 2020.

SUNDAY, MAY 31, 2020

Eleventh week after quarantine. Day 6 of protests.

So much can change in a week. Only seven days ago, people in the hardest hit parts of the country, namely the big cities on the East Coast, poked their heads out of their residential shells to see if it was safe to go outside over Memorial Day weekend. In sunnier parts of the country, where temperatures had been in the 80s for a few weeks and schools were out for the year, last weekend offered a taste of summer. Close to one hundred thousand Americans had died over the last three months, yet it still felt like we had turned a corner.

Today, however, it looks like the light at the end of the tunnel was actually an oncoming train. Street battles in the big cities. Pepper spray and tear gas. Batons and rubber bullets. Many states' governors calling up their national guard forces: Colorado, California, Georgia, Kentucky, Minnesota, Missouri, Ohio, Tennessee, Texas, Utah, Washington, and Wisconsin. Reports continue to accumulate on every form of social media that police force against protesters seems to be far in excess of what is warranted. Last night, in New York City, police drove their cars deliberately into crowds.[68] In Seattle, police pepper-sprayed children. In Columbus, police assaulted city and state elected officials—even Joyce Beatty, a member of Congress. In her words, she was "just another Black American attacked while protesting injustice."[69] Reporters are bruised; journalists are shot with rubber bullets. Taunting by protesters is met with fists, batons, unconscionable amounts of gas. Even people trying simply to march are singled out and arrested. Fox News displays different images—serene, all-white Minnesota National Guard forces, the Minneapolis police patrolling calmly, everyone striking noble poses. Then they cut to images of protesters, yelling and angry, mostly Black, with fists in the air.

Not every police force is responding in such a heavy-handed way. Officers in Camden, New Jersey—an already "reformed" police department—carried a "Standing in Solidarity" banner. The police chief of Santa Cruz, California, took a Colin Kaepernick-esque knee with his entire department. Chris Swanson, sheriff of Genesee County, which surrounds beleaguered Flint, Michigan, actually joined the assembled crowd, saying, "I took my helmet off, laid the batons down. I want to make this a parade, not a protest."[70] The crowd cheered. It is a smart move, although the time for parades has passed.

Despite the potential for violence, protests continue. Addresses and phone numbers scribbled on cards and handed to safe friends; names and emergency contacts written on arms and legs, just in case. I think of Fannie Lou Hamer in 1964 after she was beaten by Mississippi policemen. "We've given them time," she wrote. "And I've been tired so long, now I am sick and tired of being sick and tired, and we want a change. We want a change in this society in America because, you see, we can no longer ignore the facts."[71] It is a mistake to overlook how fatigue can lead to rage. Sometimes that manifests as peaceful protests. Sometimes it looks like masked men busting in store windows with hammers. Fires. Looting. Spray-painting "ACAB" (All Cops Are Bastards) on monuments and buildings and bridges. Paroxysms of fury.

Let the record show, however, by all evidence, the majority of the violence is coming from the police.[72] No protesters are shooting rubber bullets or beating cops with batons or removing cops' masks to spray into their unguarded eyes. It's Minneapolis police who shot rubber bullets at well-identified CBS reporters, hitting a sound engineer. It's police who shot freelance journalist Linda Tirado in the left eye and blinded her. Scores of journalists appear to be directly targeted by police.[73]

Unlike 1968, the crowd in 2020 is decidedly multiethnic. White people are there, holding signs, chanting "No justice, no peace!" and "Black Lives Matter." White people should not be rewarded simply for showing up. Still, it is a different level of participation than during the civil rights movement a half century ago, different even than the original Black Lives Matter protests around Ferguson, Missouri, in 2014. And, unlike in the all-white lockdown protests in Lansing, Michigan, and Dallas, Texas, a month ago, these white protesters wear medical masks and carry no weapons.

MONDAY, JUNE I, 2020

#BunkerBoy

In a year that has felt farcical almost from the beginning, today produces some of the strangest moments in American history.

In response to the protests at the National Mall, rumor has it the president retreated to a bunker under the White House over the weekend. The last president to flee to this bunker was George W. Bush on 9/11. That day, international terrorists brought down the Twin Towers of the World Trade Center using airliners. Today, American protesters marched peacefully against police brutality. A photo showing last night's darkened White House bounces around the internet with the gleeful hashtag #BunkerBoy. Social media and cable news deride or excuse this appearance of cowardice, depending on the audience. News reports later in the day attempt to clarify that the photo was doctored. Nevertheless, "BunkerBoy" memes circulate widely.[1]

Today, perhaps in some effort to reassert an image of strength, Trump first chastises the country's governors for failing to clamp down on their protesters. He threatens to send Attorney General Barr after them for negligence: "We will activate Bill Barr and we will activate him strongly."[2] What is it, exactly, that he is hoping the governors will do? He has more or less abandoned each state to its own fate during this pandemic. A number of governors remind him that protest is constitutionally enshrined and refuse to buckle under the threats.

Over 140 cities and towns across the United States stage protests.[3] Every radio show, tweet, news program, and podcast in America, Canada, Australia, and the UK—indeed, practically in the world—reflects on Floyd's murder and the pandemics of racism and police violence in this country and the European-colonized globe. Around noon in Minneapolis, at the site of George Floyd's death, his brother Terrence kneels and grieves. The protesters part. It is a moving moment of reflection for the entire world, four centuries after Europeans first sold African men and women as labor on this continent.[4]

Then, around 6:30 p.m., any hope of peace is shattered. Twitter and cable news flash with images of what look like paramilitary troops, even though they are probably police, firing enormous amounts of gas, Pepperballs, and flashbang explosives into peaceful protesters in Lafayette Park, in the center of Washington, DC. The bangs are intense. Some fear these are live rounds being fired into ordinary Americans.[5] Protesters are pushed to the ground. Meanwhile, on live television, the president declares, "I am your president of law and order, and an ally of all peaceful protesters. . . . As we speak, I am dispatching thousands and thousands of heavily armed soldiers, military personnel, and law enforcement officers to stop the rioting, looting, vandalism, assaults, and the wanton destruction of property. We will end it now."

The nation then watches as the president leaves the White House on foot, with a gaggle of advisors and generals. It soon becomes apparent authorities have removed protesters from Lafayette Park with riot gear and gas to cut a path to St. John's Episcopal Church, on the other side of the park. Once at the church, Trump holds up a Bible, as though this act alone will establish him as a man of bravery and faith. He fumbles with it like a hot potato, holding it upside down in front of him for a moment, then wields it aloft in his right hand for a photo, grimacing.

Just to be clear: the president of the United States ordered a crackdown on peaceful protesters so he could walk unobstructed to a church that he does not attend—a place that honors a Palestinian Jewish carpenter from two millennia ago whose values this president openly mocks—all for a nakedly political photo opportunity. A more flagrant trampling of the Founders' separation of church and state doctrine can barely be imagined. It feels like sacrilege to boot.[6]

In 1917, presidential candidate and labor leader Eugene Debs noted, "Every robber or oppressor in history has wrapped himself in a cloak of patriotism or religion, or both."[7] The point of Trump's exercise with the troops and the Bible was to do exactly this: to exhibit contrived "righteous" power; it was both a threat to his opponents and a nod to his supporters.

Gina Gerbasi, one of the priests at St. John's Episcopal Church, offers her eyewitness account:

> Around 6:15, the police started really pushing protestors . . . using tear gas and folks were running at us for eyewashes or water or wet paper towels . . . we were trying to help people as the police—in full riot gear—drove people toward us . . . around 6:30, there was more tear gas, more concussion grenades . . . The police in their riot gear were literally walking onto the St. John's, Lafayette Square patio with these metal shields, pushing people off the patio and driving them back . . . with SO MANY concussion grenades . . . I literally COULD NOT believe it. WE WERE DRIVEN OFF OF THE PATIO AT ST. JOHN'S—a place of peace and respite and medical care throughout the day—SO THAT MAN COULD HAVE A PHOTO OPPORTUNITY IN FRONT OF THE CHURCH!!! PEOPLE WERE HURT SO THAT HE COULD POSE IN FRONT OF THE CHURCH WITH A BIBLE! HE WOULD HAVE HAD TO STEP OVER THE MEDICAL SUPPLIES WE LEFT BEHIND BECAUSE WE WERE BEING TEAR GASSED!!!! . . . The patio of St. John's, Lafayette square had been HOLY GROUND today. A place of respite and laughter and water . . . But that man turned it into a BATTLE GROUND first, and a cheap political stunt second. I am

DEEPLY OFFENDED on behalf of every protestor, every Christian, the people of St. John's, Lafayette square, every decent person there, and the BLM medics who stayed.[8]

Today was one of those days that will go down in history, no doubt. Nonetheless, as Dr. King said, "We are not makers of history, but we are made by history." Today was "made by history," as well. For most of this country's life, its citizens have been shaped by a history that white-washed the genocide of Native Americans and downplayed the torture that supported slave labor for the global trade of cotton and tobacco, that ennobled the myth of the Confederate Lost Cause after the Civil War, and that touted a benevolent American exceptionalism as a justification for colonizing Hawaii, Cuba, Puerto Rico, and the Philippines. As scholars have been emphasizing since W. E. B. Du Bois lived a century ago, if we want to stop being destroyed over and over by the cancer of racism, the first thing we must do is to learn this *real* history. Only by facing the wrenching terror of the slave block and the tribal massacre can this nation be made into something else. Otherwise, George Floyd will be just one more statistic in a nation built on the violence done to countless Black and Indigenous bodies.

The memorialization of our history needs to be changed in order to change the future—real history instead of the shibboleths to an American mythology. Intuitively, some young people understand this. So, today, even while Trump did his memorializing stunt for cameras to create one kind of history, some are attempting to unmake it by tearing down monuments to the Lost Cause.

At last, even in the heart of Dixie.

Tonight, I drive to downtown Birmingham to watch. Mayor Randall Woodfin sends a crew to remove a Confederate monument that has stood here for more than a century. The enormous obelisk raised a generation after the war to reinforce racial hierarchies in the twentieth century is slowly pulled apart and loaded on a flatbed truck. Several of us stand in silence in the darkness on the outskirts of the park. Louder than the cranes, the sound of a woman singing "Be Still—God Will Fight Your Battle," wafting through the night air. It is an old spiritual, bearing aloft centuries of struggle, death, pain, and the promise that the God of real faith, not the kind that uses violence against innocents for a photo op, will rectify it. It took a

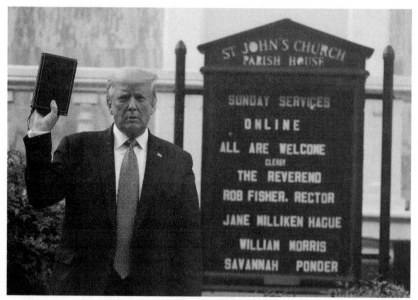

Trump holds up the Bible in front of St. John's Church, Washington, DC, June 6, 2020.
(Shawn Thew/Anadolu Images)

century to unmake this monument to false history. And these are only tiny steps. Nevertheless, be still.[9]

TUESDAY, JUNE 2, 2020

"Blackout Tuesday." Day 8 of protests.

Once he took office, President Thomas Jefferson stopped talking about noble revolutionaries and became primarily concerned with the preservation of the status quo. "Insurgents must disperse & retire peaceably to their respective abodes," he proclaimed near the end of his second term in 1808. If they refused, Jefferson commanded, "all officers having authority civil or military" could step in and break up the "insurrections or combinations" or to "deliver them over to the civil authority."[10] It was the first use of the Insurrection Act, passed by the Ninth Congress a year earlier. Jefferson's government attempted to stop smugglers who had been illegally hauling potash, pork, cheese, and grain up and down Lake Champlain to trade with the English in Canada. Jefferson demanded Vermont governor Israel

Smith call a posse, arm the state militia, build gunships, whatever it took to stop the smugglers. It failed miserably. Trade with Canada continued.[11]

Two hundred years later, the president of the United States is thinking about invoking the Insurrection Act.[12] It would allow him to call on the US Armed Forces to suppress these protests.[13] Interestingly, of the eighteen times presidents have used the Insurrection Act in the past, thirteen occurred in response to racial violence. Andrew Jackson invoked the act in August 1831 to suppress the "slave revolts" after Nat Turner's band killed a family in Virginia. Federal troops, including three companies of artillery, supported Jackson's disproportionate response, which resulted in the torture and deaths of uncounted numbers of enslaved people and even innocent bystanders in the weeks and months afterward.[14] The Insurrection Act helped quell white violence against Black people in Detroit, Michigan (1943), Little Rock, Arkansas (1957), Oxford, Mississippi (1962), and multiple parts of Alabama (1963). Lyndon B. Johnson used it four times to quash riots in African American neighborhoods during the summers of 1967 and '68. George H. W. Bush turned to the Insurrection Act during the Rodney King protests in LA in 1992. Again, it's worth nothing that these last five invocations were used against African Americans protesting white police brutality.

Vandalism is the stated reason why the government might invoke the Insurrection Act. The fear is, however, that it will shut down protest entirely. Rumors circulate on social media that vandals busting windows and threatening cops over the last few days are, on the whole, not affiliated with the protests.[15] They're opportunists at best. Perhaps even instigators, say the rumors—much like Amy Cooper attempting to trigger more violent responses from the authorities. It is true that circulating videos show smashing and stealing. Right-wing media claims BLM and Antifa leaders are paying protesters and looters to attend marches and create chaos.[16] Leftists insist white supremacists pose as Antifa to stir up a backlash.

Monitoring groups like the Network Contagion Research Institute make precisely this argument: white actors dressing in black like the fabled Antifa slip in and out of BLM marches and the white nationalist counterprotesters, like Proud Boys, Three Percenters, and Oath Keepers counterprotests. They are domestic militants organizing through the internet to incite insurrection and greater violence.[17] Groups like the Boogaloo movement, active on Reddit and darker corners of the internet and named sardonically for the 1980s B-movie *Breakin' 2: Electric Boogaloo*, have grown into a credible domestic militant threat targeting police, property, and ordinary civilians with no purpose except to sow chaos.[18]

In solidarity with the BLM protests, music corporations like Spotify and Apple Music declared today "Blackout Tuesday," agreeing either to play nothing (#TheShowMustBePaused) or to feature African American artists exclusively. Hundreds of celebrities, then millions of their followers, post a black square on their social media accounts.

These are easy ways to show the digitally connected world that one is doing one's part. It's called *virtue signaling*. Nothing real or personal is usually at stake by adding a black square, yet it shows followers one is aligned with socially astute sentiments, the trendsetters, the influencers, the platformed, without risking one's wealth or power.[19] In this case, ironically, the flood of black squares posted on Facebook, Instagram, Twitter, Snapchat, TikTok, and so on swamps posts organizing actual BLM protests. People seeking to show solidarity with the BLM movement have inadvertently hindered its progress.

Social media difficulties aside, real support for George Floyd and the Black Lives Matter movement has spread throughout the world. Millions of protesters rally in major cities and small towns around the globe, shouting the names of George Floyd and Breonna Taylor over and over again. In Los Angeles, National Guard troops kneel with BLM protesters in a show of solidarity. The internet practically broke when Gianna "Gigi" Floyd, Floyd's six-year-old daughter, sat astride the shoulders of her father's friend, NBA star Stephen Jackson, and looked out over thousands of protesters in Minneapolis. "Daddy changed the world," she said.[20]

THURSDAY, JUNE 4, 2020

Day 10 of protests. Twelve weeks since lockdowns began.

Today, Buffalo, New York, police reported that seventy-five-year-old Martin Gugino tripped and fell to the ground during a BLM protest in Niagara Square, cracking his head on the pavement. The truth is a cop knocked the Catholic peace activist to the ground, his skull smacking the concrete. On the video that emerged, while blood issues from Gugino's head, cops walk around him. When one officer offers to help Gugino get up, another grabs him by the back and pulls him away. Tonight, after the video goes viral, Buffalo police commissioner Byron Lockwood suspends the officers, pending an investigation. New York governor Cuomo is calling the actions of the police "disgraceful."[21]

Greg Doucette and Jason E. Miller are compiling documented instances of police brutality during the BLM protests into a spreadsheet.[22] Already, they have hundreds of entries. A separate tweet thread combines video evidence of over 260 instances of excessive force just during the last two weeks. The thread begins with an unarmed protester with his hands raised being tackled by jackbooted police in *the middle of his interview on live television*.[23] All the while, white men with semiautomatic weapons roam the streets of smaller cities protecting against "Antifa," completely unmolested by police.[24]

Right-wing media emphasizes that white people are killed by cops, too. But proportional to population, African Americans are at much higher risk of unprovoked attack.[25] On Mappingpoliceviolence.org, Samuel Sinyangwe and DeRay Mckesson show repeated examples of police using lethal force on African Americans with almost no provocation.[26] And, as University of Michigan political conflict specialist Christian Davenport demonstrates, dark-skinned protesters are statistically much more likely to face violence than white protesters engaged in more provocative behavior.[27] Too often, the media justify police behavior by appeals to the underlying assumption that Black and brown people are inherently criminal. *They must have done something wrong.* When a Black or Mexican or Muslim man is nearly beaten to death by a group of cops, you can count on a certain percentage of America's white population focusing not on the bigotry of the police but on the beaten man's past flaws. Whatever is needed to make it look like he deserved it—another example of ameliorating cognitive dissonance.

Meanwhile, the day is full of reactions by disgusted administration insiders. James Miller, a member of the Defense Science Board, resigns, calling out Secretary of Defense Mark Esper, who walked with Trump to Lafayette Park three days ago:

> Secretary Esper, you have served honorably for many years, in active and reserve military duty, as Secretary of the Army, and now as Secretary of Defense. You must have thought long and hard about where that line should be drawn. I must now ask: If last night's blatant violations do not cross the line for you, what will?[28]

Trump's former secretary of defense, Jim Mattis, silent since resigning in 2018, today openly condemns the president: "President Trump's actions Monday night violated his oath to take care that the laws be faithfully executed, as well as the First Amendment right of the people peaceably to assemble. . . . We are witnessing the consequences of three years without mature leadership." Trump is a threat to the Constitution, he warns.[29]

Then, tonight, President Obama releases a video with his own hopeful speech. "I want you to know that you matter," he says to the Black youth of our nation.[30] Famously measured and even-keeled, Obama agreed to speak out, not only because of the injustice and the protests, but because, "There is a change in mindset that's taking place, a greater recognition that we can do better." He later shares that he has been reading James Baldwin and, like everyone else who reads Baldwin these days, was struck by how much his words, written a half century ago, describe what we're still seeing now.[31] Millions watch Obama, if only to be comforted for a moment by the steadiness that he brings.[32]

FRIDAY, JUNE 5, 2020

Day 11 of protests

This week, Trump supporters and internet trolls have taken to Twitter and Facebook/Instagram with anti-BLM posts of a black and white American flag with one blue line (formerly used simply as a pro-police flag, now transformed into something more) with the hashtags #AllLivesMatter, #BlueLivesMatter, #WhiteLivesMatter, and the even more disturbing #WhiteLivesMatterMore. In response, millions of young people who are die-hard fans of Korean electronic pop music, or "K-pop stans," dump random music videos of dancing Korean pop stars all over social media, attempting to drown out the rhetoric through the noise. In a move that Kafka would have admired, K-pop stans have instrumentalized the absurd. These videos expose the commensurate absurdity of those who would reject the racial crisis happening in America.

The streets, filled with protesters, have become the center of political action. DC mayor Bowser issues a letter to the White House requesting federal forces be pulled back, as there is no evidence of protesters violating any laws, and she criticizes the federal forces, many of whom wear no identification. After the president senses a new political target, his thumbs get busy, tweeting threats to the Black female mayor. Meanwhile, governors from Florida, Indiana, Maryland, Ohio, Mississippi, Missouri, New Jersey, South Carolina, Tennessee, and Utah are in the process of sending National Guard units to DC. Bowser then ups the ante, saying those troops will be evicted from all DC hotels for violating the Third Amendment.[33] (I think it's fair to wager that, at the beginning of 2020, few Americans even knew what the Third Amendment was: "No Soldier shall, in time of peace be quartered in any house, without the consent of the Owner, nor in time of war, but in a manner to be prescribed by law.") It turns out many of the troops were slotted to stay in hotels already rented by the city in case of COVID overruns at hospitals, so she has the authority to deny them lodging.[34] In addition, she has ordered city street crews to paint BLACK LIVES MATTER, each capital letter 35 feet tall, over two blocks of Sixteenth Street leading up to the White House. A new street sign is hung on the corner: Black Lives Matter Plz NW.[35]

SATURDAY, JUNE 6, 2020

Day 12 of protests

Three days ago, the president claimed, in a televised phone call to Fox News, he had not gone to the bunker to hide, but to "inspect" it, despite the fact that the Secret Service already confirmed taking him there for his safety.[36] The fabrication unleashes a torrent of mockery. Playwright Eugene Ionesco noted when the world stops making sense, simply bringing attention to its absurdity can be a powerful form of resistance. Sarah Cooper, an African American woman who performs impeccable lip syncs of Trump's nonsensical rhetoric, made a parody of this absurd moment. Her TikTok rendition of his call to Fox News pulls the curtain back on an emperor desperately trying to stitch up his invisible clothes.[37]

Joe Biden has come back from the political grave to win the Democratic Party's primary presidential race. As of today, he has officially passed the nearly two thousand delegate votes needed to gain the nod at the Democratic National Convention. He promises "unity."[38]

Unfortunately, "unity" doesn't help the nation's unemployment numbers right now. Everyone applauded the news that over two million jobs have returned, bringing the unemployment rate down from 14.7 percent to a still staggeringly bad 13.3 percent.[39] However, those jobs have not rebounded evenly along race or gender lines. At the beginning of the lockdowns, the employment-to-population ratio—the metric that tracks the percentage of a particular group that are working—dropped for white men from 69.7 percent employment in May 2019 to 62.1 percent a year later. This means that around five million more white men over twenty are out of work right now than a year ago. Over the same span of time, the employment-to-population ratio for Black men over twenty is down from 64 percent in May 2019 to 54 percent today. Even more upsetting is the fact that only 50 percent of Black women are attached to the formal economy by the same metric. In other words, the African American family is suffering disproportionately. While about 1.5 million white men and another 1.4 million white women have found employment since April, only about 100,000 Black men and 70,000 Black women have.[40] Employment is looking better for millions of American white people than it was a month ago, but it's holding steady at "terrible" for African Americans.[41] Hopefully, Congress and the executive branch work out a way to extend the unemployment benefits of $600 per week. If not, we're going to have to add "catastrophic unemployment" to the list of things we're calling a "pandemic" this year.

On the other side of the economic food chain, we are witnessing one of the largest transfers of wealth in American history, according to one financial commentator.[42] Blue-chip stocks, which are the stocks of companies with reputations for reliability and profitability, have turned around and are now approaching their February heights. Meanwhile, smaller companies fall into bankruptcy at alarming rates.[43] All of this means there will be fewer and richer companies when we get out of the crisis.

A century ago, US presidents Teddy Roosevelt and W. H. Taft "busted trusts" and cut the robber baron monopolies down to size. It seems unlikely we will see that anytime soon. If the nineteenth and twentieth centuries were the age of great nations clashing for power, the twenty-first century has marked the rise of the multinational corporation and a new Gilded Age. When international companies like Amazon have a higher GDP than most Eastern European countries, the idea that a *nation* could have the power to limit the growth of a *corporation* seems increasingly remote.[44]

MONDAY, JUNE 8, 2020

Day 14 of protests. 104,000 deaths.

A 175-page report from the government-sponsored Committee on Civil Rights offers an examination of police violence against African Americans. It concludes that some defenders of the law have become "lawless," and "[R]ace prejudice" governs many interactions between the police and African Americans. Black men—even those who are unarmed or running away—are killed disproportionately because white cops believe they're acting in their own self-defense. Police departments thoroughly cover up minority deaths, especially when it's obvious a cop is to blame. This thorough government investigation reveals, at best, those extrajudicial killings by cops demonstrate incompetence. At worst, they reflect, "a callous willingness to kill."

President Harry S. Truman commissioned this report in 1947.[45]

Twenty years later, in 1968, the LBJ-era Kerner Commission on police violence concluded the same: the police "have come to symbolize white power, white racism, and white repression."[46]

It seems as if this moment happens in every generation: police violence, public outcry, marches, speeches, government report, superficial change. Rinse and repeat. For much of the last century, there has been the same analysis, the same recommendations, and the same ineffective response. After Dr. King's assassination in 1968, governments named streets after him and (two decades later) established a national holiday near his birthday. After Rodney King, in the early 1990s, police departments added "bias training." How do we stop this cycle and make real change happen?

One solution is to "defund the police," a new mantra that became prominent this weekend. Black Lives Matter protesters have painted the phrase in massive lettering on Sixteenth Street in Washington, DC, joining "Black Lives Matter." Conservatives love this phrase. It seems to show that the protest movement is fundamentally anarchistic. They label it as an agenda of that mystical "Antifa" group that seems to slide through the night like vampires in every urban area. Right-wing personalities use "defund the police" to conjure specters of convicts-at-large on the streets, gunning down police whose guns have been taken away. "No industry is safe from the Democrats' Abolish Culture," a GOP spokesman says today.

"First they wanted to abolish private health insurance, then it was capitalism, and now it's the police."[47] Tucker Carlson, the conservative TV personality, paints a vision of BLM "rioters" joining with wealthy companies
like Pepsi, Cisco, and Intel, to burn down cities and fire anyone who speaks
out against them.[48] Tellingly, D. W. Griffith adopted a similar narrative of
the Black criminal who had linked arms with financially well-connected
carpetbaggers in his homage to white supremacy, *Birth of a Nation* (1915).

In truth, "defund the police" does not mean taking away the money
that police need to enforce laws. Back in the mid-1990s, under President
Clinton, the number of police in the United States increased by 150,000,
with intense police presence focused in "high-crime"—read, minority—areas. At the same time, the GOP-controlled Congress, with Clinton's com-
pliance, redirected millions of dollars away from mental health counseling,
stable housing funding, and community support organizations—much of
which was set up after the 1960s Kerner Commission—into police departments.[49] Experts declared these actions and their follow-up policies a war
on the War on Poverty.[50]

As an unintended consequence, police increasingly became responsible
for managing pretty much any problem people might have—mental illness, housing, transportation—even if their training left them profoundly
ill-equipped to handle it.[51] Police don't even necessarily want these assignments. If taken as it's meant to, "defund the police" would mean shifting
spending away from greater militarization of the police force and toward,
as America once began to do, stable housing, mental health services, and
programs where problems can be solved without needing the police. We
have specialists for handling homelessness, mental illness, and drug addiction. Why not use them?

TUESDAY, JUNE 9, 2020

Day 15 of protests

George Floyd is today being laid to rest in Houston, Texas, where he grew
up. The Reverend William Lawson, pastor emeritus at Wheeler Avenue
Baptist Church, is speaking at the funeral this morning. Rev. Lawson acknowledges the protests surrounding the death of Floyd have turned into a
movement. Floyd's life, in becoming the tragic symbol of that movement,

is drawing comparisons with others. It began in a metaphorical "manger," says Rev. Lawson, in the "ghetto" of the third ward in Houston. But now, the name George Floyd is known, like other saints, "throughout the world. . . . You think something good can't come out of this? His death did not simply start a bunch of good speeches, a bunch of tributes. Out of his death has come a movement. A worldwide movement. And that movement is not going to stop after two weeks, three weeks, a month. That movement is going to change the world."[52]

WEDNESDAY, JUNE 10, 2020

Day 16 of protests

Protesters are defacing, beheading, and pulling down Christopher Columbus statues in Boston, Virginia, and St. Paul, Minnesota. Democrats in the House of Representatives are calling for the removal of eleven Confederate monuments in the Capitol. Many of the protests seem to have turned from addressing police brutality specifically to the larger role history plays in perpetuating structures of racism. Though protesters may not know the nuances of the stories behind the monuments they're destroying, they are less ignorant than those arguing against the removal of monuments for "destroying history." Most of those monuments were raised a half century after the Civil War as shibboleths to a false history—a history shorn of slavery, racism, and systemic injustice, meant to remain unquestioned. Monuments say more about the group putting them up than about the history they supposedly depict.

Black Lives Matter protests also take aim at academic research and higher education today. A number of Black physicists and astronomers joined to #ShutdownSTEM. They hoped to convince their white colleagues to stop work and to dwell for a day on how they would make their laboratories more diverse and hire more Black faculty. The venerable *Nature* joined the #ShutDownSTEM cause, and #BlackInTheIvory scholars broadened that charge outside of astronomy and physics.[53] The goal is to point out disparities in income, authority, and treatment by one's employer that resonate throughout education—from kindergarten teachers to endowed professors, deans, provosts, football coaches, and presidents of universities.[54]

And, in news that at any other time would have been filed under Hell Freezes Over, NASCAR bans Confederate battle flags at their races.[55]

Events are happening so quickly that in front of the House Judiciary Committee on Capitol Hill, the testimony of Philonise Floyd, a brother of George Floyd, pleading with members of the House to *do something*, is all but overshadowed. Democrats are already fashioning a bill, but the GOP stubbornly resists, lest they alienate their white base. GOP politicians have tossed around the idea of another national commission on criminal justice, apparently forgetting the Kerner Commission in 1968, Truman's group in 1947, and on and on.[56]

While we justifiably have had our attention on the deeper problems of systemic racism in our country, coronavirus isn't going away. Places like Texas and Florida and Arizona are adding thousands of cases a day, and their hospitals are filling up. Some claim that this rise is because of more testing, but this doesn't explain why there's a higher positivity rate among those tested. Even in such seemingly straightforward data, there's debate. Some claim hospitalizations are instances not of treatment, but of "hoteling" by the homeless who have no place better to go than a hospital room.[57] There is no evidence that this is true.

THURSDAY, JUNE 11, 2020

Day 17 of protests

As pastor of Greater Cornerstone Baptist Church in Dallas and president of one of the city's oldest and largest African American faith organizations, David Wilson could have been sitting on stage at a table near the president of the United States today. Trump held a roundtable with African American leaders at the huge Gateway Church in North Dallas to discuss race and policing. "I just can't do it," said Pastor Wilson, who passed on the opportunity. "I really don't want to hear the lies or be used as a prop."[58]

The stage is loaded with the president's Black cabinet members, Housing Secretary Ben Carson and Surgeon General Jerome Adams, plus Black Texas Republicans, including Will Douglas, a Dallas pharmacy owner, Scott Turner, a former Republican state representative from Frisco, now executive director of the White House Opportunity and Revitalization Council, and Robin Armstrong, physician and representative on the

Republican National Committee. Armstrong made headlines in April for using hydroxychloroquine to treat a group of patients at a nursing home infected with the coronavirus.[59]

Curiously missing from this discussion on race and policing were the city's African American police and justice officials—the very people who could have spoken with authority about race and policing. Dallas police chief U. Reneé Hall, Dallas county sheriff Marian Brown, and Dallas county district attorney John Creuzot were not even invited. The most important African American politician in Dallas, Mayor Eric Johnson, flatly refused to attend.

The megachurch where they meet is less than a ten-minute-drive down Hillcrest Road from Shelley Luther's Salon a la Mode. It's hard to know whether this is a coincidence. Much of the church auditorium audience is comprised of white folks, reportedly handpicked. Few, other than Surgeon General Adams, wear masks, despite their proximity. The moments of the president's remarks that the audience enjoys—when he says Black unemployment was the lowest it had ever been before "the plague from China" arrived, for instance—receive cheers and hoots more reminiscent of his arena rallies than a church.

At this discussion of race and policing, there is almost no talk of George Floyd, Breonna Taylor, or Ahmaud Arbery. Nothing is said of Tay Jefferson, a Black woman killed by a white police officer, while playing video games with her eight-year-old nephew, in her own home last October, just down the road from this church.[60] Instead, Trump launches into a screed against those who are protesting racism, "We'll make no progress and heal no wounds by falsely labeling tens of millions of decent Americans as racists. . . ." He pivots instead to a seemingly unrelated discussion about schools, "[W]e're renewing our call on Congress to finally enact school choice now. School choice is a big deal [applause] because access to education is the civil rights issue of our time. . . . When you can have children go to a school where their parents want them to go. . . ."[61]

Speaking about "falsely labeling" racists and "good/bad people on both sides" is Trump's standard response when addressing race and violence. It isn't shocking anymore. Yet tying his response to the old notion of "school choice" is an older, more subtle racist dog whistle. Racial integration of public schools only really began a decade and a half *after* the first *Brown v. Board of Education of Topeka, Kansas* case (1954). In *Green v.*

School Board of New Kent County, Virginia (1968), the Supreme Court found
that white politicians used "freedom-of-choice" language to keep schools
from being integrated.[62] After the *Green* decision, many white parents began clamoring for homeschooling exemptions and private schooling, still
funded by the state, of course.[63] *That's* what the president is calling "civil
rights" here during a discussion on race and policing with African American leaders.

Legendary comedian Dave Chappelle harnesses this live wire of frustration at the deep structures of American racism in *8:46*, a show recorded
in Ohio last week and released on Netflix today.[64] Near the end of the special, he recounts the story of his namesake, William D. Chappelle, a bishop
in the African Methodist Episcopal Church. In 1918, Bishop Chappelle
led a delegation from South Carolina to implore President Wilson to do
something about rising anti-Black violence spreading through the country
as African Americans moved into Northern cities for work. In a powerful,
sobering conclusion, his great-grandson Dave Chappelle reminds the audience: "These things are not old; this is not a long time ago. It's today."
Lynchings, Klan marches, Jim Crow, even slavery itself—the destruction
of the Black body was an ordinary aspect of life a mere *three* generations
ago. The destruction of Black wealth, the silencing of Black voices is ongoing. Real and lasting change will take *persistent* effort by millions, not just
these marches.

One wonders on which side of this change largely white institutions
like Gateway Church in Dallas will position themselves.

FRIDAY, JUNE 12, 2020

Three months since stay-at-home orders began. Day 18 of BLM protests.

Once you begin to see the links in the structure—how systems of wealth,
power, celebrity, and race are intertwined in America—it's hard not to
see it operating everywhere. American history, geography, demographics,
economics, education, housing, politics, voting, policing, even religious
expression makes so much more sense. White people don't have to be *bigoted*, meaning actively trying to hurt or disparage a person of color. To
be racist, we white folks just have to do *nothing*. Racism is the particular
species of coasting along, identified by that centuries-old Edmund Burke

quote: "The only thing necessary for the triumph of evil is for good men to do nothing." When a system is set up to benefit the group you're in, *doing nothing* works to your advantage. Even when it comes to something as seemingly indiscriminate as disease.

Today, I'll try to *see* a web of inequity during the pandemic by tracing the relationship between historic racism and COVID in a more granular, concrete way. I choose two counties similar in population: Lowndes County, Alabama, and Schuyler County, New York. Both counties are rural with similar age demographics. Lowndes has a population of 11,299; Schuyler County has a population around 18,000.

These two counties have had very different COVID experiences. Lowndes County has had 336 confirmed cases and 13 deaths due to COVID thus far. The raw numbers seem low, but that translates into 2,974 cases per 100,000 people. To put that in perspective, New York State, which has the highest number of cases in the country, has a per capita rate of 1,958 cases per 100,000.[65] By contrast, as of today, Schuyler County—which lies not far from New York City, the epicenter of coronavirus in America—has seen 12 cases and *no* deaths from COVID.

Why the disparity? The median household income in Lowndes County is $30,833. One in four residents lives below the poverty line, with only 48.3 percent of the population working in the civilian labor force. Only 14 percent has a college education, and less than 49 percent have internet in the home.[66] Only 19 percent of the students in the Lowndes County public school system meet national math proficiency requirements, and only 18 percent of them meet reading requirements.[67] And yet, they have a high school graduation rate of 81 percent.

In Schuyler County, New York, fewer than one in six lives in poverty. Unlike Lowndes County residents, a majority of Schuyler County citizens have health insurance. The schools are well funded, and 80 percent of residents have internet in the home. They have access to a hospital that, while small, has four ICU beds. In Lowndes County, there is not a single hospital bed, of any kind, to be found. The nearest hospital is 50 miles away.

Perhaps all of those statistics boil down to this: Lowndes County is 74 percent African American, and Schuyler County is more than 95 percent white. But why would racial differences alone lead to a depressed economic situation in Lowndes? Why, some ask, doesn't the Black community *do* anything to improve their station? After all, slavery has been over for a century and a half. Couldn't Black people just work the land like white people always have in New York, thereby increasing their wealth?

The answer is that the Black freedmen of Lowndes County *did* work after emancipation. They worked hard. They earned money. They bought land. They grew crops. They were on track to look like thrifty, white Schuyler County.

And then it was taken.

Here's just one example. On December 4, 1947, a white mob lynched Elmore Bolling, a successful Black businessman in Lowndes County, ostensibly for insulting a white woman. More likely, however, it was for being successful. He had picked himself up by his bootstraps and done everything Lincoln promised the former slaves and their descendants would do. Then white people murdered him. No one was ever convicted.

When we talk about race-based killings in the USA, we sometimes tell stories like Elmore Bolling's, then stop and shake our heads. *Such a shame about those racists*, we say. But the example of Bolling helps explain at a micro level what we're seeing today on a macro level. Often erased from these stories is what happened afterward. After Bolling's death, after his surviving family fled in the middle of the night, his land fell into the hands of the white people who remained.[68] The Bolling family *wealth* disappeared with the main wage earner's life.

Bolling was just one of the over 360 African Americans who were murdered by mobs in Alabama from 1877 to 1950, many for trying to be thrifty and hardworking, like a Schuyler County, New York, kind of American. And his story is one pebble in the landslide of wealth transfer that followed lynchings. All the possessions the families could not carry or hide were looted, burnt, stolen, or left for the forest to reclaim. Wealth leaked out.

Lowndes County granted *voting* rights to its majority African American population in the mid-1960s. But white landlords immediately pushed thousands of Black farmers and laborers from their land after they legally voted. That's *after* the "I Have a Dream" speech, *after* the march from Selma to Montgomery, *after* all the civil rights events portrayed as definitive triumphs in books and documentaries.[69] Little changed otherwise. There was no economic investment, no genuine equality, as Dr. King pointed out time and time again.[70] Consequently, Lowndes County has barely shifted since the days of Bolling. Poverty remains so entrenched across this former plantation county that the United Nations recently investigated it as a site of "extreme poverty" otherwise unseen in the "first world."[71]

For a time, voting rights offered at least a hope for change. Recently, however, Alabama passed a requirement that you must have a state-approved photo ID to vote. Simultaneously, across the largely Black counties of Alabama, the Republican-dominated government has closed the offices where one can get an official ID. This is not a coincidence. The point of these laws is to roll back the gains of the civil rights era.[72]

Even in 2020—in the middle of a pandemic that disproportionately preys upon the poor and disadvantaged—medical care is desperately absent in Lowndes County. The Alabama Department of Public Health reports a *single* COVID-19 testing center at the Lowndes County Health Department. When I call them, I learn that—three months into this pandemic—the state health department conducted *one day* of drive-through COVID tests on April 24. Then, I look at Butler County, just to the south of Lowndes. The Alabama Department of Public Health says that Butler has four testing centers. But when I call those places on the phone, they tell me they have *no* facilities to test people, symptomatic or not. They direct me to a hotline number, which connects to a hospital in the state capital of Montgomery, 47 miles away—difficult to reach when you don't own a car and can't get a driver's license.

As it turns out, this is not an urban-rural divide alone. Alabama's Jackson County, an equally rural but 90 percent white county in northern Alabama, has six COVID testing facilities. When I call, they all appear to be open and operating.

SATURDAY, JUNE 13, 2020

Day 19 of protests

Tonight, a Wendy's in Atlanta is burning. Late yesterday, police shot and killed a Black man running from them in the restaurant's parking lot. Rayshard Brooks fell asleep at the wheel and was blocking the drive-through line around 11 p.m. Friday night. Two officers arrived and, for about a half hour, interacted with Brooks. When they attempted to restrain him, Brooks fought back. They tackled him. He slipped away, grabbed one of their Tasers as they tried to use it on him, and ran across the parking lot, beside the other cars in the drive-through line. The Wendy's security camera shows Brooks point the Taser over his shoulder as he's running at full sprint and fire off an errant shot. Immediately, the officer chasing Brooks and brandishing his own stun gun in his right hand switches it to his left, grabs his gun with his right, and fires into Brooks's back multiple times. Brooks stumbles to the ground and stops moving. The drivers of the four cars still in the drive-through leave the line and begin to film the police, who rapidly put restraints on Brooks. Another cop car roars into the scene exactly one minute later. Brooks was pronounced dead by the time he made it to the hospital.[73]

This afternoon, people began protesting the killing of Brooks. After watching the available footage, which includes police body cameras, Atlanta mayor Keisha Lance Bottoms announced the resignation of Police Chief Erika Shields. But that did not dampen the protesters' ire, who gathered at the Wendy's and made their way up the embankment to nearby Interstate 75/85. They brought all eight lanes to a standstill. At some point, the Wendy's was set aflame—no one can say by whom—and now it burns a bright orange in the hot summer night.

Just when it seemed like the burst from the George Floyd and Breonna Taylor's protests was beginning to calm down, that policy changes were actually moving, police brutality explodes again, and again. It underscores what activists have been pointing to for decades: a Black man, even one resisting arrest, even one fleeing from the scene, even one with a cop's Taser, should not automatically get the death penalty without being convicted by a jury of his peers.

On the flip side, police themselves react with hostility to what they see as the unjust politicization of their work. The entire SWAT team of the Hallandale Beach Police Department in Florida resigned after Vice Mayor Sabrina Javellana and the command staff of the department knelt with BLM protesters last week. The team said they felt "openly disrespected" as well as underequipped and undertrained for their jobs. The mass resignation was largely symbolic, however, since they keep their paychecks, their pensions—and their police jobs.[74]

Millions of Americans, mostly white, want the police to retain their power without too many conditions. Without it, the fear must be, crime will run rampant. But millions of nonwhite Americans see themselves at the receiving end of the state's capricious lethal force. If anything is different this summer versus all the times this has already been stated over the years, it's that a significant number of white Americans now seem to agree lethal power given to police is all too often wielded unfairly and in defense of the wrong things. *This* is what Black Lives Matter hopes to highlight.

SUNDAY, JUNE 14, 2020

Day 20 of protests. 108,000 deaths from COVID.

> *"Black people gave you this country. We gave you capitalism because we were the first capital. We are not impatient. We are not unreasonable. We are dying."*
>
> —JOY-ANN REID, MSNBC, June 14, 2020

Today the debate is over whether Rayshard Brooks deserved to be executed for taking a Taser away from a cop and running. On network after network, show after show, the interviewers pose the same questions, focusing on whether Rayshard Brooks had "deadly intent" when he fired the Taser at the cop. I can't find any expert responding with the obvious counterquestion: How could there be deadly intent with a Taser since, according to arguments the police have made for decades, *they aren't deadly?* In fact, a Taser not being lethal is why so many cops claim they must draw their weapons and fire on already tasered suspects.[75]

The police have backed themselves into a corner. If Tasers are not lethal, then this means it is okay for police to use them relatively indiscriminately, as they often do. This also means that Rayshard Brooks's firing of the Taser could not have implied *deadly* intent. It implies the police officer who shot him knew that but nonetheless elected to use lethal force. On the other hand, if Tasers *are* lethal, this means that Rayshard Brooks did have deadly intent and the officer was justified in shooting him. This also would mean that police officers have been using a deadly weapon indiscriminately on people for minor infractions for years.

Criminal justice research seems to support this second reality: Tasers *are* lethal weapons. A comprehensive 2018 study demonstrated that police claims that the Taser was the "perfect nonlethal weapon" were wrong; over one thousand people in the US have been killed by Tasers. In Atlanta, not far from where Brooks was gunned down, police recently tasered a man to death.[76] They argue that the Taser was incidental to the cause of death in each case. Yet wrongful death lawsuits forced Axon, the Taser manufacturer, to drop the shock power emitted from the Tasers in the hope that fewer people would die.[77]

All of this is secondary to the real question: *Why did Floyd's and Brooks's infractions warrant death?* Even if those men were breaking the law (and the evidence seems to show that George Floyd did not try to pass a counterfeit note), they did not warrant the death penalty. Serving to obscure these ethical issues, the corporate media replays the same ten-second clips of Brooks running. They never show the forty-five minutes that lead up to that moment, during which the suspect and the police interact. Nor will they show the moment of execution. They won't show the cop firing repeatedly into Brooks's back as he runs, just as they won't show Minneapolis police officer Chauvin suffocating Floyd to death.

On Fox News, the death of Brooks serves two purposes. They bring on Ted Williams—an African American former DC detective—to first absolve the police of guilt for Brooks's death by calling Tasers lethal instruments. But then Williams goes on to reassure the Fox News audience that white police are guiltless of *racism* as well as murder. "A few bad apples" is repeated by multiple interviewees. All miss that the adage is "one bad apple *spoils* the whole barrel."[78] If these "bad apples" have remained on their forces or been reassigned to others, then they are not exceptions at all—they signify a much deeper problem.

After absolving the police of murder and assuring white viewers they aren't "racist," Fox News moves to the story of Sergeant Damon Gutzwiller, killed in the line of duty. They bring on his supervisor to laud him as "a great man, a great father, and a great police officer"—not one of the bad apples, clearly. This is more of the Fox News message: Introduce a replacement hero, in this case, a martyr. Yet it turns out Gutzwiller was *not* gunned down by a Black man or a BLM protester. He was actually shot over a week ago by a white Air Force staff sergeant with possible associations with the Boogaloo movement.[79] Gutzwiller's death is doubly tragic because it's being introduced to distract from the ethics of extralegal executions by police.

In Philadelphia last night, white men holding baseball bats knocked around a reporter covering their second night of spontaneous "protection" of the Christopher Columbus statue in Marconi Park. Eventually, one white "protector" slashed the tires of the reporter's bicycle. There were police present at the scene. Not only did the police neglect to intervene, they actually helped push the white reporter out of the area.[80] Later, as BLM protesters assembled in the park, none of whom were armed, the Philadelphia police, with guns and batons at the ready, circled around the white "protectors," nearly all of whom carried bats, hockey sticks, guns, clubs, and other makeshift weapons. In other words, the Philly police were protecting the armed protectors of the statue from unarmed marchers.[81]

As COVID cases climb, we see our police outfitted in the latest military gear. We even see expensive military hardware driving down the main streets of America—not everywhere, but in more than a few cities and towns. Meanwhile, many of our physicians and nurses have had to outfit themselves in plastic bags and homemade PPE to stay safe in their places of work. As Dr. David Himmelstein, Laurie Garrett, Elizabeth Rosenthal, and so many others have noted already this year, America operates a just-in-time health system that prioritizes profits. It is no surprise that our medical workers are underfunded. Whereas militarization has been a critical part of our understanding of safety and protection since the nation's inception, the idea that safety is contingent on the promotion of public health, is relatively new to our history and still largely ignored. Moreover, in a nation that prioritizes individual profits and property, we understand the value of the police, who are there to protect us and our stuff. But public health? What does that do?

MONDAY, JUNE 15, 2020

Day 21 of BLM protests

It feels like we are well into summer, even though summer hasn't officially started yet. This year, all sense of time is lost. "Summer" started back in March, when most of us were told to stay home. During a normal summer, people go on vacation. People find a pool or a lake to swim or fish. This summer, the streets are filled with protesters, and the rest of life has gone still. There is just the inside of the house. Television and internet full of protests, emails, Zoom meetings. And that's if you are lucky. For many, there's worry about work—worry over safety on the job with just a flimsy mask, worry if you're going to be able to keep your job at all, worry about what to do with your kids while you go to your job.

The marches are happening a few times a week, even in our small city in the Deep South. We gather in the stewing afternoon air, huddling under the few trees inside the square. Local Black leaders give talks, one after another telling a story of a cousin or brother or father shot or beaten by police. Officers stand on the outskirts, watching, arms folded over their chests. They congregate in little pockets beside their cars, whispering quietly to each other, avoiding eye contact.

When the speeches are over, our march begins. We walk around a city block, passing an Irish pub filled with white patrons lounging behind the pub's fence, laughing, maskless, swilling their drinks under billowing fans. They find us amusing. A handful of police officers stand along the sidewalk, occasionally opening a blue cooler to hand out cold water as we march and chant. I think I see friends in the crowd, but with their masks on, I can't be sure. My chanting starts tentatively. Maybe this is not my place. Maybe "Get your knees off my neck!" should only be yelled by Black folks. At the same time, I want the chant to be loud. I want the police officers and the people in the pub to hear us. No one can see my mouth behind the mask. Even though we are giving each other space, the group feels tight and deliberate. As we march, I think of the uncounted thousands pounding streets across the country. The outpouring is so immense the Smithsonian has started collecting BLM protest signs for its archive.[82]

There's no smashing or looting here in this small, Southern city—too heavy a history for that. Everything is orderly. We march around downtown twice. People honk. Men in pickup trucks angrily "roll coal" at us, their black exhaust curling into sooty grime, sticking to our throats in the humid air. And then it's over. We disperse to our cars, carefully stow our signs, and crank up the AC. We hang our masks on the gear shifts (these are the masks that we keep for the car). I wonder if we have made any difference.

TUESDAY, JUNE 16, 2020

Day 22 of protests

Today, I observe and transcribe a Montgomery City Council hearing on a proposed mask-wearing ordinance put forth by Councilman Cornelius Calhoun, who is African American. All the race, class, gender, and urban-versus-rural issues swirling around the middle four-fifths of the country collide in this meeting.[83] It feels momentous.

Three doctors have already reported that the Montgomery hospitals are at capacity and that 90 percent of the people on ventilators are African American. Councilman Glen Pruitt, a white man, angrily opposes the mask ordinance.

A citizen comes to the podium to make a comment. He doesn't give his name. He is African American.

> Councilman Calhoun, you need to be commended. This is not about a mask issue for certain people. The question on the table is DO BLACK LIVES MATTER?! . . . I lost six loved ones during this pandemic . . . I got a brother who is about to expire any day now. Just to watch him on that ventilator and all those patients on all those machines going beep-beep-beep. I didn't see no white people up there. . . . This stuff is attacking *our* community. [He points to his chest emphatically.] I saw six of my family go down the drain because of COVID. You don't know what it feel like, Glen Pruitt, to lose a loved one. *That's* what's happening in the Black community.

Pruitt yells from the dais, "For *you* to sit up here and call somebody out! I'm gonna take that personally!" But the man at the podium refuses to be silenced: "You don't know how it feel to lose a loved one?! The doctor said just a little mask will save people's lives, and y'all wanna make it political."

"That's enough." The president of the city council, Charles Jinright, who is white, interrupts. (I notice, so far, he's interrupted every African American speaker at this hearing.)

"No, no. I'm not through! . . . Do you know how many ordinances we have on the books that we don't enforce?!? . . . This would just be another [ordinance]." He whispers, holding up his index finger. "But this is a good one. This is about saving lives. The other petty ordinances out there that lock Black people up that are on the books . . . you were fine with those ordinances when the *previous* [white] mayor was in office. . . . If you got any goodness in your heart—anything for the citizens of Montgomery, Alabama—you will vote for this ordnance right now because *we* are dying . . . Where will we go from here?"

Ernest Clayvon, who has brought his young son to the podium with him, speaks next. This Black man makes the opposite argument, for terrifying and compelling reasons: "Mr. Calhoun, I know your heart is in the right place . . . you care, and your intentions are good, but the road to Hell was paved with good intentions." He touches his hand to his heart, and his small son reaches up and touches his father's hand. "The problem is *enforcement* . . . Birmingham had that rule—the face 'covering' rule. . . . The Black woman that was in Walmart there, do you know what happened to her?" He slams his hand down loudly on the podium. "She was thrown down while she was handcuffed in the back. Her crime was not wearing a face mask. When you pass this law, *who do you think will get arrested?* All I'm saying is we have to look at the unintended consequences."

This is a terrible choice to have to make. An ordinance requiring masks will save Black people, who are disproportionately dying from this horrible virus. But in the process, it could give the police another excuse to persecute the Black community.

Montgomery City Council votes down the mask-wearing ordinance. "I wonder if we as the council realize how serious this really is?!" says an agitated Councilwoman Audrey Graham, one of the few Black councilmembers, after the vote. "I want to be on the record that, as a council, we did *not* take this seriously enough today. When we see those [COVID] numbers continue to rise, we will have nobody to blame but us."

FRIDAY, JUNE 19, 2020

Day 25 of protests. 111,000 deaths from COVID.

"Happy Juneteenth." Like those black squares on social media a few weeks ago, this message is everywhere today. An email from Walgreens says, "This Juneteenth, we share our commitment to racial equality," then lists all that they are doing for America's Black communities. It feels egregious because Walgreens, owned by the Walton family, is among the worst violators of the spirit of Juneteenth, according to Human Rights Watch. They keep their workers just below full time so they don't have to pay benefits (pushing working employees into state welfare programs), routinely deny breaks and overtime pay, and have been accused of violating child-labor laws.[84] Black and Latinx workers make seventy-five cents on the dollar compared to their white peers in Walton-owned companies, a gap of $7,500 a year on average.[85] So, while the email is lovely, it's hard to take seriously.

Walgreens is not the only company virtue signaling for Juneteenth. Nike, Twitter, and the NFL have said they will give their employees the day off on June 19 from now on. As journalist Jamelle Bouie puts it, "Paid holidays, while nice, are a grossly inadequate response to calls for justice and equality."[86] Why has it taken over 150 years to have Walgreens, Nike, and all the rest recognize Juneteenth? The simple answer is that it's now in their best economic interests.

FRIDAY, JUNE 26, 2020

One month since George Floyd protests began. 122,000 deaths from COVID.

Another record spike in cases—39,327 reported last night, with the average age of infection now being thirty-five instead of sixty, as it was three months ago. In Austin, Texas, they are projecting that the hospitals will be overrun by mid-July. Texas, Alabama, Missouri, and Nevada all reported record daily highs in the last two days. Florida is overwhelmed.[87] The CDC says that the actual number of COVID cases is probably ten times higher than the official numbers (the official number today is 2,374,282). Based on antibody tests, it looks more like twenty-four million people have been infected with the virus—perhaps 5 to 8 percent of the population. On the one hand, it means these people have survived it. On the other hand, it means over 92 percent of the population is still susceptible.

But last week, Vice President Pence confidently declared that no "second wave" of the virus would be coming.[88] He chalked up the rise in cases in the southern half of the country to more testing. The media, he said, was fearmongering.[89] We should stop worrying and get back to normal life.

And now mask wearing is becoming thoroughly politicized. The pushback against it seems to be unique to this nation, although not to this time. During the 1918 influenza epidemic, the Red Cross declared that "the man or woman or child who will not wear a mask now is a dangerous slacker." Most people complied with mask-wearing laws. However, there were groups like the Anti-Mask League, four to five thousand strong, in San Francisco. Members from the business community claimed that masks would hurt commerce and slow economic recovery. Given that the pandemic happened at the height of the first Red Scare, others declared that the laws represented a slippery slope toward socialism and communism.

Current arguments against mask wearing undoubtedly borrow from these old tropes, but such differences as there are, I find disconcerting. An anti-masker on my neighborhood online listserv argues that mask wearing is medically unsafe: "They are literally trying to poison us to death with our own CO_2. They've gotten their 'science' worshippers on the mask train and they want it everywhere all the time. Every man, woman, and child must show their submission."

A parent steps in to say we need to wear masks so the schools can re-open in the fall and kids can be safe. The anti-masker responds that "kids can't get sick," and the whole pandemic is a "liberal conspiracy." A health-care provider leaps in to say the ICU in our city is overflowing. But the anti-masker is undeterred: "You have probably just seen bad cases of flu and pneumonia. I have never witnessed anyone with this disease. Sorry you have been misled by the liberal mainstream media. . . . If someone feels that they are in an at-risk category then I feel they should wear a mask but if others feel like they shouldn't then I think they have that right. Mandating that to me is like doing away with the bill of rights which some of you would probably think that's a good idea."

Perhaps most riveting is this man's resignation to the inevitability of death. "We all have to go sometime," he finally says. Perhaps, on some deep level, people feel like puppets on strings, angry at a world that doesn't make sense anymore, resigned to the decisions of a higher power, whether that is God or Donald J. Trump.

Then I remember that 122,000 people have died. These were people who were forced to face death alone, whose families are now broken. They had holidays and laughter and beautiful sunsets still to see. Their deaths were unnecessary, tragic, and possibly preventable.

SUNDAY, JUNE 28, 2020

The president retweets a video of a white supremacist driving his golf cart around The Villages in Florida, yelling "White power!"[90] Trump later deletes the tweet without a mention, after popular outcry. People in the future may not understand how, right now, a disturbing number of Americans in places like this commend this sort of behavior.

The Villages reveals how history shapes, reinforces, and reflects structures of class and race. It is not a town per se but a "census-designated area"—a gigantic retirement community with no elected ruling body. It represents an idealized vision of the 1950s white-flight suburbs. Over 98 percent of the roughly 110,000 retirees in The Villages are relatively affluent whites. A wave of baby boomer retirees moved there from the Midwest and the East Coast in the last twenty years. Together, they have made The Villages one of the fastest growing, least diverse "company" towns in American history.[91]

The company that owns The Villages hired a theatrical set-design company to fabricate a history for the place. They built historical plaques, photographs, and statues to honor a past that literally never happened. One placard commemorates a warehouse where a fishing and bait shop ostensibly stood back in the early twentieth century. Next door, on the wall of the radio station, you can find an old, grainy photograph of well-dressed gentlemen and ladies excitedly looking at the record-setting fish that was theoretically caught in the lake. Both the warehouse and the lake were built within the last thirty years. These plaques, statues, and photographs provide a nice ambiance—a sepia-toned sentimentality for a past that is unapologetically imaginary. It is Disney for nostalgic people who want to live in the good old days, even if it is as fake as Cinderella's castle.

A lot of people have written about the history and legacy of redlining in America. Less known is the recent trend of white, wealthy people creating de facto segregated spaces, complete with well-trimmed golf courses, tastefully designed over Native American land. Even an all-too-real African American graveyard is hidden nearby, out of sight, out of mind. These purpose-built communities do not have laws against Black and poor people living there, but they nonetheless create an entire world, with manufactured history included, that renders those populations invisible. These are make-believe spaces, keeping white people comfortable and amused until they die.

MONDAY, JUNE 29, 2020

Mark and Patricia McCloskey stand outside their opulent Gilded Age home in St. Louis, Missouri, with guns waving, screaming obscenities at peaceful BLM protesters marching to the nearby mayor's house. Given the symbolism, the story dominates all media today. Online commenters view the McCloskeys as irrational, unhinged, an overprivileged "Killer Ken" and "Killer Karen." Many Trump supporters, by contrast, see them as heroes defending their turf from delinquents, many of whom are not white.[92]

Not far away, other protestors march against poor labor conditions at Amazon warehouses, where access to PPE is difficult and employees are expected to keep working even if they are sick. Workers have been attempting to raise awareness about this for months. Unfortunately, when they do speak up, they are often fired straightaway.[93] According to an Amazon VP who resigned after learning how workers were being treated, many company execs believe warehouse workers are expendable. After all, Amazon, which will deliver to your door everything you used to buy at the local store, is turning historic profits.[94] The "human costs" of Amazon and CEO Jeff Bezos's "relentless growth and accumulation of wealth and power" are disturbing. And yet, like almost everyone else, I have an Amazon Prime account, I will admit. I use it when the alternative is impossible or dangerous. If I refuse to use Amazon, I have to go in to a store to get what I need, which, if it is even open, poses a COVID risk. If I use Amazon, I am following quarantine guidelines, but I am supporting a company that exploits its workers. We are all in difficult positions, caught in a system where we must choose between two bad options. But, as Frederick Douglass emphasized long ago, power concedes nothing without a forceful demand. Amazon is not likely to protect its workers just because we tepidly think it would be nice of them.

SATURDAY, JULY 4, 2020

Forty days since the killing of George Floyd. Sixteen weeks since shutdowns began. Two hundred forty-four years since independence from Great Britain declared.

The more things change . . . This evening, the musical *Hamilton* is streaming on Disney+. Deafening cracks and booms of fireworks resound from every direction. There are no great gatherings or large fireworks shows this year, just individual families trying to do *something* on the Fourth. I imagine all the dogs in the nation quivering and barking in unison tonight—a fitting cacophony.

What history do these fireworks commemorate? As I try to comfort my quaking dog, I ponder how history will see us in 2020. Will this year—this pandemic, these protests—have marked the beginning of something, or the end? Or neither: will the forces that have brought us to this place remain largely intact, rewriting this year into a comfortable story of American heroism that fits the old historical narrative? Will it remain a narrative that can be made into musicals; something that people will blow up fireworks in their yards over—but ultimately something that will leave the powerless still sick and poor, and the powerful still in charge?

MONDAY, JULY 6, 2020

Egg and meat prices are almost 5 percent higher than last year.[1] Food hoarding has largely ended. Supply chain problems that were so catastrophic in May are largely solved. So why are groceries so expensive?

Elise Golan, director of Sustainability at the US Department of Agriculture, helps make sense of it. Grocery store workers need PPE, and stores adopted additional safety practices, all of which costs money. Those costs are passed along to the consumer in the price of our food.

History has shown again and again that in moments of crisis, when nations need quick mobilization of vast resources and people, capitalist systems struggle to adapt. Back in 1941, when Germany invaded the Soviet Union, and Japan attacked the United States, the centralized Soviet economy allowed them to uproot entire factories almost overnight, move them to the hinterlands beyond the Ural Mountains, and put them back together. The US, by contrast, only slowly switched to a war footing, even with the advantage of no enemies on their home soil.

Today's food supply encompasses millions of farmers, processors, factory owners, and distributors, all of whom must adjust individually to the new normal. Just as with our healthcare system, the food supply chain is so brittle when disruption like this comes along, only gigantic corporations, functioning almost like states, can adjust by scaling up or down production, using their leverage with banks and even governments to keep afloat, and eat up the smaller businesses.

Or maybe, capitalism is working just like it is supposed to under the circumstances. There is no question that people in the grocery world are making a lot of money. Food companies continue to show historic profits. B&G Foods, which manages Green Giant, Crisco, and dozens of other brands, saw a 38 percent increase in sales in the second quarter of this year. Nestlé and Pepsi have stayed in the black. Publix saw a second quarter increase of $1.94 per share this year, with a 20 percent jump in sales.[2] It seems fair to say they are all passing their increased costs along to consumers, who wonder why ground beef has tripled in price.

Meanwhile, lines at food-distribution sites grow longer. They swell because unemployment remains well above the levels seen even during the Great Recession a decade ago.[3] While state and federal assistance did help staunch some of the initial hemorrhaging of paychecks, unemployment remains above 10 percent. Hunger stalks not far behind. A few months ago, people set up tiny food distribution centers in their free libraries and other small venues.[4] Now food lines stretch across parking lots outside of warehouses, arenas, churches, and stadiums from coast to coast.[5] San Francisco turned its famed Cow Palace into a food distribution center.[6] The United Center in Chicago, where the Bulls and Blackhawks play, became a staging area, stuffed with boxes of food and supplies.[7] The needy overwhelmed Houston volunteers at the Texans' NRG Stadium in April—even 500,000 pounds of food wasn't enough. The city switched to delivering directly to families via school buses.[8] The reality that the economic recovery is going to be much slower and harder is beginning to set in for millions of Americans, which means that families already at the margins are now suspended over grinding poverty by those CARES Act checks, and little else.

TUESDAY, JULY 7, 2020

We are witnessing a collision of several epidemics. Coronavirus was the most obvious, though in its wake, the fragile economic status of millions cratered. Today, I am resolved to learn what is happening with an epidemic that, until this year, was one of our major national crises—opioids. According to the CDC, over one hundred thousand people died of drug overdoses in 2017, with 66 percent of those deaths due to opioids. In 2018, the percentage of opioid overdose deaths rose by 10 percent.[9] The era of doctors writing limitless prescriptions from "pill mills" peaked in 2012 and has been declining ever since. Heroin overdose deaths declined as well, only to be replaced with the synthetic opioid fentanyl. Today, DEA agents seize fentanyl at least as much as any other opioid.

That was before the coronavirus pandemic. Now, perhaps not surprisingly, the overdoses are getting worse. Early predictions are that the

COVID-19 pandemic is contributing to a disheartening "Fourth Wave" of overdose deaths. The *Washington Post* and *Politico* report that overdoses have increased by 42 percent from this time last year.[10] The Shelby County Health Department in Tennessee reported 391 overdoses from April 7 to May 7 of this year—their highest total ever. Columbus, Ohio, showed a 50 percent increase in fatal overdoses from last year. Milwaukee saw a 54 percent increase from last year in drug overdose calls. Madison County, Alabama, not far from me, reported 22 overdoses in three days last month.[11]

All the literature points to the fact that social distancing and psychological trauma from disasters lead to a rise in substance abuse disorders.[12] "Pure heroin has gotten less and less available over the years and with COVID has become even harder to get," says Brandy Henry, a professor in the School of Social Work at Columbia University. People are mixing what drugs they can find, which is dangerous. Social distancing also means that people are more likely to use drugs in isolation without someone there to administer the lifesaving naloxone that can reverse the overdose.

Ironically, the COVID pandemic has pushed legislators to authorize reforms in addiction management that mental healthcare providers have been requesting for years.[13] Traditionally, people with substance use disorders looking for treatment had to go to officially certified opioid treatment programs to get the needed therapies. Public health professionals have argued for years putting up such access barriers is a mistake.[14] Now, because the opioid treatment programs have had to close, the Substance Abuse and Mental Health Services Administration has authorized pharmacies to distribute methadone, naloxone, and sterile syringes. A person who is trying to stop using can now get methadone for twenty-eight days instead of only two days previously, and all from their local pharmacy. One of the strangest consequences of the COVID-19 pandemic is that the United States is now in line with methadone treatment delivery in the rest of the world.[15]

Unfortunately, Dr. Henry says over Zoom, even these steps have created unforeseen problems making access to treatment harder.[16] The local opioid treatment programs play a vital role in helping people in recovery, including getting started with counseling and prescriptions. They are now mostly closed to in-person appointments, making it harder for new patients. Many of the programs are facing bankruptcy. In places where Medicaid and insurance do not cover the costs of these services, the programs make most of their money by collecting cash payments from patients. Now that is gone. How do you bill a patient for their take-home medication and telecounseling if they do not have a bank account or a computer?[17]

Henry tells me interwoven economic and political interests have made access to naloxone increasingly difficult. "Naloxone is a strangely regulated drug because people who purchase it are usually not purchasing it for themselves. You can't administer it to yourself, after all," she reminds me. And yet, in order for your insurance to bill for the medicine, you must be the one that fills the prescription. Insurance also has all these rules about how much you can buy at a time and how frequently they will pay for it. "It is all about money, really," Henry sighs.

We both nod. "And is there not also the fear that if you make the naloxone available then people are more likely to use more drugs?" I ask.

"Right," she responds quickly. "That has been a policy narrative. I think insurance companies take advantage of that narrative to justify not paying for the naloxone." On top of all this, she suggests, no new addiction and mental health practitioners can be licensed to take care of people who suffer from addiction disorders at present.

Substance abuse disorders tend to correlate with other health issues and comorbidities, which makes COVID even more frightening. Among people who smoke or have respiratory problems, COVID-19 has a fatality rate of 6.5 percent, much higher than in the general population.[18] According to Nora Volkow, director of the National Institute on Drug Abuse, people who have COVID-19 and then use opioids, methamphetamines, and other psychostimulants are at real risk of fatal overdoses because of what COVID does to lung capacity. These drugs can cause hypoxemia (slowed breathing), potentially fatal if you already have COVID.

There are more indirect ways that people with substance abuse disorders are at increased risk right now. They are more susceptible to homelessness and incarceration, both of which increase their risk of getting COVID. Not to mention that these populations are already underserved and marginalized in our healthcare system, mostly because of the persistent belief that addiction is caused by weak character, poor choices, and moral failing. All of this has been proven false for decades, but hospitals and officials still discriminate against them. One police department in Indiana is refusing to give naloxone to people who have overdosed, because they are afraid of being coughed on when the person comes back from the dead.[19]

"There is also the despair," Henry says. She looks away from her Zoom screen, furrowing her brow. "Mental health disorders and depression are on the rise everywhere, which is what happens when you have massive disasters. People try to cope with that, and they start using or they develop a disordered pattern of use, or they risk earlier death. People are more likely to be suicidal because of the collective trauma. . . . There is also mass decarcertation going on, and people who are just released from jails and prisons have astronomically higher rates of fatal overdose because they have low tolerance for drugs that may have become way more powerful while they were away." Not to mention that it is really stressful to reenter society. Even if you have been able to maintain sobriety in jail, a lot of people relapse in the real world. The rate of overdose is 140 percent higher for people who have substance abuse disorders and have been released from jail than it is for those who have not been in jail. On top of that, many people who come out of jail cannot stay with family because of COVID and end up going back to the places where drugs are available.

Big Pharma companies who produce the opioids are still in court, denying any responsibility for this nightmare. Drug manufacturers like Purdue Pharma lied in their reports and told doctors that opioids like Oxycontin were not addictive. They distributed the pills like candy, made *billions* of dollars for their shareholders, and refused to assume blame for the over half a million dead.[20] How can regular folks stand against that much greed?

SATURDAY, JULY 11, 2020

The big news of the day is the president wearing a mask on a visit to the Walter Reed National Military Medical Center (he has previously refused to mask). This same day, at the grocery store, I encounter a woman and her five children, none of whom are following the mask-wearing ordinance. Should someone say something? What is the right thing to do in this circumstance?

I turn to Julia Marcus, an epidemiologist in the Department of Population Medicine at Harvard Medical School, for advice. Marcus has been writing about such moments in *The Atlantic* for the last couple of months. Her research focuses on ways to help public health professionals overcome prejudices they often have toward populations on the margins of society.

"Anger and shaming actually prevent us from making positive changes with those people who are refusing the masks," Marcus responds. "Research has shown again and again that shaming does not change behaviors. . . . Even some of the people who understand how toxic shaming is in other areas of public health have engaged in it in 2020 because the target is perceived as being a right-wing, selfish, privileged group. But public health doesn't get to choose who it helps."

I understand her, but it *does* seem to matter that privileged people are putting their selfish needs above those of the public good.

"It's not about condoning all behavior," she interjects, her voice steady. "It's not about allowing someone to not wear a mask in the grocery store. It is about stepping back and asking *why* they're not wearing a mask. It's about not dismissing their reasons as being stupid and not shaming them and, instead, it's about coming up with ways to reach them and change their behavior. . . . I am not pushing for tolerance per se. I am pushing for compassion, which is different. . . . These days, we see everyone as *vectors for disease* before we see them as human beings."

At the end of our conversation, I ask Marcus what lessons we have to learn from this experience so that we don't make the same mistakes again. Her reply is not encouraging: "What's hard is that the lessons are the same lessons we had already learned before and we are just relearning them over and over again."

If only we paid better attention to history.

FRIDAY, JULY 17, 2020

3.5 million cases—128,000 deaths

As the infection spreads across the Southeast and Southwest, the administration moves against Anthony Fauci and the CDC, blaming them for the obvious failures in managing the epidemic.[21] The White House trade advisor, Peter Navarro, wrote in *USA Today* that Fauci "has been wrong about everything that I have interacted with him on."[22] Then, Dan Scavino, one of the president's closest assistants, posted a cartoon on his personal Facebook page portraying Fauci as a faucet whose policies are drowning Uncle Sam. At the same time, the presidential spokespeople claim that the president is "listening" to Fauci's advice.[23] In April, this group did something similar, but now with Trump flagging in the polls, it feels more serious.

The potentially most concerning aspect of this scapegoating is a new White House mandate requiring that coronavirus data no longer go to the CDC first, which has been the infectious disease information hub for generations, but to TeleTracking Technologies in Pittsburgh, Pennsylvania. TeleTracking, run by moderately successful commercial real estate developer Michael Zamagias, has overseen smaller projects in Mount Lebanon and Lancaster, Pennsylvania.[24] TeleTracking did not start as a tool for tracking outbreaks but as a patient tracker in the UK and smaller US markets to make medicine sales and distribution more "efficient." This privatization of COVID tracking will monetize access to life-changing data. Public health will be privately owned, and the use of the data will go to the highest bidder.[25] The added benefit for the administration? That inconvenient data can disappear.[26]

SATURDAY, JULY 18, 2020

John Lewis is dead.

The "conscience of the Congress" for twenty-two years, Lewis pushed for civil rights at every juncture. He wielded scars received during the first attempt to cross the Edmund Pettus Bridge in Selma on Sunday, March 7, 1965, when an Alabama state trooper fractured his skull with a nightstick. Those scars gave him credibility and standing to deliver scathing speeches over controversial legislation when no one else could. Everyone knew John Lewis had earned it.[27] Sadly, C. T. Vivian, one of Dr. King's chief strategists, also died yesterday.[28] America has lost two icons of the mid-century civil rights movement in two days.

The deaths of these two major figures again conjure associations between this year and 1968. Yet there is a better historical analogy that reveals just how deep the creases are in the landscape of America—the "Red Summer" of 1919.

In the summer of 1919, the United States experienced what Cameron McWhirter and many other scholars have described as the "worst spate of race riots and lynchings" in its history.[29] That summer, the whole world was heading home after the Great War, including many Black soldiers whose heroism set off a paroxysm of white rage. In a nation that prided itself on venerating its soldiers and degrading the Black man, the image of a Black war hero was incompatible with the established social order. White people began their reign of terror immediately after Black troops started arriving home, with hooded men lynching Private Charles Lewis, still in uniform, on December 16, 1918. It was, as one Louisiana newspaper put it, an attempt to "Nip It in the Bud," to show African American servicemen that their sacrifice for the country meant less than their permanent relegation to an inferior caste.[30] As W. E. B. Du Bois, who initially prodded African Americans to enlist in 1917, admitted two years later, "This country of ours, despite all its better souls have done and dreamed, is yet a shameful land. It *lynches*."[31]

Dozens of documented—and untold numbers of undocumented—cases of anti-Black violence engulfed the United States over the next year, killing hundreds. White mobs lynched many returning Black war veterans. Arson and looting spread nationally, through dozens of cities. And not just in the former Confederate states; some of the most destructive riots, in terms of both financial damage and casualties, occurred in major northern cities.[32] James Weldon Johnson, field secretary of the NAACP and author of "Lift Ev'ry Voice and Sing," dubbed 1919 the Red Summer for all the blood of Black men that flowed through American streets.[33] Meanwhile, city and state governments supported and even funded the construction of Confederate monuments and renamed streets and schools after Confederate soldiers, from California to Maine.[34]

2020 doesn't have the same version of coordinated anti-Black mob violence as 1919. But Americans are marching in the streets for racial justice now, just as then.[35] And, as in 1919, disease still stalks the land. Coronavirus exploits the same lines of discrimination that were set up a century ago.

In what is perhaps the most pernicious parallel between 2020 and 1919, politicians and police connected the reaction against anti-Black mob violence to "red" communist and socialist agitation. The "Red Scare" of 1919 (not to be confused with the Red Summer) connected the nascent civil rights movement to Bolshevism, Jewishness, labor unions, and immigration.[36] The Ku Klux Klan channeled these fears to grow in prominence through the 1920s. Members of the Democratic Party introduced an anti-Klan platform in their 1924 national convention, but backroom machinations allowed Klan influence to remain. The Republicans under Calvin Coolidge didn't even attempt to push back against the Klan. Back in the late 1860s and early 1870s, President Grant's Republican government had passed three Klan Acts, started the Department of Justice, and mustered Union troops to reoccupy the former Confederacy to tamp down Klan violence. Yet by the time Coolidge left office, the KKK marched confidently down Pennsylvania Avenue in front of the US Capitol, numbering in the millions nationwide.[37]

John Lewis knew that the fights for civil rights for African Americans didn't start in the 1950s, weren't resolved in 1968, and haven't truly ended in 2020, either. May he finally rest in peace.

MONDAY, JULY 20, 2020

Eight weeks since George Floyd was killed. Almost 130,000 deaths from COVID.

In San Diego, about a month ago, an unmarked van raced up to a group of protesters. Men in black and camo grabbed a woman, cuffed her, and threw her into the van. One threatened to shoot her comrades if they followed. The posse would not identify themselves. It was only after the *Los Angeles Times* got involved that the police admitted complicity. They were undercover police, including SWAT personnel, making an arrest because she had held out a BLM sign at a passing officer on a motorcycle.[38]

It's not an anomalous event. In cities across the country, groups of men dressed in paramilitary gear and armed with what appear to be assault rifles, jump out of unmarked vehicles, abduct one or more unarmed protesters off the street, and race away without revealing information about themselves or the abducted person.[39] None are read their Miranda rights. It is not clear that arrest warrants are being issued. For historians, these events conjure terrifying images of secret police in authoritarian states.[40] They remind us that constitutions are just words on paper, easily trampled in the service of power.

The BLM protests in Portland have continued unabated since May 28. On June 9, the US District Court of Oregon issued a temporary restraining order limiting the use of tear gas by the police on protesters. Police used gas anyway during the June 25 march near the North Precinct, a mostly Black neighborhood in Portland. When protesters lit fireworks on July 4 outside the Multnomah County Justice Center and Mark O. Hatfield US Courthouse, there were more arrests and more gas. Ten days ago, federal agents entered the fray, firing off "less lethal rounds" (another new term to understand this year) into crowds of protesters, injuring a few quite seriously before making more arrests.[41] Around 2 a.m., on July 16, after protesting for most of the night, two young white men were headed home when an unmarked minivan caught up to them, grabbed one, pulled his hat over his eyes, and stuffed him into the vehicle. Soon they unloaded the still blindfolded Mark Pettibone into the federal courthouse and placed him in a cell after rifling through his possessions. Finding nothing, they read him his Miranda rights, which he did not waive. Then they released him, without any record of his arrest.[42]

According to acting deputy secretary for Homeland Security, Ken Cuccinelli, these actions, which certainly *seem* like state-sponsored counterterrorism kidnappings deployed against American citizens, are completely above board.[43] The officials involved are Federal Protective Service agents, supported by CBP and US Immigration and Customs Enforcement officers. Why are these specific government agents arresting people in the middle of Portland? Why is it not an absolute violation of ordinary constitutional rights?[44] No one can say why.

The internet is flooded with videos from Portland showing federal troops beating and gassing military veterans and even yellow-T-shirt-wearing moms chanting "Black Lives Matter." The (acting) commissioner of US Customs and Border Protection, Mark Morgan, says these paramilitary forces are not identifiable to protect them from "Antifa." Never mind that there is no evidence that any government official is being targeted for retribution by Antifa, or that Antifa really exists as an organization.[45]

I watch as a hooded policeman maces an elderly veteran holding a BLM sign, as if that veteran has not earned the right to be there. "It feels like Vietnam," one veteran describes this year: "Indecisive leadership, the constant invisible threat, and feeling on edge." A veteran nurse notes how, like in war, people die alone now, far from their families.

We have been at war since 2001. We tout our military as the greatest in the world, flying fighter jets over sports stadiums and offering early airline seating to honor our men and women in uniform. We also often forget that we are at war and that those people are carrying psychological and physical burdens that shape them inexorably. Now, during COVID and the protests, it seems they are again a marginalized population at real risk.[46] According to Jodie G. Katon, epidemiologist at the Department of Veterans Affairs, veterans who struggle with PTSD and depression can be at a real disadvantage when it comes to fighting pandemics like COVID.[47] Being maced by a policeman certainly can't help.[48]

THURSDAY, JULY 23, 2020

Nineteen weeks since lockdowns began—nearing 1,000 deaths per day, again.

The Wall of Moms—mostly white, mostly suburban, mostly in yellow shirts with bicycle helmets fastened—intend to use their white privilege to stand between protestors of color and police in Portland. Federal agents have tear-gassed, shoved, and even shot rubber bullets at the moms this week.[49] Some members of the crowd have taken to shining lasers in the eyes of the federal paramilitary officers. Some throw back the tear-gas canisters. Others have knocked about the chain-link fence erected around the courthouse or shot off fireworks. But the crowd does not physically attack law enforcement.

Tonight, the tone changes. Portland mayor Ted Wheeler joins the protesters on the streets. Once they recognize him, they jeer. They hold him responsible for enabling the violence against them, calling him Tear Gas Ted. At one point, the protesters present a list of demands, one of which calls for his resignation. Then, Mayor Wheeler is tear-gassed, just like the rest of the crowd. Now it seems that he has gained some credibility. It also looks as if there is little Wheeler can do about the paramilitary presence in Portland, aside from politely asking them to leave.[50]

Last year, the Department of Justice began a program called Operation Relentless Pursuit (ORP). The program stepped up funding for police in seven American cities, cities with many minority citizens and located in political swing states: Albuquerque, Baltimore, Cleveland, Detroit, Kansas City, Memphis, and Milwaukee.[51] Though ORP launched last December, it only got off the ground this spring with a rebranding. Attorney General Bill Barr announced the launch of Operation LeGend, named after LeGend Taliferro, a four-year-old boy who was shot while sleeping in his bed in Kansas City almost a month ago, on June 29.[52] The FBI says the purpose is to "address a recent surge in violent crime."[53] Yet mayors in these cities oppose federal troops being used against protesters. Given that LeGend Taliferro was killed in a domestic dispute, his terrible death seems like a convenient prop instead of a true effort to address situations that lead to children being shot in their homes.[54] The president denies he is mobilizing federal officers as a nakedly political move or as a means to consolidate power.

SATURDAY, JULY 25, 2020

The "Battle of Portland" is in its fifty-fourth day; it is currently being fought with leaf blowers. A few nights ago, Portland dads joined the Wall of Moms and a second Wall of Veterans to protest continued crackdowns and police violence. When Department of Homeland Security agents at the Portland federal building fire tear gas, Portlanders crank up their leaf blowers and send it right back at them. Evidently, some of the federal agents are blowing the gas back with their own leaf blowers and specially created gas-blowing wands.[55]

Thousands of Portlanders are now out on the streets. Ever since Trump sent in the federal agents, numbers have swelled. Groups are color-coordinating their looks: social workers (green), cooks (chefs coats), parents (yellow and orange), and healthcare workers (blue). Others play marching band instruments. White virtue signaling is on full display, with people coming into the city from their comfortable homes in the suburbs to snap pictures of themselves protesting and post on social media. Riot Ribs, a twenty-four-hour, volunteer-driven outdoor kitchen, has set up a booth to feed people for free.[56] At one point, the volunteers were ordered by the police to move everything out of the area. When they rented a U-Haul truck to carry away their recently donated seventy grills and more than one thousand coolers, the police slashed its tires and towed it away. Eventually they were able to buy two used Sprinter vans and set up more mobile food trucks to feed people on the go.

It is not clear what both sides want out of this continuing moment. Portland NAACP president E. D. Mondaine notes in a *Washington Post* column today that there's a legitimate concern that what started off as Black Lives Matter protests and then Defund the Police protests have become just "white spectacle" now.[57] Regardless of the shifting message coming out of Portland, it does appear they have spurred other cities to restart their BLM protests. Some, like Seattle, Minneapolis, Chicago, and Columbus, never really stopped.[58]

The protests also continue because the news of violence continues. In Aurora, Colorado, protests tonight call out the chokehold killing of

Elijah McClain by police last year.[59] The Not Fucking Around Coalition (NFAC), an all-African American armed militia appeared at Stone Mountain, Georgia, earlier in the month—very intentionally chosen because it's the birthplace of the second KKK. Today, NFAC is marching in Louisville, Kentucky, to encourage the Kentucky district attorney to pursue justice for Breonna Taylor. Three hundred NFAC members are facing off against about fifty Three Percenters, an all-white vigilante group supposedly "defending" the police, who stood between the two groups. A much larger right-wing attendance was anticipated, but, as with earlier threats, most did not show.[60] One accidental shot was fired, but today, no one was hurt, no gas fired off, and everyone went home safely.[61] Online, however, the white rage is building.

WEDNESDAY, JULY 29, 2020

Donald J. Trump ✓
@realdonaldtrump

> I am happy to inform all of the people living their
> Suburban Lifestyle Dream that you will no longer
> be bothered or financially hurt by having low
> income housing built in your neighborhood . . .

12:19 PM—Jul 29, 2020

Trump came into office implicitly promising that he would take care of the white people in America. To the lower classes, he promised that he would keep open their coal mines, that immigrants would not compete for their jobs, and that they would continue to receive Social Security checks. He promised middle-class white people that no low-income housing would be built near them. Black and brown folks would be kept in their places by the police, he intimated, so that white folks could have whites-only public spaces again. He promised white people that they wouldn't have to send their sons to war and that they would make enough money to take a Disney cruise every few years. To upper-class whites, he promised that he would cut taxes and deregulate industry in a way that benefited them. You won't even have to be polite to Black people or the poor anymore if you don't want to. He promised comfort, ease, and a return to the happy days of white dominance. It makes sense that he is now promising the Suburban

Lifestyle Dream, free of Black and brown people. This is, after all, the slogan upon which he was elected.

This also explains why Trump has not been able to ask the population to mobilize for this pandemic. A president who makes these kinds of promises cannot then ask those same white people to make sacrifices. He cannot ask them to stay at home and wear masks in order to protect the same people he promised to exclude. His entire legitimacy is based on the promise that he will make white America happy and comfortable, again.

THURSDAY, JULY 30, 2020

The NBA shutdown was twenty weeks ago. Over 4.4 million cases of COVID.

In 1973, the General Social Survey (GSS) reported that 16 percent of all Republicans and 13 percent of all Democrats distrusted their government, scientists, and the press. Forty-five years later, 65 percent of Republicans and 28 percent of Democrats responded they'd lost trust.[62] Scholars such as Marc Hetherington and Jonathan Ladd at the Brookings Institution have spent a lot of time discussing how conservatives have so dramatically lost trust.[63] Mistrust is an intentional, long-term project, they suggest. Since Barry Goldwater in the 1960s, corporate-backed conservatives have pushed back every time there is a new regulation for greater protection of minority communities by casting doubt on science and the media. Now, that lack of trust has led to greater infection and death during this pandemic.

It's also undercutting the ability of minorities to vote for change. In an interview on NPR, Attorney General Bill Barr declared that "the possibility of counterfeiting" mail-in ballots in the upcoming election was a real concern.[64] He said this same thing during yesterday's hearing at the House of Representatives.[65] Later this afternoon, the president reiterates the danger of mail-in voting and floats the idea of delaying the November election.[66] This is a prime example of how one imaginary fear (the repeatedly debunked charge of voter fraud) can be amplified, while a very real danger (curbing the long-standing practice of mail-in voting in the United States in order to influence the coming election) can be simultaneously swept under the rug.

Federal authorities in Portland have been issuing ultimatums to arrested protesters, offering them lower charges if they will sign an Order Setting Conditions of Release, which bars them from returning to the pro-

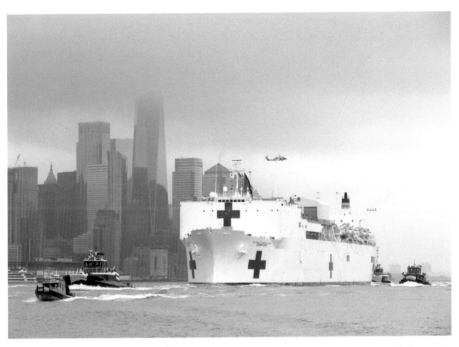

The US Coast Guard, NYPD, and NYFD provide a security escort for the USNS *Comfort*'s arrival into New York Harbor, March 30, 2020.

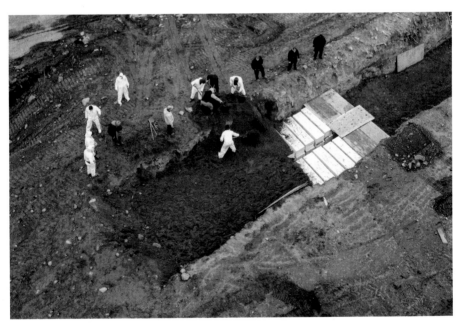

Drone pictures show inmates burying bodies on New York's Hart Island, April 9, 2020.

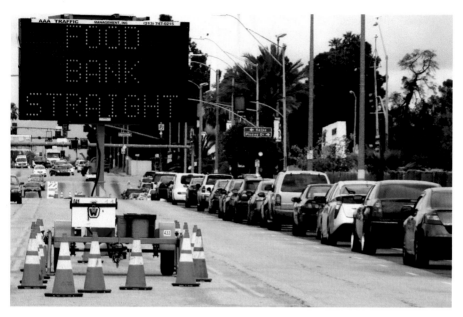

Cars line up at a free-groceries distribution in observance of Good Friday for those impacted by the coronavirus pandemic, Inglewood, CA, April 10, 2020.

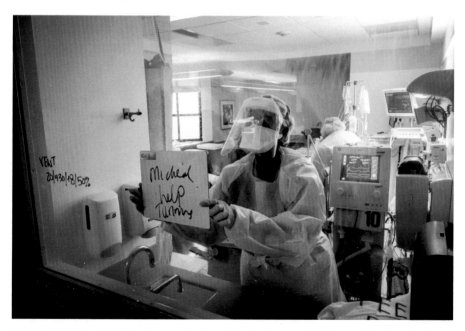

RN Linda Isidienu signals for her coworker Michael Manriquez to help her care for a COVID patient on a ventilator at the intensive-care unit at Sharp Chula Vista Medical Center, Chula Vista, CA, April 10, 2020.

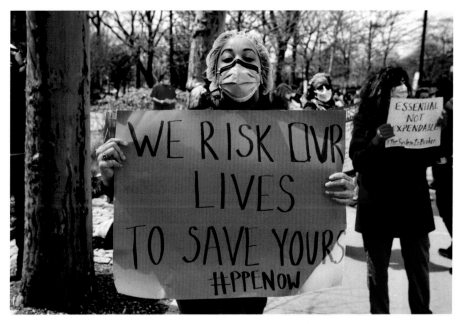

Nurses protest over PPE, Bronx, NY, April 17, 2020.

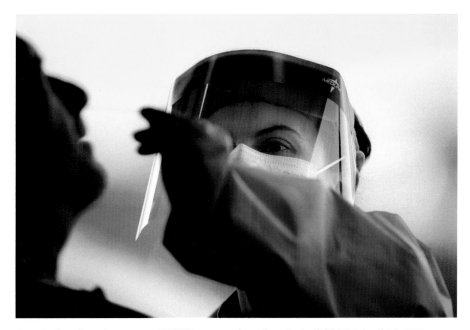

A medical worker administers a COVID test at a drive-thru, Springfield, TN, April 18, 2020.

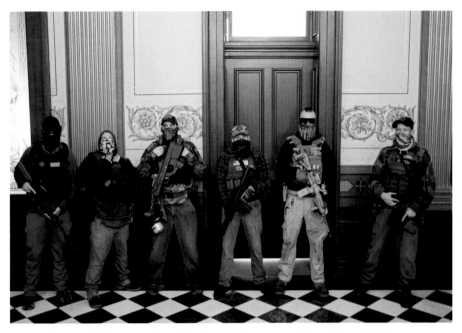

A militia group, including men charged for their involvement in a plot to kidnap Michigan governor Gretchen Whitmer, stand in front of the governor's office after protesters occupied the state capitol building, Lansing, MI, April 30, 2020.

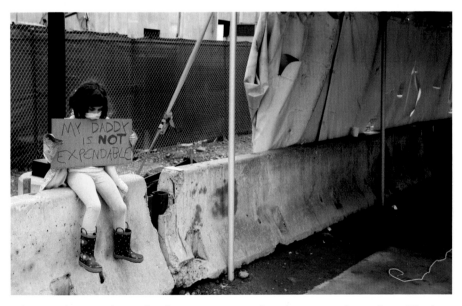

Adria Rosenberg joins her mother during a protest outside an Amazon warehouse, Staten Island, NY, May 1, 2020.

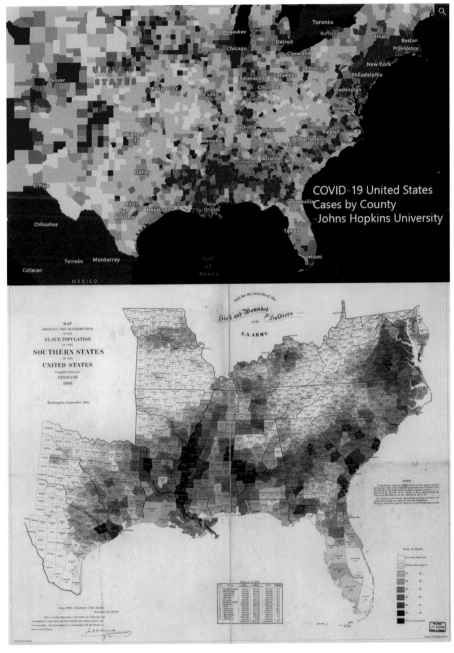

Johns Hopkins University COVID-19 map and the 1860 US Census.

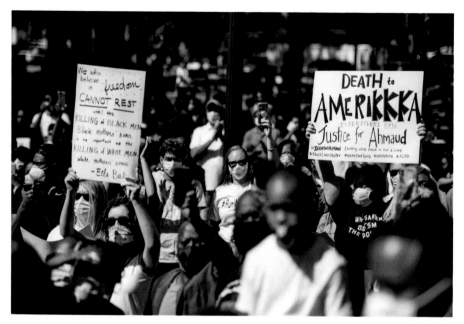

Georgia NAACP holds protest for shooting death of jogger Ahmaud Arbery, Brunswick, GA, May 8, 2020.

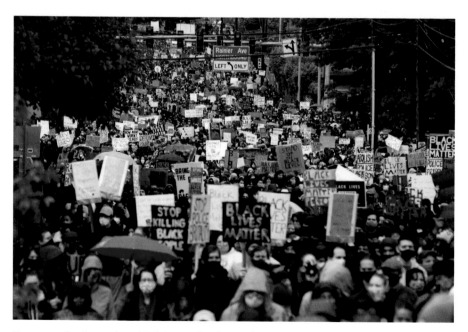

Protesters silently march up 23rd Avenue South, Seattle, WA, June 12, 2020.

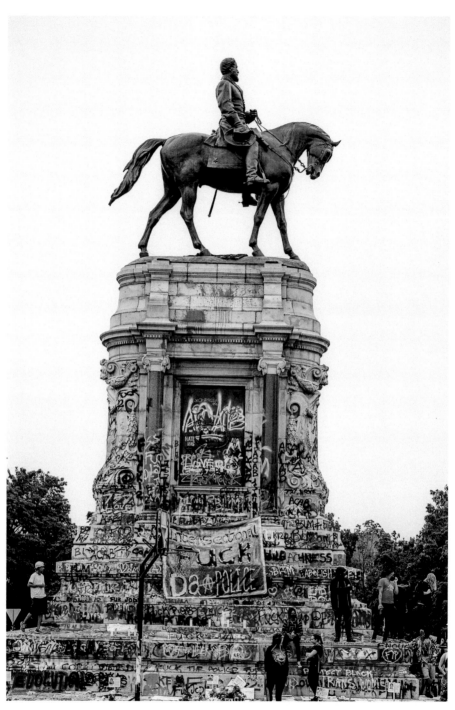

Protests continue over removal of the Robert E. Lee monument, Richmond, VA, June 20, 2020.

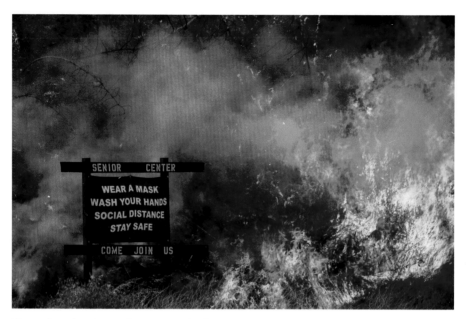

Flames from the LNU Lightning Complex fires in unincorporated Napa County, CA, August 18, 2020.

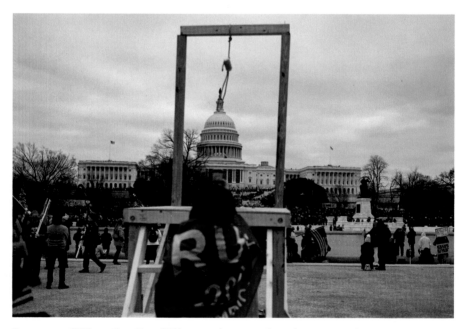

Supporters of US president Donald Trump gather across from the US Capitol, January 6, 2021. Demonstrators breached security and entered the Capitol as Congress debated the 2020 presidential election Electoral College certification.

tests. Effectively, this order would take away part of their First Amendment rights in return for not facing jail time. A third of the arrested protesters are being charged with "failing to obey a lawful order" or "inciting a riot," not vandalism or assaulting an officer.[67] DHS is using Trump's designation of Antifa as a domestic terrorist group as their justification for these actions. Notably, it is still not at all clear that Antifa even *exists*—certainly not in the way that the Proud Boys and other right-wing white nationalist groups exist, no matter what acting undersecretary for DHS Office of Intelligence Brian Murphy says about "core actors" who "show up night after night."[68]

Equally disconcerting is the news that the DHS has begun collecting information dossiers on members of the American press. Dubbed "baseball cards," these dossiers are traditionally part of the counterterrorism effort that DHS uses to target international terrorists. They've now used baseball cards targeting a reporter from the *New York Times* and the editor-in-chief of the blog *Lawfare* for allegedly reporting on DHS activities, including their seemingly unconstitutional gathering of financial information on protesters.[69] The echoes of Nixon's infamous enemies list are unmistakable.

It seems like the crackdown on the protests is entering a new phase. All of these measures represent a carefully choreographed performance meant to show that Trump is "winning." Like the awkward Bible photo two months ago in Lafayette Park, projecting the image of strength is as critical to consolidating power as controlling the armed forces is. It works. As scholar of propaganda Jacques Ellul noted long ago, such shows of force attract those who need to identify themselves with a winning side.[70] Donald Trump has cultivated a deep following based on this message, deep enough to distract from the collapsing economy and the deaths of nearly two hundred thousand Americans.[71]

Oregon governor Kate Brown has finally arranged for the removal of federal officers from Portland.[72] Hopefully, this will change the tenor of the protests.

SATURDAY, AUGUST 1, 2020

Day 68 of BLM protests

I get to see my coworkers today standing in line for our back-to-school COVID tests. Everyone looks tired and mildly shocked. We are pleasant as we shuffle forward, exchanging *hellos* and *how-have-you-beens*, each hoping to learn from the other additional information about the reopening of the university in two weeks. The administration has told us little about what it will look like to be in the same space and breathe the same air as hundreds of eighteen- to twenty-three-year-olds, many of whom will not be social distancing before entering the classroom.

The federal government has had the better part of seven months to come up with a national plan to combat coronavirus. Yet, over the summer, there has been so much chaos and so little clear communication that no one is sure what will happen if we send students, teachers, professors, and administrators back to school. Most universities on the coasts and K–12 schools where teacher unionization is strong will be online for the fall semester. Many in the interior, where unionization is weak and tax revenues barely support public schools and even "state" universities, are under pressure to be in person.

The question of whether students should return to school and how they should do it is complicated. Science journalist Laurie Garrett, who turned out to be a Cassandra, calls America's efforts to get schools going a "moral and medical catastrophe."[1] Scientists in South Korea identified the greatest spreaders as ten- to nineteen-year-olds, with adults around children this age being the most likely to be infected.[2] We have heard terrifying stories (many of which thankfully turned out to be exaggerated) of "COVID parties," where one young person with the virus comes and everyone else *knowingly* plays a kind of epidemiological Russian roulette to see who gets sick.[3] Many college students, it seems, believe they are immune. What if I pick up the virus from a student and give it to my eighty-four-year-old mother, who has diabetes and hypertension?[4]

At the same time, we really need to send our children to school. Public schools function as day care for a huge percentage of America's workforce. No alternative public infrastructure exists to provide safe spaces for children during the day. If grade schools close, kids will have to stay home, alone, which is usually a bad option, or with a caregiver. Working parents will either have to cut back on their hours, find a friend or family member, or pay for childcare. Most of these options are so expensive that many parents have had to quit working outside of the home.

Many Americans don't realize how many millions of children rely on their schools for basic nutritional needs. Joanne Guthrie and Katherine

Ralston, senior nutritionists at the US Department of Agriculture, tracked the 2.4 billion breakfasts served at public schools in 2017 and 2018. Eighty percent of those children lacked resources to get breakfast any other way.[5] Similarly, schools serve nearly *thirty million* free lunches daily. Online-only schooling is made even more complicated by the technology gap. How will students learn online if they have no computer, no internet, and no access to the public library?

One alternative would be to subsidize American workers so that they can stay home and wait out the pandemic. Dip into savings, tax the wealthy, and offer a safety net, both financially and epidemiologically. Germany, Spain, France, Italy, and Britain all have paid up to 80 percent of private-sector salaries for workers furloughed because of COVID-19.[6] Unfortunately, we are not in a cultural space as a nation to be able to consider such an option. The president and education secretary, Betsy DeVos, call on the schools to open, arguing that children need education. They may be right, yet they continue to downplay the risks of the coronavirus to school staff.[7] School reopening in the fall is now a fully partisan issue, like wearing masks, COVID-related health statistics, and nearly every other aspect of this pandemic.[8]

MONDAY, AUGUST 3, 2020

The cable television company HBO teams up with Jonathan Swan of the website and podcast news agency Axios to interview the president.[9] A sizable portion of America watches. It's immediately apparent that their exchange signals two whole conceptual universes at odds with one another, seemingly unbridgeable.

Swan starts the interview with a compliment. He notes Trump's devotion to Norman Vincent Peale's *The Power of Positive Thinking*, then asks how that mindset is suitable for handling the worst pandemic we have seen in a century.[10] Trump cites how well "we" have done in making ventilators available and "stopping very infected people from China coming in. . . . and then the ban on Europe." Swan attempts to redirect him back to the question, suggesting that perhaps what is needed instead of saying that everything is going to be okay is a consistent message rooted in reality. Trump resists. "We will never forget" how China gave us coronavirus, he blurts, voicing this repeated racialized grievance. Trump asserts that America was in the process of making billions of dollars off of Chinese losses because of "their" pandemic. But then it came here.

At one point, the president launches into a staccato chain of words, his body leaning forward in his chair. He is enraptured by his description of the crowds that he drew at his Tulsa rally last week. Three times, he repeats the sentence that his Saturday night speech had the highest ratings in Fox News history. It's a falsehood, but it is an old and effective ploy, as the CIA itself pointed out in the 1940s when investigating the popularity of Adolf Hitler: "people will believe a big lie sooner than a little one; and if you repeat it frequently enough people will sooner or later believe it."[11]

"I'm asking about public health," Swan interjects, brow furrowed. "I've gone to your rallies. I've talked to your people. They love you. They listen to you. . . . They don't listen to me or Fauci or the media. They think we are fake news. They want to get their advice from you!" Swan exclaims, "So when they hear you say that everything is under control, don't worry about wearing masks," he pauses and looks away, exasperated. "Many of these people are old, Mr. President!"

"I think it's under control—" Trump jumps in, his hands spread wide like a child's finger painting of a turkey at Thanksgiving.

Swan jumps in, "How?! A thousand Americans are dying a day!" Trump rolls his eyes. Then he locks on Swan, raises his left eyebrow, and tries again more emphatically, faster now, "They are dying, that's true, and . . . *it is what it is.* But that doesn't mean we aren't doing everything we can. It's under control as much as you can control it." He then pivots to lay blame on the governors, sloughing off any responsibility, and the conversation is derailed again.

The exchange is indicative of two contrary communication styles. Swan uses language to move the conversation along a logical path from question to answer to follow-up question, aiming for a distilled awareness of the issue. Trump's comments are not logically tied to the topic of conversation. He merely repeats variations on three themes: I am a great man; my opponents want to deny, discredit, or destroy my success; and I will be avenged for these grievances.

Tellingly, my own research shows that this is also a version of the message consistently parroted by Fox News. Having run regression analysis on over five thousand Fox News stories over the last six months, I can say with confidence that, like Trump, Fox News has a set of key messages that are not specific to the question, place, or crisis being covered: (a) suggest present near greatness for a conservative-led America, with a nod to past true greatness; (b) repeat a grievance caused by an enemy who has dragged the present away from its former glory; and (c) promise revenge against that enemy. These messages play on the core emotions of pride and fear. Much of Fox News content is subsumed beneath that trinitarian message—a message reinforcing group identity.

The real question today is: How is it that these illogical messages, which bear little resemblance to verifiable facts, resonate so powerfully with so much of America? All across the country, folks place "Trump 2020" signs in their yards. If they watched this interview, they would see Trump as the hero and Swan as the foe. In the run-up to the 2016 election, historians identified key motivations for Trump supporters: nationalism, anti-globalism, and anti-elitism.[12] These belief structures are rooted in pride. Yet their analyses did not address the role *fear* had in leading the public into the arms of Trump. People are not just afraid of losing their material possessions to people of color; they are afraid of their own historical narrative being rewritten without them as the aggrieved and triumphant heroes.

MONDAY, AUGUST 17, 2020

Another strange consequence of coronavirus: today, I was turned away at the fast-food drive-through because I couldn't pay in exact change. They are out of coins. It turns out the rumors that businesses across the country are experiencing a severe cash shortage are true.

Last month, the Federal Reserve put together a Coin Task Force (another "CTF," not to be confused with the Coronavirus Task Force) to address the problem.[13] On July 24, the Federal Reserve said the shortage is caused, at least in part, by the 128 million American households who are not paying in cash because they are doing most of their purchasing online from home using credit cards.[14] It's not a shortage at all, the Federal Reserve implies. It's our behavior: "Business and bank closures have disrupted the supply chain and normal circulation patterns of US coins."[15]

Later, I speak with Amy Burr, vice president at the San Francisco Federal Reserve. Indeed, she confirms, coins are accumulating in vast numbers in people's homes. Change jars go unredeemed. In the first few months of lockdowns, grocery shoppers were not thinking about bringing their spare change to the Coinstar machine to exchange it for cash. They rushed in and out to avoid COVID exposure. Coins didn't circulate. In a normal year, for every dollar worth of coins that the Federal Reserve reinserted into circulation, eighty-three cents of it was already circulating coins. Now, less than fifty cents are recirculated.

The shortage is in paper money as well. Last March and April, lots of people intentionally withdrew cash from the banks, just to be safe. As Burr puts it, "When people are unsure, there is always a flight to currency." When disasters hit, people go to the ATMs and put money in their pockets. Burr tells me that certain ATMs even ran out of money as people changed their money-seeking habits. In response, the Federal Reserve has been issuing money to banks.[16] Economists are saying that this does *not* mean that we are heading toward inflation. They are saying that *de*flation remains the bigger worry because people are not spending their cash.[17]

And yet, prices are consistently rising for basic consumer goods, and the purchasing power of the average American has dropped significantly. This started when Trump took over in January 2016 and has worsened

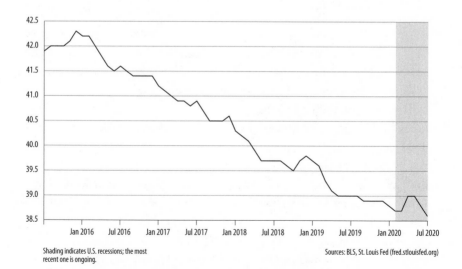

Shading indicates U.S. recessions; the most recent one is ongoing.

Sources: BLS, St. Louis Fed (fred.stlouisfed.org)

Consumer Purchasing Power, 2016-July 2020.
(U.S. Bureau of Labor Statistics and St. Louis Fed)

ever since. Perhaps there is no connection between the printing of money and the rise of consumer costs. Maybe rising prices are simply attributable to disrupted supply chains. We have cratering employment numbers; still over one million unemployment applicants week after week for over twenty weeks. I have a hard time seeing how the average American will not be on the losing end of this equation.[18]

THURSDAY, AUGUST 20, 2020

Twenty-three weeks since stay-at-home orders were first issued—162,000 deaths

Historians Deborah Cohen and Lessie Jo Frazier argue the year 1968 represented, "a long historical moment . . . an idea."[19] The year brought to a head the war in Vietnam; the civil rights movement; the Chicano/a, American Indian, and Asian American liberation struggles; student and feminist movements; decolonial movements in Africa, Latin America, and Asia; and the antinuclear movement. George Wallace ran for the presidency, with plenty of support in rural America. Dr. Martin Luther King Jr. and Robert F. Kennedy were assassinated only weeks apart. The electorate seemed irreparably divided.

On the one hand, that year marked a global outpouring of expression and freedom, what historian Gerd-Rainer Horn called "the dynamic towards personal and collective liberation."[20] On the other hand, it also rang the death knell for the old political liberalism and the Democratic Party as it had existed.[21]

At the Democratic National Convention in Chicago that August, Mayor Richard Daley's blue-helmeted police dragged from the floor those calling for an antiwar platform. Outside the convention center, National Guard troops tear-gassed protesters and beat them with nightsticks. For people like Daley, "liberals" had gone too far. "What are we coming to as a society," he posed, "if *policemen* are treated the way they've been treated—not only in Chicago, but all over the country?" He blamed the protesters for their own beatings.[22] A year later, a National Commission on the Causes and Prevention of Violence, formed one year after the better-known Kerner Commission, resolved that the police used excessive force: "There was enough wild club swinging, enough cries of hatred, enough gratuitous beating to make the conclusion inescapable that individual policemen, and lots of them, committed violent acts far in excess of the requisite force for crowd dispersal or arrest."[23]

Much like the Kerner Commission in 1967, this National Commission in 1968 resulted in a large report and little actual reform. Instead, Richard Nixon, who painted himself as the defender of law and order, harnessed the memory of that night to enlist his "silent majority" of Americans who viewed protest and civil rights as democracy gone too far. The entrenched pro-business Republican Party shifted colors to become the new defender of law and order, property, family values, the Second Amendment, and white resentment toward racial and ethnic minority groups attempting to be included in the American Dream.[24]

Given the conflict of this year, one might be tempted to use 1968 as a model for anticipating *this* year's Democratic National Convention. They are, however, nothing alike. This year's affair happens virtually, with each speaker tuning in from home. Each reads from a script in front of a carefully manicured background. It feels like one long commercial targeting people who are already sold on the product. Vice presidential candidate Kamala Harris becomes the highlight, bringing a sense of closeness and realism, substance and gravitas. Former vice president Joe Biden speaks cogently about the issues of the day, and everyone sighs with relief.[25] The fact that the two of them seem capable of compassion is a welcome change.

The most salient parts of the convention are the speeches of Michelle Obama on the first night and Barack Obama on the final one. Twelve years ago, when Obama won the presidency, it felt like a hydraulic lift had moved the nation. We *had* overcome. Then, four years ago, many white people realized we were naive, at best, in 2008. African Americans in this country were not surprised; they knew that racism hadn't evaporated with a Black man in the White House. Obama's victory was profoundly important symbolically, but it was hardly a reflection of concrete systemic change. Tonight, on the national stage again, now with gray hair, Obama's familiar smile looks weary.[26] *We were eight years in power*, says Ta-Nehisi Coates. And what happened?

If 1968 (and 1794 and 1876 and 1952 and 1980 and 1994 and 2010) have anything to teach us, it is that political moments where the comparatively powerless gain something from their governments are usually followed by Thermidorean reactions, hell-bent on the retrenchment of power in the hands of the already powerful. This year is no exception: profound upheaval, exposing the nation's weaknesses in leadership, healthcare, policing, employment, and race relations, yet little actual progress so far.

And today, with our first Black president on screens across America, the country learns there is another unarmed Black man's name to chant. Pasadena police shot and killed Anthony McClain last weekend. The cops claim McClain had a weapon, but their body cams were not on at the time.[27] For the last three days, protesters have demanded the tape, demanded an investigation, demanded their elected officials to do *something*. Without video evidence, it is still the cop's word that is believed. Marching, sure; but things don't change without sustained pressure.

In fact, there is solid evidence that even in cities where the marches were largest and loudest—cities that are supposed to be "progressive"—police are arresting people off the street using only facial recognition software, software that is famously inaccurate.[28] To add to that, while Robert O'Brien, Trump's National Security Advisor, claims that "99.9 percent of our law enforcement officers" are not racists, the FBI counterterrorism investigators have found that white supremacists fill police departments in cities big and small.[29] Law and order in 2020, much like in 1968, means a billy club and pepper spray for protesters and little if any punishment for officials who break laws or create new ones to punish and intimidate those who protest.

Will the arc of time that bends toward justice—Dr. King's metaphor that Obama was keen on invoking—keep bending and bending without ever quite getting to "justice"?

MONDAY, AUGUST 24, 2020

5.64 million cases of COVID. Thirteen weeks since Minneapolis police killed George Floyd.

Jacob Blake is still alive. A video emerged yesterday showing Blake, an African American man, walking off a lawn in Kenosha, Wisconsin, and around to the front of his gray Dodge Durango. Three white cops follow him closely, guns drawn. Blake never faces the officers and attempts to get into his driver's seat. Once he opens the door, the nearest officer grabs Blake's T-shirt with his left hand and, as Blake gets into the car, shoots him, point-blank in the back: POP-POP-POP-POP-POP-POP-POP.

The screams from family, friends, and neighbors pierce the air before shots stop ringing. The Durango's horn honks as Blake slumps against it. His children, we learn, are in the back seat.

The video is blazing across a social media landscape already littered with documentation of excessive police force. Just three days ago, Lafayette, Louisiana, police fired a dozen rounds into Trayford Pellerin after he walked away from them.[30] Not surprisingly, the news focuses on Pellerin's past criminal record, as though a justification for his murder.[31]

In an article titled "Racist Police Violence Reconsidered," John McWhorter, associate professor at Columbia University, argues that while white cops might be "overarmed, undertrained, and low on empathy," the narrative about the routine killing of "black [sic] people in tense situations [due to] racist animus" by white cops is overblown.[32] McWhorter's essay, praised as it has been in some quarters, shortchanges what is so clearly happening all around us. If it is not *explicit* racial animus that makes these officers kill (or attempt to kill) those Black men while allowing other white men in similar circumstances to walk away, then it is *implicit*. Either way, streets are stained all too often with Black blood.

TUESDAY, AUGUST 25, 2020

Today, two tropical storms move through the Gulf of Mexico simultaneously—Marco and Laura.[33] The double storm in the Gulf is a first. Shopping lines, from New Orleans to Mobile, are reminiscent of five months ago. Comically, toilet paper is in short supply again.

In the western third of the country, wildfires are even more worrying. Over one million acres of California have been consumed in just the last month.[34] Rare firenados form and touch down, just like in Australia this past December and January.[35] NASA researchers in the Bay Area describe a hazy orange sky, impenetrable for meteorological observation.[36] It has been a record-breaking fire season, caused by the highest heat in California's history.[37] What has burned already this summer is more than the previous two years combined.[38]

Down in Florida, inland and away from the opulence of Palm Beach County and the president's summer palace, Mar-a-Lago, sugar companies burn the leaves off their sugarcane so it can be harvested more efficiently. The smoke contains thick black carbon, adding to the greenhouse cycle with dangerous carcinogens that can lead to increased lung ailments. The fields butt up against schools, where children in the sugarcane growing counties have seen disproportionate cases of asthma and other breathing problems.[39] Despite protests, policies don't change, possibly because the counties to the west are less heavily populated, and the population that does live there is predominantly African American.[40] Being able to breathe sits at the core of this, too.

Whatever hope existed in April that people would stay indoors to drastically change the trajectory of the planet has burned off (grim pun intended). It is easier to deny and minimize the creeping climate disaster than to do anything about it—cognitive dissonance resolved.

WEDNESDAY, AUGUST 26, 2020

George Floyd protests started three months ago. Day 4 of Jacob Blake protests.

Last night, a seventeen-year-old white boy drove from Illinois to Kenosha, Wisconsin, where locals have been protesting the killing of Jacob Blake since Sunday, and shot a BLM protester. Several other protesters chased him and tried to yank the AR-15 he was holding out of his hands. He shot two of them after they knocked him to the ground. Then he got up and walked toward the cops, his gun still strapped on. The Kenosha police drove right past him. He couldn't even turn himself in. Not only did he walk away from the scene, but he made it all the way home to another state and went to bed. Such are the perks of being a white man in America. It took hours to find him.[41] Meanwhile, it's worth mentioning that the Kenosha police have put Rusten Sheskey, the officer who shot Blake, on leave.

SATURDAY, AUGUST 29, 2020

This week, the Republican National Convention focuses on a series of contradictory messages: framing liberals simultaneously as "stupid sheep" and "clever thieves"; the dangers of the billionaire-owned network media elite contrasted with the heroism of other billionaire-owned corporations; the laziness and criminality of poor immigrants and Black folks, who should also embrace the GOP for its job-producing capabilities and open-armed acceptance of them; the defense of law and order, prosecuted through extralegal force; and the potential undermining of the November election alongside the guarantee that Trump will win it completely legitimately.[42]

The Republican platform is the same as it was four years ago. Not similar—*the exact same*. They defend their choice to keep their old platform by arguing that they "enthusiastically support the president's America-first agenda." It is shocking that, in the middle of a health disaster and the education and economic crises following from it, a major political party would not update their platform to address these issues.

The message of the 2016/2020 "America First" platform is rooted in a belief in American historical exceptionalism, the indivisibility of political and economic freedom, peace through strength, free financial markets, a "pro-growth tax system" that encourages "investment," locally controlled zoning for housing and schooling (meaning no compulsory racial integration), free commodification of all aspects of the environment, and large military spending. There is also a robust negative component to the platform: stopping an "activist judiciary." It has undermined traditional marriage, religious liberty, free speech, gun ownership, and the electoral college; it has allowed abortion and illegal immigrants to ruin the country and the Affordable Care Act to stand.

Ironically, the preamble in the 2020 Republican platform, which is copied verbatim from 2016, declares that "our economy has become weak and stagnant. Our standing in world affairs has declined." All true. When these words were written in 2016, they were written as a criticism of a Democratic president. Now, I assume they are aimed at the current administration? Clearly, no one in GOP bothered to proofread this.

In response, David Frum, a former speech writer for George W. Bush, publishes what he considers to be the real, unpublished GOP platform.[43] While continuing to lower taxes and regulations for the wealthiest, he argues that the Republican Party will mock fear of coronavirus, climate change, and Russian interference with our political system. China is the real enemy. They will disregard post-World War II alliances with European powers. The healthcare industry can do whatever the healthcare industry says it should do. Voting should be restricted to the "deserving," who also happen to be white.

Frum goes on to assert that Republicans believe racism is no big deal, except for a few "bad apples." Abortion should be basically eliminated, even if that means women don't control their own bodies between insemination and delivery. Frum says the real GOP platform sees immigration as usually bad, especially when in involves Spanish-speaking people crossing into the USA to work. A physical wall is a good solution to this. Blue Lives Matter, but Black Lives Matter strays into domestic terrorism. The true enemy of our nation is the "socialist" or the "Antifa" or the "Deep State" within.

We are now rounding the final corner into this presidential election with two diametrically opposing worldviews. The winner will frame how future generations understand the significance of 2020.

TUESDAY, SEPTEMBER 1, 2020

Over the last few years, people on social media have "canceled" celebrities, politicians, journalists, and university professors after they behaved or made statements that were considered racist, sexist, or otherwise culturally unacceptable. In 2017, Pepsi aired a commercial showing "it girl" Kendall Jenner bringing together police and BLM protesters by giving them a soda.[1] This advertisement, a clear homage to the iconic photographs from the 1960s of protesters giving flowers to riot police, felt as if it made light of police brutality. Social media called them out, and Pepsi removed the ad. More recently, Twitter, Facebook, and Instagram put warning labels on posts bearing false or offensive information, often because avid users flag the content. Sometimes, these social media giants will disable the account—in this day and age, the ultimate shunning.

"Canceling" is not new. Societies have always shunned members of their community for failing to abide by cultural norms. Who gets rejected and why is a barometer for the changing boundaries of a culture. As sociologist Pierre Bourdieu noted, cultural standing is a kind of capital. The more of it you have, the more powerful your position in society.[2]

The new wrinkle started this last decade, due to the rise of social media. There, cultural capital is measured in ephemeral clicks, likes, reposts, shares, and follows. "Platform" can determine who listens to you, gives you grant money or even a book contract. The anonymized court of social media opinion is displacing older ways of proving your worth, like your training or expertise.

Yet, some argue, cancel culture in its current state is a threat. John McWhorter writes in *The Atlantic* that the vitriolic world of social media has turned canceling into a weaponized, secular religion.[3] There is a kind of collective snowballing of people on the internet who, by virtue of the noise they can create, adjudicate the cultural capital of others.[4] Like the 153 writers, actors, academics, and journalists who signed a Letter on Justice and Open Debate in *Harper's Magazine* this past June, McWhorter warns that, like any practice of shaming, sometimes it becomes the very beast it was intended to slay.

On the one hand, it is admirable when people speak up in the millions to denounce behaviors they find offensive. And yet McWhorter and others claim that anti-racist cancel culture has a way of "dehumanizing" Black Americans, stripping them of agency.[5] He asserts that books like Robin DiAngelo's *White Fragility*, Ibram X. Kendi's *How to Be an Antiracist*, and even some of Ta-Nehisi Coates's writing places the fate of the Black world completely in white hands. Black people, Latinx people, and Indigenous people, by implication, says McWhorter, cannot alter their positions in American society, since they are only victims, and, therefore, cannot be held responsible for the position America has placed them in.[6] More than this, McWhorter worries that cancel culture shuts down dialogue.[7] Even asking the wrong question could lead to being canceled.

Over this summer, we witnessed "canceling" become another form of virtue signaling, "Outrage theatre," exposing another's misstatements on social media, is mistakenly equated with justice. Historian Barbara Benedict argues exhibitions of outrage and sentiment, in fact, draw us *away* from the moral difficulties of the world around us, turning the act of being a spectator and judge into a substitute for honest dialogue.[8] While it may feel cathartic to cancel offenders, it is merely an aesthetic act that ignores the deeper causes of the perpetrator's actions, including the extent to which the perpetrator is neither exceptional nor fanatical.

On a more practical level, cancel culture does not work. For example, a few years ago, Jeffree Star, a famous YouTube makeup artist, was canceled after videos emerged of him using profane, racist language. The efforts to cancel him were remarkable, but it has made no difference in his popularity or profit margins. It may have even improved his brand. Once the thirst for punishment and redemption is slaked, everyone goes back to their daily business, and the power structures that profit from the process of cancelation remain very much in place.

WEDNESDAY, SEPTEMBER 2, 2020

Historian, activist, and politician Michael Ignatieff has spent much of his career trying to understand how to foster truth and promote reconciliation in war torn parts of the world. People on different sides of a conflict must find a shared truth and understanding of the past, he argues, to serve as a basis for reconciliation. Each side carries with it a version of the past that sits at the core of its identity.[9]

The year 2020 has revealed once again the extent to which Americans live with two versions, two truths, of our past. In one, we are a society that was "stamped from the beginning" by its legacy of slavery, that still struggles to be something other than the inheritor of Jim Crow and institutionalized discrimination.[10] In the other, we are a nation created by plucky idealists and revolutionaries who created the freest nation in the world and who are still working to make it more perfect. A critical part of this second past depends on forgetting our founding crimes and glossing over the parts that do not fit the glorious narrative of freedom and progress. Denial becomes the defense of everything we Americans hold dear. Both of these truths shape who we are now, and in this sense, the past is not past. It is here all the time; it defines everything we do. As long as we remain in the twilight of what Ignatieff calls "collective illusion," we will never be able to put our past in its proper context to move toward healing.

Ideally, we would try to find a shared truth, a shared past, that lies somewhere close to verified historical accounts. This could allow us to let go of the past, to apologize, make amends, and move forward. But, as Ignatieff notes, there often is no "in between" when it comes to how we understand the past. For Americans, either we acknowledge how the brutality and horror of the African American and Indigenous experience is *the* core contradiction in this country's history, or we don't. There is not a lot of middle ground to be found there.

Moreover, even when leaders occasionally do proclaim the ugly truth of our national DNA, it is not likely to be accepted by those in power. As Ignatieff observes, those with actual power in any society, like the police and military, hold fast to their own truth: "people in uniform, do not easily or readily surrender the premises upon which their lives are based."[11] Acknowledging the real truth of our nation's past can be purgative for victims, but until the perpetrators and those who profit from that unexamined history come to terms with the real version, we will never move far as a nation.

So, then, how do we carve a path toward reconciliation? How do we break from the cycles of anger, grief, and revenge that continue to dominate us? How do we make it so that our history is not our future? For Ignatieff, the answer is that we will not be changed simply by being confronted with facts that contradict our mythical version of the past. *It is when our need for that mythical past ebbs away that we will be able to move on.* And for this to happen, we need, at minimum, a public discourse that gives permission for it to happen.

SATURDAY, SEPTEMBER 5, 2020

"Last night I was arrested" was how one contributor, a middle-class, educated professional who I'll call Rob, started his messages. Since May, he has been involved in the BLM marches in a large city in the middle of the country. Now Rob is caught in the currents of accusation and arrest.

While in custody, police pressured him to divulge any information he had on "Antifa." He laughs sardonically over our Zoom call. "Antifa?!" He has neither seen nor heard anything of Antifa in the weeks that he's been protesting law enforcement brutality. "It's absolute nonsense," he says, "it's actually worse than that. It's just a lie." But I press him. *Someone* has to be smashing the windows. Can the police call that "Antifa"?

"'Antifa' is not an organization," he makes air quotes. "In fact, we protesters talked explicitly and repeatedly about how any criminal acts or escalatory noncriminal acts could result in police violence being dealt out to Black/brown folks at a protest. So, our overwhelming and explicit choice was always emotional deescalation, coregulation, and nonviolence. We didn't scream at the cops or break windows or throw things at police, and when we saw a [protester] doing any of those things, we grabbed them and told them to stop . . . We stood with our bikes *between* cops and other protesters and between traffic and protesters and remained as emotionally neutral yet vigilant as we could be."

Rob was arrested anyway, and now he is facing serious charges. His case is now quite typical. Last month, *The Guardian* reported that over ten thousand peaceful protesters had been arrested during BLM marches.[12] That number will be much larger by now. Each of those people's lives has been turned upside down in the search for "Antifa."

Later in the day, I ask an attorney with twenty years of experience at the local, state, and federal levels as both a prosecuting and defense attorney—I'll call him Abe—to join another Zoom call and speak with Rob. Rob tells me and Abe that now the police have informed the human resources director at his job that he was thrown in jail. Now he is worried that he will be fired. Abe is nonplussed. "Going directly to your employer is a common intimidation tactic, even if it has nothing to do with the reason you're arrested," he shrugs. "Maybe they figure that, if they can't get you through the ordinary legal means, they'll get to you in other ways."

Rob responds, scratching his hairline with worry. "Well, I'm intimidated, man." He has been charged with rioting, which is a first-degree misdemeanor. This is the same classification that is given to domestic violence and driving while intoxicated. "My health insurance . . . ," Rob's voice fades, realizing what being fired might mean during a pandemic.

"Typically," Abe continues, "if the police are being unfair in their arrests, the prosecutor's office can act as a brake on them. And if the prosecutor's office and the police are aligned in an unfair way, the court system acts as a check to weed out unfair treatment. So, assuming you did nothing wrong—and you know the right people—you should be okay at the municipal level," he laughs.

Rob resumes his story. Once taken into custody, he realized that the police orchestrated his arrest in order to make him turn over his plans with "Antifa." They urged him to divulge the organization's structure, to name names. "You can't be a leader of a thing that does not exist," he remarks. "Sometimes I wished we *could* get coordinated . . . but these are just regular folks protesting against state violence used unnecessarily against regular people."

His night in jail "was really, really bad," he says, his eyes foggy with fatigue and stress. "Just the complete lack of bodily autonomy, being given nothing, in this room with all these other people you don't know. No mattresses. No blankets. No water, unless you count the three small Styrofoam cups that were set in the middle of the room for the thirty-plus people in the cell to share. One exposed toilet." Overnight, Rob curled up in a corner of the concrete cell, using his jail-issued sandals as a pillow. He was fortunate enough to be bailed out early in the "lottery" the next afternoon.

After a pause, Abe the lawyer, replies, "Not a single bit of that was news to me. Relationships are 95 percent of the legal system at the municipal level," Abe says when Rob asks what he should expect moving forward. Again, he stresses, at the local level, it is all about who you know and what favors you can summon. Justice works for those who have social connections.

Adding even more worry to the already rotten experience, there is the ever-present threat of COVID. The nurse in the jail stood too close, her mask dangling below her chin, free to cough directly on Rob.

This nonchalance regarding COVID is typical behavior in jails as well. Marianne Rosenzweig, a forensic psychologist who works with jailed populations across the Southeast, tells me that the "hygiene theater" Rob experienced seems to be widespread, though the level of COVID precautions in jails varies widely by jurisdiction. None of her stories sound positive, though. In one jail, Rosenzweig reports, guards handed inmates a single-use disposable mask in May—to use indefinitely. At a different facility, another inmate, who has been in a county jail for the last three years awaiting trial, says that, when the first person in his dorm tested positive for COVID, they quarantined that man for a single night. The next day, the jailors brought the COVID-positive inmate back into the dorm. "There are no sick days in jail," they told the other inmates. Within weeks, nearly everyone tested positive.

Though they work in different parts of the country and in different facets of the legal world—from rural to urban, local to federal, Abe in one region and Rosenzweig in another—they paint similar pictures of a justice system that is far from blind. Who you are, where you are, and who you know have always been life-and-death matters in the American justice system. Now, with COVID, the stakes are even higher.

TUESDAY, SEPTEMBER 8, 2020

Many of the largest school districts in the country resume instruction today. Chicago, Dallas, and districts in northern Virginia are off to a bumpy start as they struggle to navigate full-time online learning.[13] Many more K-12 schools are already running, especially charter schools.[14] While all the evidence seems to show that individual educators and schools did not spend the summer wasting time or vacationing, no national educational mitigation strategy emerged from Betsy DeVos's Department of Education. It barely updated its website.[15] Millions of students of all ages, abilities, and circumstances will have to rely on whatever resources their districts, teachers, administrators, and families can muster.

In the absence of federal help, most public schools convert to online classes, with in-person instruction to come later, when the virus subsides. Social distancing saves lives, and schools could create thousands of small outbreaks across the country; it's not ideal for anyone, but it makes sense. Superintendents turn to software companies like Schoology to develop curriculum and provide centralized spaces for teaching.[16] This perhaps was the easiest way for districts to offer relatively standardized instruction with limited resources and uncertain budgets.

Online schooling makes effective pedagogy very difficult. It requires far more parental involvement than is advertised or available. Moreover, when children don't physically attend school, parents have to stay home. When parents cannot go to work, they cannot make money to pay the rent. As the *Lancet* argued back in March and April, school closures lead to increased "dropout rates, child labor, violence against children, teen pregnancies, and persisting socioeconomic and gender disparities." Plus, they exacerbate food insecurity and contribute to declining student health.[17]

Some schools, perhaps in an attempt to make home learning as close to normal school as possible, require their students to be on Zoom or some other video conference tool from 8 a.m. to 3 p.m. It is exhausting for everyone. Parents of younger children must sit beside their child the entire day to make sure they are learning and to help navigate the online tools. Other schools limit live instruction to three hours, with greater homework expectations. This ameliorates some of the fatigue for teachers and gives them more time to prepare and adapt lessons. But students miss out on real instruction. Whether they are kindergarteners learning how to read or high school seniors learning calculus, instructional time with a teacher is critical.

One contributor admitted that his thirteen-year-old son is struggling in math. After walking the dog, doing the dishes, and finishing up his own work, he watches YouTube videos about Euclidean geometry proofs under the covers in bed at night. With his son receiving minimal instruction and a mound of homework, it's up to him to help his son meet the high school math requirement. "It really seems pointless to crush students with this," he says, a little embarrassed.

While upper-class families can hire tutors and nannies, many middle- and lower-class parents have to go to work. And then what do they do? Maybe they can drop their kids off at a "schooling pod" with another family. More than likely, though, they will send their kids to school as soon as it opens. This keeps the children occupied while parents work, but it comes with the risk of contracting COVID-19. The alternative is keeping children in remote school. Everyone stays safe-ish from the virus, but an adult has to remain at home. Children will continue to receive on-line instruction in isolation, made worse from watching their "in-person" friends have a social life. Parents all over the country are weighing impossibly hard choices.

WEDNESDAY, SEPTEMBER 9, 2020

Eighteen days since the shooting of Jacob Blake. Twenty-six weeks since the Jazz-Thunder NBA shutdown. 6.23 million COVID cases.

The White House is being roiled by a new controversy today—legendary journalist Bob Woodward's new book *Rage*. In it, he shares taped interviews with the president. Trump knew in January that the coronavirus was going to be bad. On March 19, Trump told Woodward he didn't want to tell people the truth about coronavirus, lest they "panic."[18] Trump lied and *tens of thousands* died, Woodward argues.

FRIDAY, SEPTEMBER 11, 2020

Nineteen years after 2,700 Americans died in a terrorist attack. The equivalent of sixty-seven 9/11 attacks have died of coronavirus in America.

A letter arrives from the poet, Chrystos, who lives in Tacoma, Washington. She worries about the "abusive landlords" who are trying to evict her and her partner. On July 23, Washington's governor extended the moratorium on evictions for the state. It will not last forever. In fact, as the Eviction Lab at Princeton University has shown, in every state where the moratoriums have lifted, evictions have skyrocketed.[19]

Take Milwaukee, Wisconsin, for example, the subject of Matthew Desmond's *Evicted*. On March 27, the governor declared an eviction moratorium. When it ended on May 26, evictions resumed in force, skyrocketing to 17 percent above last year's average. This is the average for all of the neighborhoods in Milwaukee. When you look more closely, eviction rates are up 150 percent in Lindsay Heights and Walnut Hill, the same places that were groaning under the weight of eviction and poverty in 2016. It was not until the CDC imposed a federal moratorium on evictions that they again stopped, but it is only a temporary salve. Given the unemployment rates that rack these cities (13.6 percent in April, according to the Bureau of Labor Statistics), the tenants are not likely to have the many months of unpaid rent ready to pay when it comes due.[20]

We have all heard the adage that you should never spend more than 30 percent of your income on housing. And yet even in non-pandemic years, when people do have jobs, they spend closer to 70 percent of their salary on housing. Small economic setbacks can mean that you have to choose between feeding your family and housing them. As Desmond shows, being evicted is profoundly destabilizing for the adults and millions of children who experience it every year. Eviction means loss of home, school, neighborhood. It means loss of possessions—books, furniture, clothes—and they take a long time to replace. It means the loss of employment and access to government aid. It also means that families have to accept whatever they can find, even if it is dangerous and substandard, even if it means moving into a scary part of town. "Then there is the toll eviction takes on a person's spirit," Desmond says.[21] It is a violent experience that leads to depression, anxiety, suicide, and trauma. If there is another crisis that this pandemic has revealed, it is rooted in the lack of affordable housing for families that just want to work and raise their children in safety.

At the logical end of this sad story are the unhoused, the rough sleepers, and the homeless of this nation. This massive group is made up of "battered and abandoned women, single mothers, evicted families, single unemployed and older women, deinstitutionalized mental patients, illegal immigrants, street youth, drug addicts, alcoholics," as well as veterans.[22] According to the Department of Housing and Urban Development and the National Alliance to End Homelessness, the number of unhoused people in America peaked in 2007 at almost 650,000. That number steadily declined for the next eight years, falling to 550,000 in 2016. Since then, the number has slowly risen again, totaling 567,715 in 2019.[23] All of these numbers are tentative, since the problems with counting the homeless are famously "legion."[24] And, as Jonathan Kozol poignantly put it in his 1980s study of the unhoused: "Any search for the 'right number' carries the assumption that we may at last arrive at an acceptable number. There is no acceptable number."[25]

No one knows what COVID has done to the numbers of homeless people in the nation. On the one hand, they have suffered inordinately and are likely to see a rise in their population as evictions resume in the coming months. If you think about it, everything that we have done to mitigate this virus has required that you have a home. Those without housing cannot obey a shelter-in-place order. Maintaining social distancing in a homeless shelter is nearly impossible. Testing presents problems for the homeless, since those without a permanent address or even cellphones lack a reliable way to receive their results. Shelter is its own basic need, but in a society where communication and distribution of resources are centered around a permanent residence, those without housing are dangerously marginalized.

Paula, a homeless woman in Savannah, Georgia, remembers how, in the first few weeks of the lockdown, "it was impossible to get stuff that we need. You know, we use hand sanitizer all the time because, well, you've got no real way to wash your hands out here. We live by the stuff . . . Toilet paper! We need it too."[26]

WEDNESDAY, SEPTEMBER 16, 2020

Forty-seven days until the presidential election. 6.5 million COVID cases.

Hurricane Sally lashes the Alabama-Florida coast and wildfires are blazing across the West Coast. L. J. Weaver, an anthropologist who specializes in global health inequalities at the University of Oregon, writes of her family's decision to evacuate from Eugene. For weeks, the sky has been so thick with smoke that it felt like a dome was hovering overhead, like they were sealed within a snow globe. Outside, nothing but "raining ash and the smell of burning." Two centimeters of soot coated every tree and plant. Sweeping it only created clouds. She prudently taped up her doors and windows, but the outside made it inside anyway. When she drove to the store, all the ash whirling made her feel disoriented and nauseous. Today, with the air quality at a level never seen in Oregon, she felt compelled to leave. She's going back to the Midwest to her parents' house, thankful that they can still accommodate the whole family.

"Birth certificates, the deed to the house, favorite stuffed animals" made it into a hastily packed suitcase, along with a paper map in case the GPS died on the way out, instant coffee packets, and sleeping bags.

All these disasters signal to her something even more unnerving. She sees unmistakable parallels between the impoverished populations she studies in India and Brazil and the chaos happening around her in the United States. "It's clear that we as a country are only injuring ourselves." It's not just the fires, it's the rumors that "Antifa" set these fires. "Even natural disasters push us apart," she says, noting that the Portland BLM protests continue even in the face of fires and smoke, that even in her neighborhood, people are divided over who is responsible for what. Should we blame the cops, the protesters, the "white extremists" who do the looting or the "white extremists" who fire off the tear gas at the protesters? This is what her neighbors debate. Underneath those worries, she wonders "will my kids have an ordinary lifespan?" If we cannot handle something straightforward like a killer virus—if even *pandemics* divide the country into two roughly equal, opposite chunks—how will we address the heat that's coming, heat that will start fires sooner, that will make hurricanes wetter?

FRIDAY, SEPTEMBER 18, 2020

Forty-six days until election. 6.6 million cases, 2.23 million of which are active.

Supreme Court justice Ruth Bader Ginsburg died today. Her passing escalates the avalanche of news going from really bad to horrible. "Not RBG" and, simply, "No. No. No." reverberate across social media.[27]

Scholars and journalists have churned out books and documentaries—there was even a feature film—about Ginsburg. They marvel at her tenacity and resolve; they chronicle her work as one of the few female professors of law at Rutgers, and later, Columbia University. She became a cultural icon after issuing a dissenting opinion in the 2007 *Ledbetter v. Goodyear Tire & Rubber Co.* case. After the court dismissed Lilly Ledbetter's suit alleging employment discrimination based on her sex, Ginsburg wrote, "The Court does not comprehend or is indifferent to the insidious way in which women can be victims of pay discrimination." It was a profound moment when a female justice publicly chastised her male colleagues for their blindness and prejudice.

Just as no one seriously expected the Republican-controlled Senate to vote to convict the impeached Trump earlier this year, no one expects Mitch McConnell (R-KY) and the GOP to follow their own precedent in replacing Ginsburg's vacancy on the court during an election year. Four years ago, McConnell blocked Merrick Garland, President Obama's choice to replace the late Antonin Scalia on the Court. But this time, McConnell moves forward with filling the vacancy. Highlighting the hypocrisy, Senate Minority Leader Chuck Schumer (D-NY) tweets McConnell's 2016 tweet verbatim: "This vacancy should not be filled until we have a new president." When confronted, McConnell replies by arguing that might basically makes right.[28] McConnell believes "politics is for power."[29]

There is a larger backstory here than just realpolitik. The rift between our two major parties has become stark, intractable. Yet, polarization into two sharply divided camps did not occur overnight. Stephen S. Smith, director of the Weidenbaum Center on the Economy, Government, and Public Policy at Washington University in St. Louis, has tracked the contours of Senate debate since the 1950s. Like many, he decries the spiral of increasingly obstructionist rules and the mounting impetus to break the obstructionist logjam with new Senate rules. The "parliamentary arms race between the parties," says Smith, has made the once well-functioning, congenial Senate into a quagmire. Why has this happened? Party leaders like McConnell are actually guided by what Smith calls "a consensus view" among voters in their parties that centrism and compromise is itself wrong. They then pursue strategies that, according to Smith, "perpetuate the obstruct-and-restrict syndrome of the modern Senate."[30] A self-destructive positive feedback loop.

Smith's observations about this "Senate Syndrome" correlate with another trend in American politics. As revealed in *White Rage* by historian Carol Anderson (2016) and the recent confession by former GOP strategist Stuart Stevens, *It Was All a Lie* (2020), the GOP has shifted inexorably toward the weaponization of white grievance since the civil rights era of the 1960s and '70s. While Democrats attempted to extend voting rights, integrate schools and neighborhoods, provide low-income housing, hold public authorities accountable for equal justice, and level the economic playing field for nonwhites by raising taxes to pay for these programs, Republicans pulled back, dug in their heels, called for "massive resistance," and stood for "No."[31] This stance became most apparent when Barack Obama gained the presidency in 2008. McConnell and other Republican insiders resolved not to "give" on anything for any reason.[32] "The way it was characterized to me," said Joe Biden, the newly elected vice president at the time, "was, 'For the next two years, [Republicans] can't let you succeed in anything.'"[33] After fifty years of piecemeal white backlash, a Black man had broken the barrier to the highest office, and the established white-controlled power structure in the Senate locked up. The result? He would get nothing from them. The GOP would block Garland from the Supreme Court and install conservative Neil Gorsuch, then conservative Brett Kavanaugh. And in this case, the GOP will almost certainly install a conservative successor to RBG—their own stated justifications for doing precisely the opposite in 2016 be damned. Even if every single GOP senator would swear they lack racial animus individually, it just so happens that their tactics draw water from the same well of obstruction that has worked against the expansion of a more racially equitable society for generations.

MONDAY, SEPTEMBER 21, 2020

J and his friend, L, have agreed to speak with me, but I am thirty minutes late because the road that J lives on does not appear on Google Maps. I finally nudge my little van down a gravel road, so narrow the tree branches scratch the windows on both sides. A few hundred yards in, the driveway turns steeply downhill, etched with huge gullies where the rain has washed out the red clay. Then I see J and L and a couple of additional friends standing outside, shirtless, smoking cigarettes, enjoying the beautiful day.

J has cobbled his house together from found objects and abandoned construction materials, his toilet carved from an old tree trunk. In one corner sits the disarticulated front and back ends of a FEMA trailer left over from Hurricane Katrina. After a friend overdosed in it six months ago, he cut the trailer into thirds so that no one would try to come and live in it. He has welded the middle third of the trailer to an old RV, where he sleeps and eats.

J was a meth user but is in recovery. I am not sure if L is still using. Both men have done time. I came to them because they can talk to me about how the COVID-19 pandemic has affected the meth world.

"The market shriveled up completely in March," L begins, "just as the lockdown was happening." He wipes his hands and takes a long drag off his vape. "The government cracked down on the three Mexican cartels that cook most of the meth for Alabama down here."

"If everything was closed down, how did people manage their habit?" I ask.

"We shook a bottle," L replies, lying on the bed inside and talking through the open door. They explain to me that, to shake a bottle, you have to get someone to "smurf" some pseudoephedrine (PSE) from a pharmacy for you. You shake the PSE with some common household chemicals in a two-liter bottle and *voilà!*—you have some low-quality methamphetamine. "It's shit," L says, "but it's better than nothing." What they don't mention is how dangerous it is. The bottle could explode; the formula could be toxic.[34]

L gets off the bed and comes to the doorway.

"How long did you have to shake a bottle for?" I ask.

L thinks for a moment, "Up until April or so. After that it was only being sold by the narcs. Every narc had it and every narc was selling it."

J sees my astonishment. He smiles, "Narcs will sell to small-time buyers with no intention of arresting you. They just want information. You have to be desperate though."

L nods, "I never buy from the narcs because then you owe them."

"You didn't know that the government runs its own drug cartel, did you?" J asks me, resting his left foot on his right knee and taking a sip of lemonade. "The government needs people like us to stay addicted." I don't know how to weigh this claim.

"It's not hard to find now," L interjects. "Oh God—Florida, Louisiana, and here are flooded. Everyone is also looking for ketamine."

"Okay, but what about heroin and fentanyl?" I ask, recalling the conversation I had with Brandy Henry at Columbia University in July. "Why do you think fatal overdoses are up by 42 percent since the shutdown?"

J has an answer ready. "Two reasons. One, it is really hard to get heroin. We don't grow heroin in this country. It has to be shipped in. . . . When the government shut down all the supply chains because of COVID, the only thing that we got left is fucking fentanyl. And that's what you're going to get, is fentanyl sprayed on Sheetrock, or whatever. And people will shoot it up and rave about it." Pausing, he looks knowingly at L. "And they are trying to die. That's the shit to them. That is the goal." He says this part more slowly and with a little bite: "If it kills you and someone has to *bring you back*, that's the shit you want."

"And the second reason?" I manage, trying not to let my eyes go too wide.

"You can't get naloxone," J replies with a shrug.

Just as Henry said last month, J confirms that the price of naloxone has skyrocketed, and the life-saving intervention has become nearly impossible to get. "And when there is no naloxone," L continues, looking away, darkly, "there is no way to save you."

WEDNESDAY, SEPTEMBER 23, 2020

The US passes a grim milestone: two hundred thousand Americans dead due to coronavirus. It took the country from February 29 until June 3 to hit the first one hundred thousand deaths—just over thirteen weeks. One hundred thousand additional Americans died over the next sixteen weeks while mandatory stay-at-home orders and shutdowns were in place. That averages out to a death from COVID about every ninety seconds.[35] Cases of coronavirus have dropped significantly in the large cities in the Northeast and Northwest, where the virus theoretically first entered the country. Nursing homes and convalescent care facilities are no longer the epicenters. But coronavirus lingers in the cities of the Midwest and the South.

THURSDAY, SEPTEMBER 24, 2020

In the early months of the pandemic, cases of child abuse appeared to decline across the country. Indiana Department of Child Services saw child abuse reports decrease by 35 percent compared to 2019.[36] Children's Medical Center of New York found a 50 percent drop in the first three months of the lockdown.[37] Washington, DC's Child and Family Services saw a 62 percent decline.[38] It is the same story in California, Virginia, Massachusetts, Texas.[39] Sadly, this did not mark a decline in abuse.

Jamye Coffman, director of the Center for the Prevention of Child Abuse and Neglect at Cook Children's in Fort Worth, Texas, believes these numbers are deceptive. She has had glimpses over the last five months of the real catastrophe under the surface. While child abuse reports were much lower, the cases they did see were far worse than anything Dr. Coffman has experienced in her long career.

"Initially, in the first six weeks after we went into our lockdown in March, we had four child abuse deaths . . . in six weeks. To put this in perspective, we normally get five or six *a year*. Some had been placed with CPS [Child Protective Services], where they were supposed to be safe, and they ended up being killed. Some had no CPS history. Some were killed at home. Normally our child abuse deaths are infants, but these were pre-schoolers." She pauses for a moment. "It is harder to kill an older kid, remember. And these were horrible, horrible cases. Horrible cases."

In other words, because of the shutdowns, mandatory reporting, which comes mostly from teachers and doctors, dropped. Abuse did not. Doctors' offices shut down or reduced staff, which meant seeing fewer patients each day; hence, fewer opportunities for clinicians to catch child abuse. In tele-medicine appointments, nurses and physicians attempted to see the tell-tale signs in a child (like being withdrawn, anxious, or uncharacteristically aggressive). But, of course, discovering child abuse over a computer screen is next to impossible. Coffman nods. "When the person who is presenting the child is the one doing the abusing, they aren't going to show you what's happening. With abuse, you must check every inch of a child's body, and we can't do that on a screen." Neglect, an even more common kind of abuse, almost certainly remained hidden. This was the case all over America. In Pennsylvania, doctors saw far more severe injuries than normal, with particularly high incidences of head and abdominal trauma.[40] A recent article in the *Journal of the American Medical Association* observes the same, with "brain bleeding and skull fractures" among children on the rise.[41]

"Something else happened," Dr. Coffman adds. "We saw this unexpected change in [the tone of] our interactions with children and their families. Usually, when families come in to be evaluated for abuse, pretty much, they are nice, and they cooperate. We treat them with respect, even if we think they are the perpetrator, and things run smoothly. Now, I don't know if it is because of the pandemic and everyone's overall stress, but parents and caretakers are much angrier. Their world is in such upheaval." She looks up at me. "You can imagine, our real concern is that this anger will ultimately be taken out on the *child*, because they can't really take it out on us."

As spring turned to summer and families headed back into public settings, reports of child abuse rose dramatically. For instance, the Indiana Department of Child Services reported that 22,994 children had been abused in the month of July.[42] In 2019, the number was 14,672.[43] In Indianapolis alone, sexual abuse rose by 35.5 percent, neglect by 32 percent, and physical abuse by 46 percent, compared to 2019. Predictive models estimate that child abuse may have risen by 1,493 percent from previous years.[44]

I ask Dr. Coffman if they have seen any changes in the demographics of children being abused. She answers that they have seen more children from higher socioeconomic groups than usual. But the biggest determinant, she says, seems to be families who have lost jobs. "With almost all of our families, there has been at least one parent that lost a job." Coffman puts her hand up to make an important point. There is a common bias that poor minority families are the most likely to be abusive. They are policed and stigmatized. It is often an overreporting of that population and an underreporting of white people. I think of the minority families who are torn apart by overreporting and the white kids who are not protected. She continues, "There are regular instances where we see *white* children whose abuse has been missed because they are from white, educated, middle-class, married, 'nice' families. Those were preventable, but our bias got in the way."

I look down at my hands, overwhelmed by the brokenness that I see everywhere I look this year. "But there is some hope," she interjects. Given what she does for a living, Dr. Coffman's brightness and positivity are breathtaking. The pandemic has precipitated a system-wide reevaluation of their program. They have worked with other public health experts to issue statewide guidelines so emergency room workers will have standardized training and reporting mechanisms. Ironically, those horrible deaths in April forced professionals to take action. Like with George Floyd, it seems to have required the death of four preschoolers to get statewide reforms in place.

"How do we stop the kids from getting abused in the first place," I ask her, leaning on my hand as I stare into the screen.

"That's the million-dollar question, isn't it?" she looks me dead in the eye. "Primary prevention all goes back to social determinants of health. It's not going to be fixed by CPS and Child Welfare. By the time they are involved, the abuse has already happened. It has to start early in the game with an all-encompassing model of public health." This means fixing poverty, addressing drug and alcohol abuse, providing mental health services to parents, reducing teen parenting, offering family planning support, providing good education and women's access to healthcare. All of these factors, when left unattended, increase child abuse and neglect. This "silent pandemic" will have a lasting impact on the children who have lived through this year.[45]

SUNDAY, SEPTEMBER 27, 2020

6.9 million COVID cases

Unexpectedly, the *New York Times* just located and released a partial copy of several of Trump's tax returns. They reveal that Trump has not paid any taxes for eleven of the last eighteen years, and in each of the last two years, paid only $750 in taxes.[46] Trump, true to form, denies the newspaper has seen his taxes and claims all of it is fake. Some of his supporters concede these likely are his taxes but then applaud him for figuring out how to cheat the system. Others express disgust at what this says about our president. Many point out the rank unfairness, contrasting his life of luxury to the small stimulus checks that Americans received during the pandemic. Trump spent $70,000 on hair care alone last year, as much as a middle-class family's salary.

This news will not change the political landscape. We have become inured to scandal, collectively agreeing, like the citizens of the decaying Roman Empire, that power and platform matter more than character and conviction. Right now, Fox News has six pundits on air defending Trump for knowing how to game the IRS and avoid paying his taxes. The *Federalist* tells its readers that Trump's taxes are not out of the ordinary. "Tax evasion is different than tax avoidance," announces Ryan Ellis at the Center for a Free Economy, "and tax avoidance is smart."[47] If only we all had the money to avoid paying taxes. The most disconcerting part of this whole story is how common it is. As WNYC and *ProPublica* have shown, the current White House occupant is a part of a much wider network of people and transnational corporations that protect a small group of the world's wealthiest.[48] They have used those positions to enrich themselves, their families, and their personal connections—the very behavior against which decades of American legislation and norms were supposed to defend. All of this has been exacerbated by the pandemic. While six million people filed for unemployment this year, the nation's billionaires saw their net worth jump by over $500 billion.[49]

On the news, images of a party celebrating Amy Coney Barrett's nomination to the Supreme Court, only eleven days after Ruth Bader Ginsburg's death, flash across the screen. Powerful white people who pull the levers of power in this country crowd together inside the White House, shaking hands, laughing, hugging—without masks in the middle of our nation's greatest pandemic in a century, believing they're immune from consequences.

WEDNESDAY, SEPTEMBER 30, 2020

Last night's debate between President Trump and former vice president Joe Biden was arguably the worst in American history.[50] Pundits and journalists in other countries, the intellectual political-right, and even Fox News agree the performance debased the entire idea of a presidential debate.[51] It showed a new level of pugnaciousness from this president. It felt like listening to conservative talk radio or watching second-rate reality television.[52]

The night was an exercise in interruption, with Biden largely unable to finish a sentence before being cut off by a belligerent Trump.[53] The content of those interruptions was even harder to stomach. The news headline of the night came when Fox News moderator Chris Wallace, son of the late legendary journalist Mike Wallace, asked the president about white supremacists:

> WALLACE: Are you willing, tonight, to condemn white supremacists
>   and militia groups and to say that they need to stand down and not
>   add to the violence in a number of these cities as we saw in Keno-
>   sha and as we've seen in Portland? Are you—
> TRUMP:—Sure, I'm willing to do that—
> WALLACE:—prepared to do that specifically?
> TRUMP: But I would say—
> WALLACE: Go ahead, sir—
> TRUMP:—I would say almost everything I see is from the *left* wing,
>   not from the right wing.

WALLACE: So what do you— What are you saying?

TRUMP: I'm willing to do anything; I want to see peace.

WALLACE: Well, then do it, sir.

BIDEN: Say it. Do it. Say it.

TRUMP (gesturing to Wallace): Do you want to call 'em—what do you want me to call 'em? Give me a name. Give me a name. Go ahead . . .

WALLACE: White supremacists and right-wing militia.

TRUMP:—Who would you like me to condemn?

BIDEN: The Proud Boys.

TRUMP: Who?

BIDEN: The Proud Boys.

TRUMP: Proud Boys? Stand back and stand by! But I'll tell you what, I'll tell you what. Somebody's got to do something about Antifa and the left, because this is not a right-wing problem.[54]

Within an hour, the Proud Boys were marketing "Stand By" material on Amazon.[55]

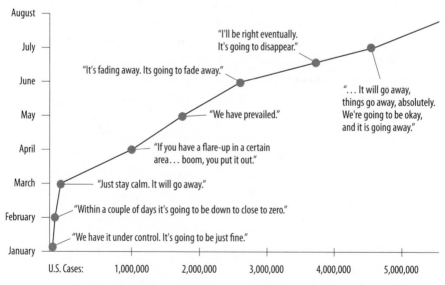

Trump says, "It will be fine."
(RCraig09, CC BY-SA 4.0, Wikimedia Commons and additional data)

Toward the end of the debate, Chris Wallace gave Trump the opportunity to say that he would abide by two centuries of American presidential behavior and accept the results if he loses the election. Trump spouted the discredited fear that there will be millions of fraudulent ballots cast.[56] Already, the GOP seems poised to challenge a loss.[57]

The only real takeaway from this debate is that it should never happen again.[58] In the background, Americans query Google in large numbers about moving to Canada.

FRIDAY, OCTOBER 2, 2020

The Trumps test positive for coronavirus.[1] Immediately, the entire world reacts, with leaders sending telling correctives. "Now, he is suffering himself and he should be compassionate for his people," a Myanmar pastor writes. "I suggest you do not try to treat yourself with bleach," a former foreign minister of Poland tweets.[2] One wonders if hydroxychloroquine will be part of Trump's treatment.

The whole White House is a hot spot for coronavirus. Hope Hicks, Trump's aide, has it.[3] Eleven employees tested positive at the Secret Service training center in Maryland recently.[4] We all watched the unprotected hugging and back-patting (which feels alien now) during the Amy Coney Barrett nomination party. Barrett, who already had COVID-19, seems well enough.[5]

The president's health is consuming most of the nation's attention. In left-wing circles, there's a theory circulating that this could be "crying wolf"—in other words, that for Trump's "October Surprise," he is pretending to be sick so that when he recovers, he will look strong, and COVID-19 will seem inconsequential. That sentiment, though easily discreditable, reflects the deep wariness among many in this country that our president's sycophants would devise such an underhanded plan. After the disinfectant comment—combined with Woodward's revelations that Trump refused to warn the country after early knowledge about the spread of the disease—it is perhaps not surprising that there is skepticism in the wake of this announcement about his health. And other evidence supports their skepticism. Scholars at the Cornell Alliance for Science publish a study today showing that Trump has been the single largest spreader of disinformation about coronavirus.[6]

Risk experts at Cambridge University say that Trump's age and comorbidities give him a 4 percent "notional risk" of death.[7] And his behavior—not wearing a mask, mocking the disease—is actually consistent with findings from the National Bureau of Economic Research that older folks, who are more susceptible to bad outcomes from COVID-19, nevertheless consistently underestimate both their risk of contracting it and their chance of real harm from it.[8] For the moment, no one has said whether there will be a temporary transfer of power to Vice President Pence while Trump is treated.

Assuming Trump survives and returns to full capacity by the election, how will this affect him? We have Boris Johnson as a data point; Britain's prime minister had a "rally around the flag" effect after he came down with COVID early in the pandemic. Yet he also emerged a changed man and, consequently, the UK's policies around coronavirus changed.[9] Another data point is Ronald Reagan, who received an overwhelming jolt to his ratings after surviving an assassination attempt in 1981.[10] Whether or not the illness is real, should Trump recover without much of a struggle, we might see him become more popular in the buildup to the election.

MONDAY, OCTOBER 5, 2020

198,000 deaths from COVID

In the 2004 book *Trump: Think Like a Billionaire*, the president revealed that his favorite musical was the Andrew Lloyd Webber and Tim Rice masterpiece *Evita*. He and his wife at the time, Ivana, saw the performance on Broadway six times.[11] Indeed, similarities between the stories of Trump and Perón abound. One was a reality star who became president, the other a radio star who became a powerful first lady. Both used antiestablishment messages to mobilize a working class that launched them into power.[12]

This evening, the president stages an iconic scene as he emerges from his helicopter after his three-day hospitalization at Walter Reed. He marches slowly but deliberately up the steps of the White House, clearly weakened from the virus, hands shaking as he turns to face the photographers. Around 6:15 p.m. (EST), he rips off his mask with a flourish, takes a few long, painful breaths, and with a stern countenance, salutes an imaginary American public for an awkward thirty seconds.[13] It is a clear homage to the famous moment in *Evita* when Eva Perón stands at the balcony of the presidential palace and declares her calling as the voice of Argentina's dispossessed *descamisados* (shirtless ones). The reference to *Evita* is so obvious that Patti LuPone, the famous mezzo-soprano who played Perón on Broadway, trolls Trump with a tweet: "I still have the lung power and I wore less makeup."[14]

Regeneron Pharmaceuticals supplied the monoclonal antibody cocktail for the president's treatment. The antibodies perhaps helped kick-start his immune system against the spike protein that gives coronavirus its halo, according to Jeanne Marrazzo, director of the Division of Infectious Diseases at University of Alabama at Birmingham, who has been monitoring the development of COVID-19 therapies this year.[15] Predictably, this news boosts Regeneron stock to over $605 per share today, almost double its per share price of $333 in late January. There are several more established pharmaceutical companies producing monoclonal antibodies for SARS2; Eli Lilly and AbCellera started testing their antibody treatment in humans a full month before Regeneron. Nonetheless, Regeneron is receiving the president's sponsorship. Perhaps not surprisingly, Regeneron CEO, Dr. Leonard S. Schleifer, has a relationship with Trump through the Westchester, New York, golf club.[16] The appearance of corruption, channeling government patronage to businesses via wealth-and-class-based personal connections—the *Evita* moment continues.

And it's just one of many eyebrow-raising connections. The Regeneron-made monoclonal antibodies that Trump claimed saved his life involved HEK 293T cells harvested from kidney tissue originally belonging to a fetus that was aborted in the 1970s.[17] A Gallup poll from last July found that 30 percent of Americans consider abortion a key voting issue and will vote for Trump based on his support of the pro-life movement.[18] A critical part of the pro-life movement is its opposition to the use of cells taken from aborted fetuses for scientific research. Yet, when push comes to shove, Trump, his "conservative" political party, and his supporters in the media, remain completely silent about the inconvenient science behind his miraculous recovery.

TUESDAY, OCTOBER 6, 2020

Today, the CDC says that coronavirus may remain airborne for long periods of time, not only following sneezes and heavy breathing.[19] A number of scientists are frustrated with the slow pace at which the organization is releasing this information. They have trumpeted this fact for months, repeatedly stressing ventilation as one of the most important factors in mitigating the virus' spread.[20] "Can we still trust the CDC and FDA (and other federal agencies, like the NIH, ostensibly dedicated to upholding policy based on good science)?" asks David H. Gorski, MD, PhD, FACS. Though he agrees that these federal agencies can provide guidance and support on "most topics," Gorski fears that, "for COVID-19 increasingly the answer is no."[21]

Some of the concern from scientists comes from the large numbers of political appointees, chief among them, HHS communications director Michael Caputo. Originally a Trump campaign official, Caputo directed his assistants to adjust official CDC reports, including an effort to alter retroactively published reports that didn't line up with the president's view on coronavirus.[22] Caputo is now on leave after a cancer diagnosis.[23] Before leaving, however, Caputo pushed conspiracies that undercut the CDC's authority. On a Facebook video, he said CDC employees were political hacks and predicted Biden would refuse to concede after Trump wins re-election. Then, "the shooting will begin," he threatened.[24] He deleted his entire Twitter account after these incendiary comments earned him internet scorn.[25]

Gorski reserves his most potent concern, however, for Operation Warp Speed, the administration's push for a coronavirus vaccine. The White House has put intense pressure on the FDA to issue an Emergency Use Authorization (EUA) for a vaccine before the election. The president himself claimed last month that a vaccine before Election Day would be possible.[26] He has personally pressured companies like Pfizer to act *as if* they're going to have a vaccine ready, or at least make the announcement before Election Day.[27] Whether or not a vaccine by early November is possible remains uncertain. Also unclear is how much real mobilization is happening to distribute the vaccine once it is ready—equally critical to actually vaccinating the country.

In order to address that pressure, nine pharmaceutical companies leading on vaccine development promised in a joint statement last month they would only conduct "large, high quality clinical trials that are randomized and observer-blinded, with an expectation of appropriately designed studies with significant numbers of participants across diverse populations."[28]

Nevertheless, Gorski fears the first vaccine that the FDA approves using an EUA would make finding a safer vaccine less likely. "Once a vaccine is issued an EUA, the ethics of continuing a placebo control group in other ongoing vaccine trials becomes problematic," he explains. "[T]he EUA would result in a de facto standard of care, and clinical trials cannot ethically deliver care that is below the standard of care." With this shifting standard, other vaccine developers would be under pressure to discontinue placebo control, since it would be unethical not to offer the newly approved vaccine to everyone. Newer trials, Gorski warns, would shift into comparison mode. Newly developed vaccines wouldn't be measured against a placebo (the scientific standard) but against the original vaccine developed under the EUA (the FDA ethical standard). Ultimately, according to Gorski, the rush to be first "would make it difficult to tell which vaccines are the safest and most efficacious."[29] Ironically, the FDA's desire to vaccinate ethically could undermine public trust in the ethicalness of the FDA.

WEDNESDAY, OCTOBER 7, 2020

Almost 7.4 million total cases

In Washington, DC, Democrats and Republicans wrangle over whether working Americans should be given another "handout" of $600. Meanwhile, lines of mostly women and children wrap around relief centers, asking for basic assistance in the face of yawning poverty. It's an under-acknowledged crisis that single mothers are experiencing across America—problems rooted both in the precarity of women's work and in the now-constant obligations of childcare.

Women held 58 percent of service jobs before the pandemic hit. Among all women, 17 percent have lost their jobs since March, 5.7 million women, compared to 3.2 million men. But for single mothers, the drop is 22 percent.[30] Tim Henderson of the Pew Charitable Trust says that these disparities are rooted in the kinds of work that single mothers tend to do— jobs with flexible hours that often pay poorly. In mid-April, 83 percent of waitresses lost their jobs; 72 percent of single moms who are cleaners, 58 percent of single moms who are cooks, and a third of those who had jobs as personal care aides were also out of work.[31] These losses are far higher than married couples with children or single fathers. Far more single-parent households are now receiving or seeking assistance through the Supplemental Nutrition Assistance Program (SNAP) (34.1 percent versus 13.1 percent for households with children) or unemployment benefits (24.5 percent versus 18.4 percent). Even with this support, 11.5 percent of single parents still cannot find enough food to eat or have kids who are missing meals.[32]

Melissa Radey, a professor in the College of Social Work at Florida State University, set out in May to see how the pandemic had impacted vital social networks for single moms. The first point she makes when we talk over Zoom is that low-income single mothers have always struggled and are adept at finding ways to survive. "For people like us who have relative wealth and safety, this virus has made leaving our homes dangerous. But for those who live in a neighborhood with lots of crime, going out has always been dangerous." Radey reminds me that not having easy access to food and supplies made life difficult for many of us in the early months of the pandemic, but for others, constantly juggling rides to the grocery store and struggling for steady money, dealing with food insecurity is common. For many of us, relationships nonessential for daily life had to be closed off until coronavirus recedes. But the extended friend and family networks had to remain in place for moms who needed to get to an essential job. Because of this, some low-income single moms seem more resilient right now—our crisis *is* their normal.

Not surprisingly, what Radey found was a population of single moms who were navigating the pandemic in a variety of ways. Some moms never left their houses, some lamented that their nightlife was not as good as it had once been, some ventured daringly to the drive-through at Dunkin' Donuts as their form of escape. One mom worked as a transport driver for troubled and violent foster children. She had no choice but to take her four-year-old along with her to work every day, sitting in the back seat next to the kids being transported.

Like in my conversation with Harvard Medical's Julia Marcus in July, Radey argues that everyone builds their own boundaries and rules for how to navigate crises like this pandemic. "How we understand and interact with the world shapes how we form those boundaries and rules." For some, drive-through is okay but going inside is not. For others, leaving the house is unthinkable.

Not only that, but the rules change over time, giving way as necessity, experience, fatigue, and desperation bear down upon us. I would not have believed this in the early months of the pandemic. I was convinced that I had a set of rules that I simply would not violate: I would order my food, I would not go into someone else's house, I would only see my mother outside, my children would go to school virtually, and absolutely never would I eat in a restaurant or go into a public space. But now I can say with humility, and perhaps some shame, that I was wrong, and my rules have changed. I go into the store now because delivery is expensive and a part of me loves to walk the aisles. I pick my mom up at the nursing home and we sit in my car every week, eating a sandwich from Arby's. I know it is dangerous, but I miss her, and I know that there isn't a huge amount of time left for us to have those moments together. I marched with thousands of people for Black Lives Matter because it was a risk worth taking. I will send my daughter back to school in the spring because school-on-screen this fall is so hard for her, and she needs to see her friends.

We have all been beaten down and humbled by this.

Even with all of these survival strategies, Radey notes the desperation and confusion that single mothers face each day as they try to be the breadwinner and the caregiver in a locked-down world. Single parents of special needs children are in particularly troubled positions. Many lost access to the support systems that make education as well as mental and behavioral health care possible. Mothers who relied on schools and specialists to help manage severely autistic children, for instance, found themselves on their own and at times unsure what to do in moments when they felt that their child's health, or their own safety, were at risk.

There is a pencil-thin silver lining; some single moms have had a rare chance to spend extended time with their kids. In their pre-COVID routine, they had, in Radey's words, "fifty balls in the air at all times. And then, suddenly, they were able to let some balls drop . . . They have some time, for the first time in their lives." I hear so many complaints from middle-class parents who are chomping at the bit, impatient to send their kids back to school in person, to get back to their in-person career routines. (No judgment; I feel this, too.) "But for the single moms, it is now or never. They are not going to be able to be with their kids like this when they return to work."

TUESDAY, OCTOBER 13, 2020

"Back in January," Bertha Hidalgo, an epidemiologist in the School of Public Health at the University of Alabama in Birmingham says, "I distinctly remember thinking, 'We've got this! There is a plan in place and there are people who are trained to respond to this. This is not going to be something we are going to need to worry about." She meets with me over Zoom today to pinpoint where the response to the pandemic first broke down.

"People talk about the fog of war and how we didn't fully understand the risks and consequences. Partially, this is true," Hidalgo admits. "I was concerned about the opioid epidemic and the oncoming flu season, but we were all wrong. We overestimated our nation's preparedness for this virus in part because we simply had no information. We didn't fully understand early on that the disease could spread asymptomatically. Moreover, all that was published at the time said that cloth masks were ineffective. . . . We also believed that masks could not protect the wearer and would only protect others. We have since learned that it *does* confer some protection for the user, but we didn't know that then. We also believed at the time that N95 masks *were* likely to work, but we also knew that there was a limited supply of those, and we needed to make sure that health professionals had access to them."

"Then was our current situation unavoidable?" I ask.

"No. It was definitely avoidable," she replies. "We made some critical, preventable mistakes in the early months of the pandemic. Always the idea in risk communication for epidemiologists and infectious disease professionals is that you do not incite panic. You tell the facts. You do it in a measured way. You try to get people all the information they need in order to make decisions. The critical information in this case was that COVID-19 was a highly efficient virus that could spread asymptomatically."

We talk about the Woodward book and the fact that Trump knew by the end of January this virus was deadly and efficient. He had been told that this would be the greatest test of his presidency. And yet, all through March even, he repeated the mantra that the flu is worse. "They knew that this crisis was coming, and they did not share that information with the rest of us," Hidalgo shakes her head. Instead, Trump and Limbaugh pushed the narrative of a Deep State conspiracy hell-bent on undermining Trump's reelection bid. Their conspiracy got in the way of hearing and acting in a way that could have saved thousands of lives.

But even if we didn't know that the virus could spread efficiently and asymptomatically, "then at minimum," Hidalgo declares, "what we needed was a coordinated message calling for collective unified action from all governors in all states so that we didn't have this patchwork of responses happening all across the country. Instead of having a nationally coordinated plan, what we got were fifty-plus states all bidding against each other, working on fifty-plus plans to stop something that does not respect borders."

"Also," she continues, "once we realized how important mask wearing was, we needed a recognition from our leadership that getting people to put on masks was going to require serious advertising. Mask wearing is not an endemic cultural practice in the United States." Indeed, as so many scholars have shown, mask wearing has negative associations for many Americans, whether they connect them with criminals or the Muslim hijab. "Based on that, we needed to develop a health belief model that would reach early adopters and eventually bring the majority of Americans on board. This includes making sure that the messaging to populations is done in languages that they understand."

When I ask Hidalgo about the consequences of these early mistakes, she shakes her head, "incalculable . . ." People with other sicknesses are also going to suffer. "When COVID hit, epidemiologists all over the world had to drop what they were doing and become experts in coronaviruses. As a consequence, there has been a huge loss of scientific progress in each of their individual fields as we have had to turn our attention to handling what should have been managed at the government level.

And then, just as I launch into a new question about the difficulty of projecting uniform public health messaging in the age of Twitter, Hidalgo's face turns ashen as her eyes clearly move to another screen on her computer. Her hand goes to her face. "Oh no," she says quietly.

"What's wrong?" I ask. There is a pause. She swallows and puts her hand to her chest, her eyes filling with tears.

"My uncle just died of Covid," she says. "Um, I have to call my dad. They have been calling me, and I ignored it because we were talking."

We end our call quickly. I find myself crying too, unexpectedly, for her loss, for the weight of listening to and reading about all these stories of loss, day after day, for everyone who is alone and hurting because of this nightmare.

THURSDAY, OCTOBER 15, 2020

After the mess of the last presidential debate and Trump's recent encounter with COVID, it was not surprising the Biden camp offered to hold the next debate over Zoom. When the Trump campaign refused, Biden scheduled a "town hall" in its place. Unlike debates, town halls allow a candidate to speak directly to constituents, and while Biden may not be adept at the made-for-TV zingers, townhalls play to his strengths. He conveys a sense of empathy and concern that translates well in that looser forum. News then broke that NBC would be airing a competing Trump townhall during the same time slot.[33] Many in politics and the entertainment industry see this as a crass move by NBC to boost ratings.[34] "Why not a new Bill Cosby special while we're at it?" mocked late-night host Jimmy Kimmel.[35]

These townhalls are supposed to be populated by undecided voters with real issues to ask candidates. Biden makes his townhall as warm as a socially distanced, nationally broadcasted political event can be, speaking directly to his questioners, turning his body to face each person, looking them in the eyes and saying their names, attempting to persuade them. It is a little boring—delightfully, refreshingly, presidentially boring.[36] So ordinary, in fact, that it brings people to tears.[37] A Trump advisor pejoratively compares it to *Mr. Rogers' Neighborhood*, as if that were a bad thing. Social media goes supernova: We want *much more* Mr. Rogers in our lives right now.[38] Biden sticks around to speak with people long after the crew breaks down the set, fielding tough questions from these undecided voters on the Muslim travel ban, the economy, how to handle the small but continuing BLM protests.[39]

In contrast, NBC's Savannah Guthrie and Trump spend most of their time sparring with each other; he barely makes an effort to persuade anyone in the audience. In fact, much of the townhall is spent with Guthrie pushing back against the president's falsehoods, such as when Trump claims that "85 percent of the people that wear masks catch it."[40] At one point, she urges Trump to say point-blank that he denounces white supremacy. He shakes his head while saying it, jutting out his hands as though he is about to catch a football. "I have denounced white supremacy for years—you always do this," he says indignantly. Guthrie starts to speak but he interrupts her, "You didn't ask Joe Biden whether or not he denounces Antifa . . . I denounce white supremacy. Frankly, I denounce Antifa and these people on the left that are burning down our cities that are run by Democrats." Guthrie asks Trump also to say for the record that the growing QAnon conspiracy theory positing Satan-worshiping Democrat pedophiles is false. He refuses, saying he knows nothing about it, and that he respects the QAnon opposition to pedophilia. He says in the next sentence that Democrats do kill people. Guthrie reminds him that he is "not just someone's crazy uncle who can just retweet whatever." "No, no," he replies.

It could be, in our "politi-tainment" world, that the only thing that matters tonight is television ratings. If so, the first polls suggest Biden won.[41] But if the last few years hasn't disabused us of the notion that "ratings" or "likes" translates to political competency, I don't know what will.

MONDAY, OCTOBER 19, 2020

"When the pandemic hit, there was just wild uncertainty." Tim Keller, mayor of Albuquerque, New Mexico, leans forward in his chair. I reached out to him because Albuquerque displays elements of each of the sticking points that we've seen in many American cities during 2020: elevated COVID rates, poverty, unemployment, immigration issues, high crime, and a history of police violence against minority citizens. I specifically want to get Mayor Keller's perspective on the early days of the lockdowns, the BLM protests, and the insertion of federal troops in his city this summer.

Albuquerque is known for its troubled policing history. Six years ago, the Obama Justice Department put the city under a consent decree after concluding that officers in the Albuquerque police department too frequently use deadly force against people who posed minimal threat. Moreover, the city has an infamously huge backlog of never-processed rape kits.[42] Under Keller's leadership, the city had improved slowly in these areas.

And then came the pandemic. At first, everything was as chaotic for him as it was for everyone else. "Every morning I would wake up and get in as many briefings as I could," the mayor says. "In the afternoons, I would meet with all the department heads from police, fire, our health department, and just try to figure out what do we have to do for *tomorrow*." It was touch-and-go like this for six straight weeks, "all we could think about was a couple of days ahead."

Without federal guidance, each mayor had to decide what constituted an "essential worker" and a "necessary store," when to mandate masks, and how to keep people from starving. Albuquerque decided to pay many businesses to stay closed. Yet, unlike many other cities, they kept the outdoor parks open. They fed thousands with drive-through food distributions. They deputized the fire department, food inspectors, and code inspectors to make sure that grocery stores and other establishments deemed essential stayed at safe capacities. They realized early on that they had a homeless population that could not shelter in place, so they converted some community centers to homeless shelters.

This summer's BLM protests were the city's big test. In response to calls to "defund the police," Albuquerque successfully piloted a program where they redirected ten thousand 9-1-1 calls away from the police to medical professionals and social workers. "For decades, we have asked the police, who are already understaffed, to do more," admits Keller. "This idea is actually about sending certain 9-1-1 calls to *unarmed* professionals. Sometimes it is a mental health professional. Sometimes a paramedic if someone is passed out. Sometimes it is a city worker who can give someone a ride to a homeless shelter." By their estimates, they kept six thousand people out of emergency rooms and jails. This was a better result even than they anticipated, and it makes sense as a long-term strategy. It is cheaper. It fights the mass incarceration problem. It gives people the response that they need at the right time. And the police like this idea. "They will tell you that they just want to be police officers," Keller emphasizes. "They were never trained to do all this other stuff. It is naive to expect them to be mental health professionals. We are not just following through on the defunding idea, but we are also fighting crime better."

When I ask Mayor Keller lessons we should take from Albuquerque's experience this year, he pauses. "The federal government should have just done that with the whole country. That was an instance where no one was stepping up and taking leadership." The response of Albuquerque's local leadership to the pandemic was, he feels, a powerful example of the good that government can do in times of public crisis. Unfortunately, we can only wonder what could have happened if such policies had been federally mandated and supported across the country. In other words, while Albuquerque might have been a small success story, it also signifies something sadder. "I think there is a real need for a shared collective identity that would bind us together. Wouldn't it be great if we had that as a country?" he says as he looks down. "When you don't have it as a country," he says, opening his hands, almost apologetically, "I guess you have to look locally. It would be better, though, if we were all doing it together."

WEDNESDAY, OCTOBER 21, 2020

8.1 million cases—209,000 deaths

COVID cases are rising again, over sixty thousand just yesterday. The pundits and politicians speak of the virus as moving in waves, but this is not an accurate metaphor. Waves rise and fall. We rise and then plateau for a bit, and then rise again, like the coming of a tsunami. Rural areas are now being hit the hardest. Health professionals complain of "mask fatigue," a lack of energy that results from prolonged wearing of a mask.[43] Many believe that coronavirus is not a real danger. Resentment and case numbers rise simultaneously in rural areas.[44]

Sadly, a certain portion of the media landscape supports the rejection of masking and social distancing orders.[45] On October 4, three prominent men from Harvard University, Oxford University, and Stanford University signed the Great Barrington Declaration. It asserts that people are not statistically likely to die by this virus should just expose themselves to it.[46] Its promotors, anti-regulation financiers backed by Charles Koch, call this approach "focused protection." The Trump cabinet is now promoting it.[47] As author Nancy MacLean and others have shown, these same elites have battled quite successfully against any measures that might impact their accumulation of wealth, including regulations that might benefit minorities, since the 1980s.[48] The Great Barrington Declaration looks a lot like a move to protect wealth, couched in the language of personal freedom. It ignores findings that almost four out of every ten Americans are in the "more vulnerable" category, given their underlying health conditions.[49]

The *Lancet* just published a counter-declaration: the John Snow Memorandum.[50] The *scientific* consensus, say its signatories, is that the actions proposed by corporate leaders in support of Great Barrington would increase the danger for everyone and wouldn't even help the economy much. We cannot do what Great Barrington insists we can, since many viral spreaders show no symptoms. "Such a strategy," the John Snow group warns, "would not end the COVID-19 pandemic but result in recurrent epidemics, as was the case with numerous infectious diseases before the advent of vaccination. It would also place an unacceptable burden on hospitals and healthcare workers, many of whom have died from COVID-19 or experienced trauma as a result of having to practice disaster medicine."[51] Great Barrington, in other words, would be a step in the wrong direction.

MONDAY, OCTOBER 26, 2020

Eight days until Election Day. 8.5 million cases of COVID.

A line for early voting stretches down the steps of the courthouse and down the sidewalk. Of the fifty-one people in the line with me, forty are African American. I ask the young woman standing behind me why she is here. "I have to work all day on Election Day," she says. The older man standing behind her wears a Southern Christian Leadership Conference pin on his lapel. He is voting early because his wife is in the hospital; he isn't sure he will be able to get to the voting center next Tuesday. We wait ninety minutes outside in the sun as they slowly allow people into the courthouse, a person roughly every seven minutes.

When we are inside, a massive crowd fills every available space in the long, narrow hallway. I reflexively take a step back—these are more people than I have seen in one place since the pandemic began. At the end of the hall, a solitary woman sits at a desk writing successive numbers on yellow Post-it Notes and handing them out to each person who approaches, letting them know where they sit in the queue. I look at the numbers written on the notes of the people around me: 247, 350, 144.

"When did you get here?" I ask an elderly woman sitting on a bench whose Post-it reads 250. "9 a.m.," she responds drowsily. It is now 2 o'clock in the afternoon, and she is still waiting.

"What number are they on now?" I inquire.

"137," she answers. I crane my neck to see a small door open at the end of the hall and a single worker poking her head out. Everyone turns as she yells out the next number. "One thirty-eight! One. Three. Eight." They hand me a Post-it with the number 411 written on it.

My first instinct is to believe that this is a phenomenon specific to Alabama, but my experience today is happening all over the country—especially in neighborhoods and towns that are poor and Black or Hispanic.

Around 20 percent of all US polling locations have been closed during the Trump administration. This alarms Leigh Chapman, voting rights program director at the Leadership Conference on Civil and Human Rights. "Fewer polling places can lead to longer lines, longer wait times," she says. People with disabilities, those who cannot drive, and those who rely upon public transportation—all of these groups are going to suffer from these closures, Chapman insists.[52]

When I cross-reference the most recent US Census data with published wait times at early voting sites from the last two weeks, a clear pattern emerges: the districts populated by ethnic minorities experience longer waits. For instance, all of the neighborhoods in Miami-Dade County with wait times have median yearly incomes of under $35,000, the poorest in the city. The John F. Kennedy Library in Hialeah, Florida, which is 95.1 percent Hispanic, has a four-hour wait time. The North Miami Public Library, which is 43.8 percent Black and 44 percent Hispanic, is the same.[53] It is a similar story in Maryland, where people wait in line for four hours to vote in Gaithersburg, which is 63.2 percent nonwhite.[54] Georgia and Texas tell comparable tales.[55]

This research is troubling, but it may also speak to a possible unprecedented outpouring of political participation in the neighborhoods of America most devastated by the pandemics of this year. People are *waiting* in the lines. That means they are voting, and in record numbers. Michael McDonald, who runs the US Elections Project at the University of Florida, reports a monumental increase in early voting.[56] Already, Americans have cast 46.6 percent of the total votes cast in the entire 2016 election, particularly in swing states like Florida, Texas, North Carolina, Georgia, and Nevada.

We are eight days away from this election. If Trump captures the most votes—despite the hundreds of thousands dead, despite the revelation he knew how catastrophic this virus would be and failed to act, despite the rampant corruption, despite paying only $750 in taxes, despite "stand back and stand by," despite the "bleach speech," despite millions of protesters being pepper sprayed in the streets—what, if anything, could alter America's course?

This week, the United States reported a staggering 488,498 new cases of coronavirus and 5,658 deaths—April levels of viral spread. As unusually cold weather descends on the northern half of the country, enormous fires still rage through the Mountain West, and the Gulf states prepare for, un-believably, yet another hurricane (the most on record). The Republican-controlled Senate confirms a new conservative judge, Amy Coney Barrett, to the Supreme Court. It is the first time since 1869 that a Supreme Court judge has been confirmed without a single vote from the minority party, many of whom regard this confirmation as illegitimate.

MONDAY, NOVEMBER 2, 2020

Voting day is tomorrow.

Walmart pulls guns and ammo from their shelves, given the credible fear that there will be civil unrest tomorrow. High-end retailers board up store windows.[1] A UK poll finds that three-quarters of Americans believe there will be large scale riots on or after election day.[2] Daniel Byman and Colin Clarke at the Brookings Institution argue that election-day violence is most likely to come from "accelerationist" groups whose ultimate aim is to destabilize the country so much that it devolves into civil conflict.[3]

We have seen some evidence of this all year. And there was an omi-nous sign just last Friday, when a caravan of trucks waving Trump flags surrounded and delayed the Biden-Harris bus as it drove down a Texas freeway. The Democrats on board were so intimidated that they canceled the rest of the day's events. Trump, true to style, tweeted that "these patri-ots did nothing wrong." Both the FBI and the Justice Department begin to investigate these groups.[4] In the meantime, the president calls on the FBI to investigate anarchists and Antifa groups who, in his words, "run around burning down our Democrat run cities and hurting our people!"[5]

TUESDAY, NOVEMBER 3, 2020

9.3 million COVID cases—226,000 deaths. Election Day.

At polling stations across the country, citizens show up in record numbers. Thankfully, the predicted violent uprising never materializes. People stand in long lines, respectfully waiting their turn. I volunteer as a poll worker and am stationed in a suburban part of deeply Republican Alabama. At least where I am, officials act professionally and are kind to everyone, regardless of race or political affiliation. The man running my polling place is probably a Republican, and he spends thirty minutes tracking down the records to allow a special-needs African American woman to vote.

Quite a few people seem new to voting and ask me to show them how to vote for Trump. One elderly man asks me to steady his hand while he fills in the bubble beside Trump's name. He thanks me with a smile, a WWII veterans' hat lodged firmly on his gray head, "I would vote for the devil if he was running against a Democrat." I help him to his feet and show him how to feed his ballot into the machine.

At 8 p.m. (EDT), early polls seem to show a Biden lead in key states like North Carolina, Pennsylvania, Michigan, and even Florida and Ohio.[6] Everyone paying attention knows this is an illusion, however. Most early votes were cast for Biden. Trump supporters showed up in person, believing Trump's rhetoric against mail-in balloting. One by one over the course of the evening, so-called battleground states drift into the Trump column. As the night wears on, the tally of votes for Biden-Harris grows overall, but it remains close. On social media, the fear from Democrats that 2020 will be a repeat of 2016 grows palpable.

Then, at 11:21 p.m. (EDT), Fox News calls Arizona for Biden. *Arizona*—a reliably Republican state, a state that refused to honor the Dr. Martin Luther King Jr. holiday for seven years after it was adopted nationally.[7] Also, *Fox News!* As scholars at the Berkman Klein Center for Internet and Society at Harvard University have shown, Fox News blows the weeds of right-wing extremist misinformation across the lawn of the American people more effectively than any other source; the network may not construct the conspiracy theories, but it certainly spreads them.[8] This moment feels like a critical moment in American media history; ever so slightly, Fox News has shifted the media landscape. The president tweets twenty minutes later, "They are trying to STEAL the election." Twitter immediately flags Trump's tweet as "disputed" and "misleading." By the end of the night, the election is too close to call. These swings between Democratic early voting, Republican day-of voting, and millions of largely Democratic absentee ballots still to count over the next days and weeks had all been predicted. Yet it still feels tense.

The real question driving pundits tonight is, how—given all his failures and his consistently low polling numbers—could Trump still have done so *well?* If you look at the votes of white evangelicals, Trump's unwavering base, it's not difficult to find the answer.[9] As J. D. Vance suggested in *Hillbilly Elegy*, Trump and the GOP offer a measure of self-respect and an appealing mantra of economic self-sufficiency that resonates with the poor rural white folk of America.[10] I would also argue that the promises of the progressive left: more equity, inclusion, and fairness, feel profoundly threatening to much of white America. Resources for the poor are already limited, and an increase in equity for nonwhites seems like it means even more personal loss to poor white people who don't want to be grouped with other marginalized citizens. Trump promises to defend American traditions, which is really a thinly veiled pledge to uphold a status quo where Black and brown people are treated as second-class citizens.

One might imagine that a nation as rooted in Christianity as ours would reject Trump's repeated refusal to feed the hungry, welcome strangers, and care for the sick and imprisoned, no matter the color of their skin or their country of origin.[11] Evangelicals respond that Trump, while imperfect, is nonetheless a vessel for God's will, whether it is in support of Israel or in the crusade against abortion. Others believe that he will help to usher in the end times. Even more importantly, says Andrew Whitehead, a sociology professor at Clemson University, evangelicals feel drawn to Trump's white Christian nationalism.[12]

In short, Trump offers a justification for keeping the world just as unfair as it ever has been. The utter failure of evangelical Christianity to challenge this complacency—to "comfort the afflicted and afflict the comfortable," as the old pastoral saying goes—says more than almost anything about America, a so-called Christian nation.[13]

Donald J. Trump ✅
@realdonaldtrump

> *Some or all of the content shared in this Tweet is disputed and might be misleading about an election or other civic process.* Learn more
> We are up BIG, but they are trying to STEAL the Election.
> We will never let them do it. Votes cannot be cast after
> the Polls are closed!
> *! Learn about US 2020 elections security efforts*

11:49 PM—Nov 3, 2020

WEDNESDAY, NOVEMBER 4, 2020

Just after 9 a.m., news outlets announce that Biden's lead over Trump in Wayne County, Michigan, which includes Detroit, has pushed him over the top. "Detroit Absentee Ballot Counting Chaos, Blocked Windows and Observers," Trump tweets, citing right-wing website *Breitbart*.[14] Crowds of white Trump supporters gather just outside the space where election workers count absentee ballots in downtown Detroit.[15] They want to "challenge" ballots in the mostly Black city. Dozens more assemble outside the ballot-counting center chanting, interchangeably and without irony, "Stop the count" and "Count every vote." Inside, some pound on windows surrounding the ballot counting space, shouting "Let us in!" Police push them back. Workers paper the windows inside to keep those outside from photographing and identifying them. In the counting space, registered ballot challengers meander around the tables all morning: 134 Republicans, 134 Democrats, and 134 not affiliated with either party.

By mid-morning, Trump's campaign files legal challenges to stop vote counting. According to the *Detroit Free Press*, a few GOP challengers inside the ballot counting space, some of whom are attorneys, stop poll workers from counting votes, claiming that the mere filing of the lawsuit should be enough to stop the count (which it is not). Police eventually remove these challengers, who took off their masks, crowded the poll counters, attempted to take pictures of ballots and workers, or were verbally aggressive.[16] Nevertheless, and despite constant right-wing news reports to the contrary, Republican ballot challengers remain inside the facility, vociferously challenging ballots well into the afternoon.

The swing is inexorable, though. This evening, Biden's lead grows in Detroit.

THURSDAY, NOVEMBER 5, 2020

A record 114,000 new cases in one day

Joe Biden and Kamala Harris have now received more votes than any American candidates in history—close to 74 million counted by tonight with many thousands still outstanding in Democratic strongholds of New

York, California, and Illinois. Obama-Biden picked up 69.5 million in 2008. Yet Trump-Pence 2020 has *also* exceeded Obama-Biden's 2008 total with about 69.6 million votes so far. As election workers count the mail-in ballots, especially in and around Atlanta, Phoenix, Las Vegas, Philadelphia, and Pittsburgh, Trump's lead shrinks and shrinks in the swing states of Georgia, Nevada, Pennsylvania, and Arizona.

Some Trump supporters protest, including armed groups in Arizona insisting that the vote counting continue (because they expect Trump to win there).[17] Meanwhile, in Detroit and Philadelphia, Trump supporters attempt to storm counting facilities and *stop* the counting of votes.[18] A now-banned Facebook account called "Stop the Steal" briefly appears this morning to organize these nakedly partisan efforts.

At 6:45 p.m. (EDT), Trump emerges in the White House briefing room to repeat that mail-in ballots are fraudulent. "If you count the legal votes, I easily win," he says.[19] Surprisingly, perhaps for the first time in American history, major networks MSNBC, ABC, NBC, and CBS all stop airing the president. Only Fox News and CNN play Trump's speech.[20] He accuses the media of airing fake "suppression polls" that show Biden far ahead in the race in order to discourage Republicans from voting. "They want to find out how many votes they need, and then they seem to be able to find them," he says of the polling places where votes are still being counted. "That's why they did the mail-in ballots, where there's tremendous corruption and fraud going on." This is the same message he and his followers have been pedaling since the spring.

Every major media source and even some conservative politicians denounce Trump's claims as "dangerous."[21] An emotional Stephen Colbert, recording his late-night talk show, notes that no major Republican "statesman" has publicly come out against the president's blatantly anti-Constitutional claims. Where is former president George W. Bush, for instance? Where is Lindsay Graham, senator from South Carolina? Senate leader Mitch McConnell? "*Qui tacet consentire*," Colbert intones, gravely, "who is silent gives consent" to the tearing down of our democracy—potentially the most historically astute judgment spoken on air this year.[22]

In the background, the pandemic rages. Research reveals high infection rates correlate with counties where Trump performed well.[23] Of the

376 counties across the country that have the most devastating COVID rates, 93 percent of them went to Trump—his misinformation has a tangible impact on his people.

SATURDAY, NOVEMBER 7, 2020

"'Madam Vice President' is no longer a fictional character," tweets actress Julia Louis-Dreyfus, who played that character on the TV show *Veep* (2012–2019). At 11:25 a.m. (EDT), the Associated Press announces that Kamala Harris and Joe Biden have accumulated enough votes in Pennsylvania to overcome the 0.5 percent threshold that would have instigated a vote recount. Of the remaining outstanding ballots, more than two-thirds are expected to be for Biden-Harris. Even if this prediction is wrong, it would not overcome their lead. Pennsylvania officially makes an Electoral College upset an impossibility for Trump.[24]

Celebrations erupt on the streets of many cities in America as the major news sources proclaim the win. It is a moment of happiness and relief. World leaders send their congratulations to Biden and Harris who, in turn, thank their supporters. Democrats around the country note that Stacey Abrams, minority leader of the Georgia House of Representatives, and her New Georgia Project made an invaluable contribution, turning out African American voters in a Southern state dominated by Republicans for a generation.[25]

Then, a truly astonishing moment happens. The president tweets that he is giving a press conference at the "Four Seasons." Embarrassingly, it seems the person in charge of scheduling press conferences accidently reserved the Four Seasons Total Landscaping company in Philadelphia instead of the famous New York City hotel for the press conference. The lawncare service is located in an industrial part of Philly, far from population centers, between an adult bookstore and a crematorium. There is nothing wrong with having a press conference at a site of working-class life, but holding the first press conference since losing an election in 2020 next to stores that sell death and pornography is a bold choice. To many, it is a lasting metaphor for living with a president who failed to address the deaths of thousands and has a history of "grab[bing] 'em by the pussy."[26]

Aaron Rupar
@atrupar

The Trump campaign accidentally booking a press
Conference at something called Four Seasons Total
Landscaping in Philadelphia instead of the Four Seasons
hotel they intended is such a perfectly dysfunctional way for
this to end. The writers really outdid themselves.

5:39 PM—Nov 7, 2020

Even more appropriately, Trump skips the press conference altogether
to go golfing. Given how fiercely he criticized President Obama for golfing—and yet golfed at his own resorts around 247 times, or two out of every seven days he has been in office—it is somehow fitting that he would be
on the thirteenth hole when word arrived that Biden-Harris had clinched
the election.[27] In his absence, Rudy Giuliani, the now disgraced former
mayor of New York City, emcees the strange event at Four Seasons Landscaping. By the end of the afternoon, the president returns to DC to find
Biden supporters lining the streets, jubilantly celebrating his defeat.[28]

SATURDAY, NOVEMBER 14, 2020

The election might be over, but coronavirus continues to spread like this
summer's wildfires. People just keep dying; it has become tragically normal. El Paso, Texas, called four additional mobile morgues into service.[29]
Inmates from a nearby prison move bodies to refrigerated semitrucks, a
version of what we saw in New York in early April and in Detroit a few
weeks later.[30] Hospitals in the Dakotas, Iowa, Wisconsin, Minnesota, Mon-
tana, and rural Illinois are in danger of being overwhelmed.[31] Nebraska
healthcare workers plead with people to take the virus seriously.[32] Even the
vaunted Mayo Clinic system is almost crippled. Around nine hundred staff
members came down with COVID in just the last two weeks.[33] COVID
patients occupy all dedicated ICU beds.[34]

The videos of desperate healthcare workers appear regularly on social
media. I remember these videos were so shocking in China in January, Italy
in February, New York City in March, Detroit in April, Houston in July,
and Los Angeles in September. The exhausted nurse or physician, cheeks

creased by cinched-down PPE, eyes bloodshot, over and over again. Now that they're being filmed in Bismarck, Sioux City, Topeka, and Lincoln, they seem sad and tiring rather than shocking.[35] It's now a traumatically ritualized part of 2020.

Strangely, much like the virus, the drama surrounding the presidential election lingers on. The Million MAGA March in Washington, DC, today drew a few thousand supporters to wave Trump flags and cheer "four more years."[36] They firmly believe that Biden's victory is fraudulent. In the middle of the day, Trump has his motorcade drive through the crowd of his adoring fans. They shout in support of the president and his refusal to concede the election. Counterdemonstrators collect around the fringes of the pro-Trump group. Some splash water on the MAGA people. One detonates fireworks. Trump's supporters respond. Drunk men wearing the iconic red Trump hat stab a counterprotester, who is kneeling, in the back.[37] Police intervene, charging twenty-one people and confiscating eight unregistered firearms from Trump supporters, most of whom came to DC from out of state.[38]

While journalists, pundits, and politicians wring their hands over the violence, it's worth noting that right-wing violence around elections is as American as apple pie. Trump's party was prefigured by the Know-Nothings 170 years ago, when white groups in the frontier cities like Cincinnati, Nashville, and St. Louis organized against incursions on their power from immigrants. They posted armed guards around polling stations and, in Louisville, Kentucky, on Election Day, August 6, 1855, Know-Nothings ventured into neighborhoods filled with German and Irish immigrants, killing at least twenty-two people and leveling dozens of churches and other buildings. In other cities, they targeted free Blacks and Native Americans, many of whom were their neighbors.[39]

Sadly, the election of Biden-Harris does not mean Trump-style "know-nothingism" will go away. History suggests that American "nativist" violence does not require Trump's leadership.

MONDAY, NOVEMBER 23, 2020

Judges across the country spent the weekend independently dismissing Trump's many election lawsuits contesting election results. This does little, however, to stop rumors and accusations about a rigged election. Trump and his allies claim that "votes are being cast on behalf of dead people" and that "poll workers gave specific writing instruments, such as Sharpies, only to specific voters to cause their ballots to be rejected."[40] They are claiming that an unnamed man smuggled ballots into the polling places from a van on November 4. A journalist at WXYZ-TV in Detroit debunked the claim, showing it was just his videographer unpacking camera gear. The conspiracy has nonetheless permeated right-wing social media.[41] Trump's own appointed head of DHS's Cybersecurity and Infrastructure Security Agency, Christopher Krebs, counters the rumors, stating publicly the election was secure.[42] His group has consistently declared Trump's claims about voter fraud false.[43]

We shouldn't be surprised, I suppose, that Trump just fired Krebs.

Unfortunately, these repudiations of Trump's accusations have little effect on the belief among many Republicans that Trump rightfully won. Polls show that almost half of all Republicans believe "widespread voter fraud" enabled Biden to take the victory.[44] Trump partisans surrounded capitals in Arizona and Georgia this weekend, still chanting "*Stop* the vote" in places where absentee votes are still waiting to be tallied and "*Count* the vote" in counties where there may be outstanding votes for Trump. Inside, by all measures, election officials methodically certify results. They do their job, without fanfare, regardless of their own political affiliation. That is what democracy looks like.

THURSDAY, DECEMBER 3, 2020

Today, the lame-duck Trump administration quietly alters the citizenship test that immigrants must pass in order to become naturalized. Many of the questions are problematic, either because they are written in a convoluted style that will confuse nonnative English speakers or because they demand that the applicant subscribe to an inaccurate or oversimplified version of American history.[1] For instance, in questions regarding why the United States fought in Korea in the 1940s and '50s and in Vietnam in the 1960s and '70s, "To fight the spread of communism," is listed as the only acceptable answer. Forty years of historical research has proven this answer insufficient. They've also embedded a number of other historical inaccuracies in these questions that could determine the immigration status of real people.[2]

This new test reflects broad transformations in immigration under Trump. And, in 2020, the experiences of the nation's undocumented immigrants grew only more brutal. To help explain what happened with immigration this year, I reach out to Sarah Pierce, a policy analyst for the US Immigration Policy Program at the Migration Policy Institute in Washington, DC.

Trump "took the handcuffs off" of Immigration and Customs Enforcement (ICE). He promoted and televised arrests of immigrants at home, on the street, in stores, even in sensitive places like domestic abuse centers and schools. The Trump administration also leaned into worksite enforcement actions. "Do you remember the 7-Eleven [convenience store] raids that happened last year?" Pierce asks. "It turns out a nationwide raid is a really *inefficient* way to raise your arrests and deportations, but it is a very *good* way to raise the visibility of immigration enforcement."

The irony, she points out, is that most Americans—at least prior to the pandemic—*favored* legal immigration. Not Trump's base, however, who assume "globalization" plus "demographic changes" in the United States are bad for them. Trump may not be able to make any truly draconian alterations to our broken immigration system, but he can terrorize vulnerable populations who cannot fight back, Pierce points out. It makes a great show for his fans.

In March 2020, the administration released a torrent of increasingly controversial policies on asylum at the country's southern border. When the pandemic happened, in Pierce's words, "the Trump administration got to implement their dream policy at the southern border that completely shut off asylum applications." Not surprisingly, now that the asylum system is no longer an option for the vast majority of adult migrants, they are seeing a lot more people attempting to evade detection by crossing the southern border illegally, which is extremely difficult and dangerous. Pierce tells me they are also seeing an increase in unaccompanied children seeking asylum, as this loophole is still open.

I try to imagine the kind of desperation that would lead me to send my child alone to the border of a country, guarded by men with guns, that does not want them. Pierce reminds me that this desperation is real. Many people are running from violence or from regions that have just recently been ravaged by hurricanes, floods, and landslides.[3] "If there's a system in place that doesn't allow you to claim asylum as a family but allows your child to enter the United States and claim asylum, then that is what people are going to do."

WEDNESDAY, DECEMBER 9, 2020

Another "shot heard 'round the world." Today, the British successfully administered the Pfizer-BioNTech coronavirus vaccine to first patient and "super-gran" Margaret Keenan, followed by a man named William Shakespeare.[4] The vaccine, in other words, is coming.

In the US, however, the news brings only abstract comfort. We are now at the highest daily death toll since the pandemic began—over three thousand deaths a day. Epidemiologists suggest the "Thanksgiving surge" is only beginning, since it takes about two weeks from infection to hospital admission, and an additional two weeks till death.[5] Health experts also worry the spread is likely to grow even more severe. As Olga Khazan, a senior reporter for *The Atlantic*, has noted, Americans aren't actually quarantining much anymore, and no state or local government seems to be enforcing stay-at-home orders.[6] Masking remains contentious. Hospitals are still understaffed nationwide.[7]

The vaccine is coming, though it might be a while before most of us get it. History suggests we are likely to face distribution problems. Julie Swann, a healthcare supply chain expert at North Carolina State University, stresses that the goal will be to "distribute some 510 million doses." By comparison, during the H1N1 pandemic in 2009–10, the US moved around ten million doses per week, maximum, and ultimately injected a total of eighty million doses.[8] This challenge is unprecedented. Even if we have an adequate supply of vaccine, how will we organize and administer it to millions of at-risk people?[9]

So, yes, the vaccine is coming. But first we have to get through the winter, and we have to hope that people will take the medicine when it comes.

MONDAY, DECEMBER 14, 2020

Approaching 300,000 deaths

I'm in a suburb north of Birmingham, stuck in the middle of a massive traffic jam. There is no obvious reason for it, no accident or police sirens, just a long line of cars standing still on the highway, filled with people waiting. The front of the line winds its way toward the massive parking lot of a 1980s-era Pentecostal church. I turn the car around and pull into a nearby gas station. "Food line," the clerk behind the counter says when I ask about the line. "Monday is when they do these now."

"A food line all the way out here?" I ask in disbelief. There are *hundreds* of cars in this line in suburban Jefferson County, each to pick up a box of food. Some vehicles are barely road-worthy; more than a few look in nearly the same condition as my own. These are not just the nation's poor. These are middle-class folks out of work, out of options. Hundreds of folks willing to wait for hours in this . . . well, breadline.

Around 40 percent of Americans experienced an income disruption during the last nine months.[10] With the slow and very uneven job recovery, unemployment is creeping back up again, bringing the total number of Americans receiving government support of one kind or another to over 19 million people versus 1.5 million last year.[11] So, while it's true that many of us experienced lonely Thanksgiving meals, millions more had to worry about where their next meal was coming from.

Food banks, pressed throughout this pandemic year, saw a surge like no other during this holiday.[12] Feeding America, the largest hunger-relief organization in the United States, projected in April that between ten million and seventeen million more people would experience food insecurity this year than usual.[13] Their October analysis confirmed that their most negative projections were becoming true.[14]

Of course, poverty is devouring unequally. Cities and states in the southern half of the country have been hit especially hard. Even in cities like Houston, which had one of the lowest food insecurity rates in the country before 2020 and took steps to increase food distributions from five hundred thousand pounds in the summer to eight hundred thousand pounds this fall, lines are getting longer, volunteers fewer.[15] The national media has not focused on the pandemic of poverty to the same extent as the drama playing out in hospitals and political arenas. Yet it could be the invisible story of 2020: how the haves got richer, the have-nots sicker, poorer, hungrier.[16]

As of this week, three hundred thousand Americans are dead due to coronavirus—more than the combat deaths of American soldiers over four years of involvement in World War II. It took just over thirteen weeks to initially reach one hundred thousand deaths, then one hundred thousand additional Americans died over the next sixteen weeks. Another one hundred thousand have died over the twelve weeks between September 23 and December 14. According to WHO, pandemics are not supposed to happen this way.[17] The "aftershocks" are supposed to be less intense than the initial outbreak. Of course, they predicated this idea on the belief that, in the face of great calamity, people will take great precautions.

MONDAY, DECEMBER 21, 2020

Throughout 2020, numerous states have instituted new laws and updated procedures concerning police conduct while little has happened at the federal level.[18] California, New York, Connecticut, Iowa, Colorado, Minnesota, and New Jersey limited or banned chokeholds entirely.[19] A handful of large cities including Seattle, San Francisco, and Washington, DC, prohibited the use of tear gas and other "less lethals" by police.[20] Others instituted reforms like citizen advisory boards and forcing body cameras on all units.[21] Dozens of smaller municipalities, usually with significant populations of racial minorities, made adjustments to policing as well.[22] Earlier this month, Virginia governor Ralph Northam signed Breonna's Law banning no-knock police warrants. Florida and Oregon have enacted similar laws.[23]

At the national level, the House of Representatives passed the George Floyd Justice in Policing Act of 2020 by a 236–181 margin back in June, but Mitch McConnell wouldn't even allow it a hearing.[24] Senator Cory Booker (D-NJ) condemned McConnell's obstinacy: "This moment is being failed right now by someone who . . . has no interest whatsoever in addressing the injustices that we see in policing in America."[25]

At the same time, cities in the middle of the country are unveiling anti-protesting ordinances that make punishments more severe, even for protesting police misconduct. According to the International Center for Not-for-Profit Law, forty states have considered 142 bills cracking down on protesting since Trump entered office.[26] While representatives initially crafted this anti-protest legislation at the behest of fossil fuel industries, they've aimed their recent flurry at Black Lives Matter.[27] The Ohio House of Representatives proposed a bill imposing punitive measures on protesters for blocking traffic.[28] Tennessee instituted several new anti-protest provisions against anyone camping out on government property or instigating "extremely offensive or provocative" contact with police.[29] New Jersey, Virginia, New York, and Oklahoma are considering similar bills. Missouri's proposed H.B. 56 goes a step further, blocking civil and criminal liability for drivers who hit protesters with their cars, so long as the drivers state they believed they were in danger.[30]

Potentially the most farcical and discouraging post–George Floyd development has taken place in Detroit. In response to suits against police brutality, Detroit is suing Black Lives Matter for what they're calling "civil conspiracy."[31] These anti-protest actions are happening all across the country against a backdrop of police gunning down Black men—Casey Goodson Jr., Joshua Feast, Rodney Applewhite, and Andre Hill, just in the last few weeks.[32] At the same time, white groups, often armed, attack Black spaces like churches or protests with apparent impunity.[33]

WEDNESDAY, DECEMBER 23, 2020

While Trump spends his last weeks in office pardoning accomplices like Roger Stone and Michael Flynn, thousands of inmates who applied for compassionate release during the spread of coronavirus continue to sit in prison.[34] High-profile prisoners like Michael Cohen, Trump's former "fixer," were granted compassionate release after serving around a third of his three-year sentence. Another Trump associate, Paul Manafort, also served less than a third of his seven-and-a-half years before being released early this past spring. Neither met the federal criteria for early release.[35] Those well-heeled felons bucked the trend, however. While almost 11,000 prisoners applied for early release due to health conditions that made them especially vulnerable to COVID this spring, only around 170 had their requests granted. Wardens and the Bureau of Prisons together blocked over 9,200; they didn't even respond to 1,500 requests.[36]

Inmates requested early release because they feared prisons would turn into coronavirus incubators. New evidence corroborates their fears. While around one in twenty Americans has tested positive for coronavirus this year, the rate is four times that for inmates of state or federal institutions. Not surprisingly, rates of infection and death are much higher in prisons than even the communities surrounding them. So far, upwards of 1,700 inmates perished from coronavirus in state and federal prisons, and that's

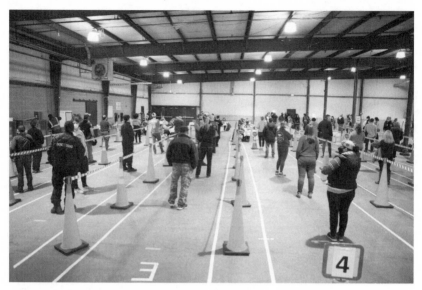

Health officials distribute the Moderna COVID-19 vaccine to frontline health workers
and first responders in Baltimore County, Maryland, on December 23, 2020.
(Baltimore County Government, Wikimedia Commons)

likely a vast undercount.[37] The cruel irony is that inmates sentenced for a
minor drug charge—now decriminalized in many areas, given the results
of votes in last month's elections—could die from coronavirus before tast-
ing freedom.

FRIDAY, DECEMBER 25, 2020

We try to make the best out of Christmas Day—a quiet meal followed
by two hours of Zooming with family. Our Christmas tree, purchased at
Thanksgiving (we were so desperate for cheer) has turned to straw, dropping needles everywhere. We have watched a holiday movie every night
this week. People we interview tell similar stories, regardless of their reli-
gions or holiday traditions.

All of this feels desperately nostalgic, as though our seasonal rituals can
somehow protect us from the darkness outside—a darkness echoed nationally this morning when someone detonates a car bomb in downtown Nashville. There were positive moments in 2020, of course, individual actions
of kindness and solidarity. But, with more than three hundred thousand

people lost to coronavirus and millions more still out of work, these individual actions seem fleeting in the face of a broken structure.

An anecdote, but not a positive one: cars with out-of-state license plates lining my street, while large families gather inside my neighbors' houses. We should not be surprised, I suppose, that Americans would violate all health advice to commiserate indoors on this holiday, prioritizing relational health and gambling that they won't catch the virus. If the predictions of health authorities around the world are correct that the virus is an aerosol and accumulates indoors without ventilation, we will see a resulting spike of new cases in the next two weeks, around January 8, 2021.

I keep my children close. I really wish I could hug my mom, who is shut in this Christmas. Until we are vaccinated, we're not taking that gamble.

THURSDAY, DECEMBER 31, 2020

We (Peacock and Peterson) drive across the Edmund Pettus Bridge on the road out of Selma to follow the celebrated path through Lowndes County that civil rights marchers traversed all the way to Montgomery in 1965. Fifty years after that march, we watched President Obama speak here on this sacred, rusting bridge, his very presence a testament to the promise of moral progress and racial redemption. Three years after that, we crossed with the crowds, pressed up against the late representative John Lewis and the soon-to-be vice president, Kamala Harris, remembering the sacrifice of Dr. King in 1968.

Today, we cross a quiet bridge, heading south and east, looking for answers to what went wrong, hoping for inspiration to close this first "history" of 2020.

After crossing a valley once fleeced in cotton, we bump along barely paved roads to seek out the bones of this land's American story. We stop at the Holy Ground Battlefield, known as Econochaca to the Red Stick Creek Indians, who once called it their home and worship center. In 1813, white settlers came in the night, razing their sacred space, murdering and enslaving its inhabitants. Legend says Chief William "Red Eagle" Weatherford rode his horse off the high bluff into the Alabama River to escape the ransacking Americans two centuries ago. A few decades ago, the National Park Service refashioned it into a campground, complete with a sign marking the spot where Red Eagle supposedly took his leap. Like the marches and speeches that took place on the Edmund Pettus Bridge, the sign is meant to redeem the space, tithing a new history, duly marked on a plaque.

And yet, this land before us, so beautiful, so seemingly reconciled with history, is not redeemed. Like the weathered picnic tables and flaking fiberglass play structures fading in the ruins of a native ghost town, the deep wounds of this place lie just under the surface. Beneath the promises of progress and the symbols of redemption, structures of racism, violence, and corruption still grip the region in large ways and small. Lowndes County is mostly African American; its population suffered among the highest COVID cases per capita in the country. And less than a year ago, a white teen, the son of a police officer in a neighboring county, shot and killed John Williams, the African American sheriff here, after Williams asked the teen nicely to turn down the music in his truck.[38]

Before 2020, most Americans would have been content to imagine that this rural southern county, with its poverty, illness, and continued bigotry, built on a soil that witnessed genocide and slavery, is an out-of-the-way exception to an otherwise uplifting American history of increasing prosperity and opportunity.[39] But here, on the last day of 2020, with well over three hundred thousand dead of coronavirus, with millions of voters and their congressional representatives falsely claiming the election was stolen, and with white police officers still gunning down unarmed Black men and facing few if any consequences for it, we must come to terms with the uncomfortable truth.[40] This country was built from broken pieces. And roughly half of the country wants it to remain broken.

We delude ourselves with a false image of who we are and how we got here. Having a Black president permitted us to believe that we were on our way to being redeemed from our history of genocide, displacement, slavery, and Jim Crow, moving into some sort of post-racial future. Yet, when we watched the murders of Ahmaud Arbery and George Floyd, many of us knew there was still such a long way to go. We proclaimed that our system of profit-driven, privatized healthcare was the best in the world. But when we saw nurses cloaked in garbage bags, the caskets stacked in a trench on Hart Island, the checkpoints arrayed around Sioux Nation, the media furor around hydroxychloroquine, and the extended debacle of the White House Coronavirus Task Force performances, we knew something fundamental in our system was broken—something deeper than Trump.

The last year has ripped away many illusions, revealing painful paradoxes that began before America's founding. We are a nation committed to the ideals of equality for all, built on the backs of slaughtered and enslaved people whose wealth and possessions often transferred to the killers and enslavers.[41] We are a nation that promises opportunity, based on an economic system that leaves increasing millions in precarity. We are a nation with high educational ideals, held hostage by the millions who willingly buy the disinformation of demagogues. We are overfed, and yet our food lines stretch for miles. We are overworked, yet unemployment numbers remain disproportionately high for nonwhite people. We see ourselves as believers in peace, equality, and order, yet the police violence continues, alongside unheeded pleas for Black lives to be treated as though they matter. We take pride in our audacious hope for change, and yet we remain fundamentally committed to an unequal status quo. We are a nation that forgets its true past so it can celebrate a fabricated history.

On July 3, 2020, Donald Trump stood in front of Mount Rushmore and spouted exactly this sort of mythologized history. After weeks of protests toppling monuments to Confederate rebels across the South, he implored his audience: "For the sake of our honor, . . . our children, . . . our union, we must protect and preserve our history, our heritage, and our great heroes."[42] They needed to believe his "true stories" of "great heroes" because, as he reminded his almost entirely white audience, they lived in "the most just and exceptional nation ever to exist," a place forged by courageous men like the four carved into the rock behind him. Trump intoned his heroic stories on land seized from the Sioux in violation of numerous treaties signed by Congress and affirmed by the courts, telling his supporters they were part of America's "Manifest Destiny," a term coined to justify the extermination of the same Sioux.

The irony that no one there recognized is this decades-old American exceptionalism that Trump conjured is the very thing distracting us from the peace and justice Trump's speechwriters assert. Mythologized praise for American wealth and power is, as Dr. King warned in one of his final sermons, "Why America May Go to Hell."[43] Believers in this false exceptionalism, wrote James Baldwin decades ago, "have been caught in a lie, the lie of their pretended humanism; this means that their history has no moral justification, and that the West has no moral authority."[44]

Perhaps the great lesson of this year is that while true American history reveals great violence and injustice, our honest acknowledgment of that history is the only thing that might begin to save us, if we can just reckon with it. Perhaps redemption will come if we can look honestly at the etiologies of our sickness. We might choose to act out of our professed religious and civic ideals and own up to our messy, difficult, uncomfortable, convicting history—from genocide through the torture-based slave economies, and the social, political, and economic systems built upon them that continue to marginalize millions for the gains of many fewer. Without that commitment to understand and reckon with real history, the peace and justice that Trump and other devotees to false American history evoke will remain an illusion. We will continue to amuse ourselves to death—one tweet, post, snap, binge-watch, drink, and Amazon package at a time.

EPILOGUE

The "Christmas surge" resulted in the highest cases (225,000)
and deaths (2,700) of the entire pandemic so far.

The day is historic even before the sun rises. One hundred fifty-one years
after white congressmen objected to seating the first Black senator, Hiram Revels, Reverend Raphael Warnock, the senior pastor of Ebenezer
Baptist, Dr. King's church in Atlanta, emerges victorious from the Senate
runoff election in Georgia. His opponent was Kelly Loeffler, a senator who
profited from her insider knowledge about the spreading coronavirus to
make millions in the spring, spending more than $20 million of it to try to
keep the seat.[1] Rev. Warnock will be the first African American senator in
Georgia's history and only the tenth since Revels became senator in 1870.
Democrat Jon Ossoff, the first openly Jewish senator in Georgia's history,
also flips the second runoff seat, bringing Georgia's Senate representation
to the left side of the political spectrum for the first time in 140 years.[2] Yet,
the narrative of racial progress must be qualified: today, white congressmen again object to the seating of the first Black vice president while white
nationalists storm the Capitol—an ominous coda to a dark year.

Trump's "Save America March," publicized for weeks, commences
early in the day with thousands of attendees bearing their iconic MAGA
hats. It's around noon when Trump bellows to them: "If we allow this
group of people to illegally take over our country, because it's illegal when
the votes are illegal, when the way they got there is illegal, when the states

that vote are given false and fraudulent information. . . . But now the caravans [from Central America], they think Biden's getting in, the caravans are
forming again. They want to come in again and rip off our country . . . and
if you don't fight like hell, you're not going to have a country anymore."
It's the same threat he leveled when he announced his candidacy in 2015,
that nonwhite peoples were gaining power in America. In other words, it's
a perfect bookend to this presidency. Yet, also like 2015, corporate media
caricatures him as an obvious buffoon peddling a message that few Americans support rather than as the oft-repeated chorus of an old white American song.

Trump follows his white-grievance rhetoric with a call-to-arms: "We're
going to walk down Pennsylvania Avenue . . . and we're going to the Capitol and we're going to try and give . . . our Republicans, the weak ones . . .
the kind of pride and boldness that they need to take back our country."[3]
And then it happens—his simmering lie about election fraud dating back
months and months boils over into an angry white mob.

Though they had been filling the steps in front of the Capitol even
before Trump finished, his "protesters" overwhelm and violently shove
their way into the building around 2 p.m. (EDT) in a last-ditch attempt
to keep Congress from affirming the election of Biden-Harris. A carpet of
flags and insignias blaze from every major white nationalist group. Among
other chants can be heard, like the Know-Nothings of old, "This is *our*
America."[4]

Over the next two hours, they wander through the Capitol, smashing
windows, scaling walls, ransacking the offices of Democratic senators and
representatives, threatening to lynch Vice President Pence, who refuses
to overturn the election, planting for the first time the Confederate battle
flag into the heart of the Union. Members of Congress and their aides hide
under desks and report out, terrified as the rioters steal memorabilia and
snap photos of themselves with statues and portraits. A few members of the
mob invade the very spaces where votes had been taking place moments
before, some in ridiculous costumes, other suited in tactical gear and bearing hostage-taking implements; personifications of the right-wing internet
where "we're only joking" quickly transmogrifies into real violence. Capitol police shoot one woman. Several rioters are trampled. Others suffer
various injuries from the chaos. Given how few wear masks, we can antici-
pate the coronavirus will soon take its insidious toll.

The president himself does not attend this insurrection attempt as he promised he would, preferring to watch events unfold on television from the White House. Staffers plead with him to stop the madness, but he says little publicly until around 4 p.m., when he tweets a confusing message saying that the election results should be thrown out—peacefully. He does not demand the rioters leave the Capitol building. As a result, Twitter, Facebook, and YouTube shut the president out of his account for twelve hours.[5] In our media-saturated, "platform"-obsessed, amusing-ourselves-to-death society, this is a mortal wound.

By the afternoon, law enforcement marches the last of the rioters out of the Capitol and establishes a perimeter. Still, a wave of incredulity floods social media. We see with our own eyes the painful discrepancy between how gingerly cops treat these profaners of our Capitol compared to the fierce retaliations against nonviolent BLM protesters on ordinary city streets. Federal law enforcement sprayed copious amounts of pepper spray and beat protesters in Lafayette Park so Trump could get a photo awkwardly wielding a Bible on June 1. Yet, for hours, they seemed unable to pry these actually violent white nationalists from the Capitol.

At 8 p.m., the rattled Senate reconvenes to certify the results of the election in favor of Biden and Harris. An hour later, the House does the same. A new president and vice president, thankfully.

But the work is just beginning. And it will not go smoothly. Even violence in that very chamber earlier in the day does not dissuade 139 GOP representatives and 8 GOP senators from voting to overturn the election results. They genuflect to Trumpian disinformation, calling into question the votes of hundreds of thousands of minority voters in Phoenix, Philadelphia, Detroit, and Atlanta—communities which have suffered disproportionately from disease, violence, and poverty all through 2020. For those who had eyes to see them, the signs were there since February, when Rush Limbaugh promoted the coronavirus-as-Democratic-hoax conspiracy, and April, when white nationalists descended upon statehouses in the Midwest, bearing nooses and rifles.

Or perhaps far earlier. These Republicans repeat a pattern set back in January 1870, when white congressmen objected to seating Hiram Revels—the man whose legacy the new senator Raphael Warnock will soon extend. Perhaps, as we surmise after having written this journal of a pandemic year, this is just part of America's historical landscape.[6]

ACKNOWLEDGMENTS

Our deep gratitude to experts of all stripes magnanimous enough to share their time, their stories, their research and writing, their warmth and laughter, and sometimes their despair with us over 2020: Buster All-away, Jim Bindon, Chad Brown, Kate Brown, Amy Burr, Matthew Chipman, Chrystos, Jamye Coffman, Holly Kyle Dixon, Evelyn Figueroa, Tom Flannigan, Larry Fox, Gina Gerbasi, Xabi Granja, Hilary Green, Corey Hebert, Brandy Henry, Bertha Hidalgo, David Himmelstein, Tim Johnson, Tim Keller, Zachary Levine, Lillie Lodge, Bob Lyman, Julia Marcus, Zsofi Marcus, Joshua Mason, Michelle Meyer, Cherrie Moraga, Tegan Murrell, Michael Oldstone, Sarah Pierce, Dayna Polehanki, Ann Powers, Ru Prasad, Melissa Radey, Richard Rosenfeld, Shelly and Marianne Rosenzweig, Sharon Sanders, Erin Schmidt, Lindsay C. Sidders, Avery Smith, Craig Spencer, Carter Stewart, Heather Thomas, Joseph Uscinski, Jo Weaver, Mari Webel, Jesse Weston, Hannah Wexner, and Brian Phillip Whalen. A number of others worked with us in both large and small ways but wished to remain anonymous, given the sensitivity of their accounts and fragility of their situations. Please accept these thanks for your willingness to put yourselves out there. We hope you're pleased with the results.

Thanks also to the Beacon Press group for developing this final product: Haley Lynch, Helene Atwan, Travis Cohen, Marcy Barnes, Susan Lumenello, and Emily Dolbear. We're overwhelmingly grateful for the incomparable shepherding skills of Jane Dystel and thankful that the whole Dystel, Goderich & Bourret family took us under its wings. And enough cannot be said in appreciation of Sonya Spillmann's friendship and editing talents amid so many challenges.

A small host of research assistants breathed life into the *Deeper Sickness* project, both on paper and online: Sylvia Cervino, Mikayla Jones, Lauren Tustison, Kenzie Wilbourne, and, especially, Jackson Foster, Emerson Jackson, Jack Mittenthal, and Jade Teel. T. Mills Kelly, Anne Ladyem McDivitt, and Chris Crawford graciously stepped in with programming and design help. The University of Alabama History Department and the College Academy of Research, Scholarship, and Creative Activity at Alabama kindly helped with funding.

Finally, to Barbara, Brooke, Greta, Will, Tracy, Erin, Hudson, D. Jay, Amelia, Mira, Sylvia, and Dorothy, with love for your research help, time, hugs, caffeine, listening ears, long-suffering, and lots and lots of encouragement.

NOTES

All cited sources, and thousands more,
are available at http://deepersickness.com.

INTERVIEWS

Jim Bindon, professor emeritus of physical anthropology, University of Alabama (in-person conversation, March 8, 2020)

Amy Burr, vice president, Federal Reserve Bank of San Francisco (Zoom interview, March 10, 2021)

Chrystos, Menominee two-spirit poet (diary entries and written letters exchanged during the summer of 2020)

Jamye Coffman, medical director, Center for the Prevention of Child Abuse and Neglect, Cook Children's, Fort Worth, Texas (Zoom interview, October 28, 2020)

Larry Fox, restaurant owner, Destin, Florida (phone interview, August 13, 2020)

Brandy Henry, professor, School of Social Work, Columbia University (Zoom interview, September 25, 2020)

Bertha Hidalgo, epidemiologist, School of Public Health, University of Alabama at Birmingham (Zoom interview, October 13, 2020)

David Himmelstein, specialist in internal medicine, New York's Albert Einstein College of Medicine, and lecturer, Harvard Medical School (phone interview, October 9, 2020)

Tim Keller, mayor of Albuquerque (Zoom interview, October 19, 2020)

Zachary Levine, director of Archival and Curatorial Affairs, US Holocaust Memorial Museum (Zoom interview, June 8, 2020)

Julia Marcus, epidemiologist, Department of Population Medicine, Harvard Medical School (Zoom interview, September 22, 2020)

Michael B. A. Oldstone, professor of immunology and microbiology, Scripps Research, La Jolla, California (Zoom interview, October 22, 2020)

Sarah Pierce, policy analyst, US Immigration Policy Program, Migration Policy Institute, Washington, DC (Zoom interview, December 16, 2020)

Dayna Polehanki, Michigan state senator (Zoom interview, February 4, 2021)

Ru Prasad, Portland emergency medical aide (Zoom interview, September 29, 2020)

Melissa Radey, professor, College of Social Work, Florida State University, Tallahassee (Zoom interview, November 13, 2020)

Sharon Sanders, founder, FluTrackers.com, Florida (personal diary and email interview, July 5, 2020)

Avery Smith, podcaster, *Blessed Are the Binary Breakers* (Zoom interview, May 17, 2020)

Craig Spencer, director, Global Health in Emergency Medicine, New York-Presbyterian/Columbia University Medical Center (email and shared tweet string August 9, 2020)

Lesley Jo Weaver, associate professor of anthropology, University of Oregon, Eugene (Zoom interview, September 16, 2020)

Mari Webel, assistant professor of history, University of Pittsburgh (Zoom interview, December 14, 2020)

JANUARY

1. Notes based on Sharon Sanders's personal diary and recollections.

2. FluTrackers.com, Qui (reporter) Ting and Xu (interviewee) Jianguo, "Experts Say Preliminary Progress Has Been Made in the Etiology Identification of the Unexplained Viral Pneumonia Epidemic of the New Coronavirus Wuhan," Xinhuanet, January 9, 2020, https://translate.google.com/translate?sl=zh-CN&tl=en&u=http%3A%2F%2Fwww.xinhuanet.com%2Fpolitics%2F2020-01%2F09%2Fc_1125438971.htm.

3. On January 10, 2020, Erik Peterson started keeping track of the virus for an upcoming course on the history of epidemics. Margaret Peacock, whose father was a world-renowned epidemiologist, and who has worked in the field of the history of Soviet science, began following the story of the virus separately. They decided to join projects in mid-February.

4. Centers for Disease Control and Prevention, *Weekly U.S. Influenza Surveillance Report (FluView)*, 2019/2020, https://www.cdc.gov/flu/weekly/index.htm; Elizabeth Cohen, "Northeast Struck by Flu as Virus Sets Tragic Record for Children Around the Country," CNN, January 7, 2020, https://www.cnn.com/2020/01/07/health/northeast-flu/index.html.

5. Michael Coston, "Avian Flu Diary: CDC Issues Level 1 (Watch) Travel Notice for Unidentified Pneumonia—Wuhan, China," *Avian Flu Diary* (blog), January 6, 2020, https://afludiary.blogspot.com/2020/01/cdc-issues-level-1-watch-travel-notice.html.

6. FluTrackers.com, https://flutrackers.com/forum/forum/-2019-ncov-new-coronavirus/china-2019-ncov/821830-china-original-covid-19-coronavirus-news-thread-weeks-1-4-december-30-2019-january-25-2020/page11. Current thinking is that actual case numbers were far higher. This is what we knew at the time, however.

7. Z. Zhao et al., "Description and Clinical Treatment of an Early Outbreak of Severe Acute Respiratory Syndrome (SARS) in Guangzhou, PR China," *Journal of Medical Microbiology* 52, no. 8 (2003): 715–20.

8. Emmie de Wit, Neeltje van Doremalen, Darryl Falzarano, and Vincent J. Munster, "SARS and MERS: Recent Insights into Emerging Coronaviruses," *Nature Reviews Microbiology* 14, no. 8 (August 2016): 523–34, https://doi.org/10.1038/nrmicro.2016.81.

9. World Health Organization, "WHO Advice for International Travel and Trade in Relation to the Outbreak of Pneumonia Caused by a New Coronavirus in China," January 10, 2020, https://www.who.int/news-room/articles-detail/who-advice-for-international-travel-and-trade-in-relation-to-the-outbreak-of-pneumonia-caused-by-a-new-coronavirus-in-china.

10. Adam Smith, *The Theory of Moral Sentiments: To Which Is Added, a Dissertation on the Origin of Languages* (Edinburgh: A. Millar, A. Kincaid and J. Bell, 1767).

11. USA Headline News Staff, "C.D.C. Identifies First U.S. Case of Coronavirus in Washington State," *USA Headline News*, January 22, 2020, https://mfamediagroup.com/archives/865391.

12. Joshua Berlinger, Steve George, and Ivana Kottasova, "US Has Its First Case of the Wuhan Coronavirus," CNN, January 22, 2020, https://www.cnn.com/asia/live-news/wuhan-coronavirus-china-intl-hnk/h_36a5d9a3ba3a46753adb7d9a5a26b6b8.

13. "Wuhan Lockdown 'Unprecedented,' Shows Commitment to Contain Virus: WHO Representative in China," Reuters, January 23, 2020, https://www.reuters.com/article/us-china-health-who-idUSKBN1ZM1G9.

14. Natsuko Imai et al., *Report 1—Estimating the Potential Total Number of Novel Coronavirus (2019-NCoV) Cases in Wuhan City, China* (Imperial College London, January 17, 2020),

http://www.imperial.ac.uk/medicine/departments/school-public-health/infectious-disease
-epidemiology/mrc-global-infectious-disease-analysis/covid-19/report-1-case-estimates-of
-covid-19.

15. Donald J. Trump (@realdonaldtrump), Twitter, January 24, 2020, https://www.the
trumparchive.com/?dates=%5B%222020-01-24%22%2C%222020-01-25%22%5D.

16. Centers for Disease Control and Prevention, "Second Travel-Related Case of 2019
Novel Coronavirus Detected in United States," January 24, 2020, https://www.cdc.gov
/media/releases/2020/p0124-second-travel-coronavirus.html.

17. Chris Woolston, "SARS: The Epidemic That Was Halted," *HealthDay*, December
31, 2020, https://consumer.healthday.com/encyclopedia/diseases-and-conditions-15/misc
-diseases-and-conditions-news-203/sars-648365.html.

18. Jon Cohen, "Chinese Researchers Reveal Draft Genome of Virus Implicated in
Wuhan Pneumonia Outbreak," *Science*, January 11, 2020, https://www.sciencemag.org/news
/2020/01/chinese-researchers-reveal-draft-genome-virus-implicated-wuhan-pneumonia
-outbreak.

19. Sharon Begley, "DNA Sleuths Read the Coronavirus Genome, Tracing Its Origins," *STAT* (blog), January 24, 2020, https://www.statnews.com/2020/01/24/dna-sleuths
-read-coronavirus-genome-tracing-origins-and-mutations.

20. Michael B. A. Oldstone, *Viruses, Plagues, and History: Past, Present and Future*, rev. ed.
(New York: Oxford University Press, 2009), 227–28.

21. Begley, "DNA Sleuths Read the Coronavirus Genome, Tracing Its Origins"; Nectar
Gan, Yong Xiong, and Eliza Mackintosh, "China Confirms New Coronavirus Can Spread
Between Humans," CNN, January 21, 2020, https://www.cnn.com/2020/01/19/asia/china
-coronavirus-spike-intl-hnk/index.html.

22. Newsploy Staff, "Was Kobe Bryant Just Assassinated? If So, Why and Who Did
It?" *State of the Nation* (blog), January 27, 2020, http://stateofthenation.co/?p=5694; Kelly
Tyko, "Google Search for 'When Did Kobe Bryant Die' No Longer Lists Jan. 26 as 'Date
of Assassination,'" *USA Today*, January 27, 2020, https://www.usatoday.com/story/tech
/2020/01/27/kobe-bryant-death-listed-assassination-one-google-search/4586160002.

23. This number includes websites I could locate and certainly is not complete.

24. "Coronavirus in China: 23 Million QUARANTINED, 2.8 Million Infected;
112,000 DEAD," *Hal Turner Radio Show*, January 23, 2020, https://halturnerradioshow.com
/index.php/en/news-page/news-nation/coronavirus-in-china-20-million-quarantined-2-8
-million-infected-112-000-dead; Ratna, "Fact Check: Bloated Casualty Figures Linked to
Coronavirus Leave Netizens in Panic," *India Today*, February 4, 2020, https://www.india
today.in/fact-check/story/fact-check-bloated-casualty-figures-linked-to-coronavirus-leave
-netizens-in-panic-1643257-2020-02-04.

25. Soroush Vosoughi, Deb Roy, and Sinan Aral, "The Spread of True and False News
Online," *Science* 359, no. 6380 (March 9, 2018): 1146–51.

26. Daniel Defoe, *A Journal of the Plague Year* (1722) (New York: Penguin, 2003), 11.

27. "HHS and CDC Supporting Safe, Expedient Departure of US Citizens," Centers
for Disease Control and Prevention, January 28, 2020, https://www.cdc.gov/media/releases
/2020/s0128-wuhan-departure.html.

28. "Novel Coronavirus Press Conference at United Nations of Geneva," World
Health Organization, January 29, 2020, https://www.who.int/docs/default-source/corona
viruse/transcripts/who-audio-script-ncov-rresser-unog-29jan2020.pdf?sfvrsn=a7158807_4.

29. Weier Wang, Jianming Tang, and Fangqiang Wei, "Updated Understanding of the
Outbreak of 2019 Novel Coronavirus (2019-NCoV) in Wuhan, China," *Journal of Medical
Virology* 92, no. 4 (January 29, 2020): 441–47.

30. "Transcript of CDC Telebriefing for the Update on 2019 Novel Coronavirus
(2019-NCoV)," Centers for Disease Control and Prevention, January 30, 2020, https://
www.cdc.gov/media/releases/2020/t0130-novel-coronavirus-update-telebriefing.html.

31. "CDC Confirms Person-to-Person Spread of New Coronavirus in the United States," Centers for Disease Control and Prevention, January 30, 2020, https://www.cdc.gov/media/releases/2020/p0130-coronavirus-spread.html.

32. Mike Hixenbaugh, "Scientists Were Close to a Coronavirus Vaccine Years Ago. Then the Money Dried Up," NBC News, March 8, 2020, https://www.nbcnews.com/health/health-care/scientists-were-close-coronavirus-vaccine-years-ago-then-money-dried-n1150091.

33. Jason A. Tetro, "Is COVID-19 Receiving ADE from Other Coronaviruses?" *Microbes and Infection* 22, no. 2 (March 2020): 72–73.

34. Sarah Boseley, "142,000 Died from Measles Last Year, WHO Estimates," *Guardian*, December 5, 2019, https://www.theguardian.com/society/2019/dec/05/142000-died-from-measles-last-year-who-estimates.

35. Maryn McKenna, "Amid Coronavirus Fears, a Mask Shortage Could Spread Globally," *Wired*, February 4, 2020, https://www.wired.com/story/amid-coronavirus-fears-a-mask-shortage-could-spread-globally.

36. Laurie Garrett, "Trump Has Sabotaged America's Coronavirus Response," *Foreign Policy* (blog), January 31, 2020, https://foreignpolicy.com/2020/01/31/coronavirus-china-trump-united-states-public-health-emergency-response.

37. Warwick Anderson, *Colonial Pathologies: American Tropical Medicine, Race, and Hygiene in the Philippines,* new ed. (Durham, NC: Duke University Press, 2006).

38. Erika Lee, *At America's Gates: Chinese Immigration During the Exclusion Era, 1882–1943* (Chapel Hill: University of North Carolina Press, 2003).

39. Wilbur Ross, "Coronavirus Will Bring Jobs to US, Mexico: Ross," *Fox Business*, January 20, 2020, http://video.foxbusiness.com/v/6128248662001.

40. Camilla Rothe et al., "Transmission of 2019-NCoV Infection from an Asymptomatic Contact in Germany," *New England Journal of Medicine* 382, no. 10 (March 5, 2020): 970–71.

41. Eric Levenson, "The TSA Is in the Business of 'Security Theater,' Not Security," *Atlantic*, January 31, 2014, https://www.theatlantic.com/national/archive/2014/01/tsa-business-security-theater-not-security/357599.

FEBRUARY
1. Donald G. McNeil Jr., "Wuhan Coronavirus Looks Increasingly Like a Pandemic, Experts Say," *New York Times*, February 2, 2020, https://www.nytimes.com/2020/02/02/health/coronavirus-pandemic-china.html.

2. Megan Henry, "Amid Outbreak News, Don't Forget About Flu—Coronavirus Is Scary but Influenza Is Deadlier and More Widespread, Doctors Say," *Akron Beacon Journal*, February 1, 2020, https://infoweb-newsbank-com.libdata.lib.ua.edu/apps/news/document-view?p=NewsBank&docref=news/178D76513AA48ED8; Grace Hauck and Megan Henry, "Coronavirus Is Scary, but the Flu Is Deadlier, More Widespread," *USA Today*, February 1, 2020, https://www.usatoday.com/story/news/health/2020/02/01/coronavirus-flu-deadlier-more-widespread-than-wuhan-china-virus/4632508002; "Our View—Virus a Cause for Concern, Not Panic," *Abilene Reporter-News*, February 1, 2020.

3. Lenny Bernstein, "In the U.S., Flu Is a Much Bigger Threat Than the New Coronavirus," *Seattle Times*, February 1, 2020, https://www.seattletimes.com/nation-world/flu-is-a-much-bigger-threat-than-coronavirus.

4. Shen Wu Tan, "'Real and Present': Risk from Influenza Is Far Greater Than Coronavirus, Health Experts Warn," *Washington Times*, January 29, 2020, https://www.washingtontimes.com/news/2020/jan/29/flu-risk-far-greater-coronavirus-health-experts-wa.; Bob Herman, "Why We Panic About Coronavirus, but Not the Flu," *Axios*, January 29, 2020, https://www.axios.com/coronavirus-influenza-disease-china-united-states-64311582-2031-40af-8ec3-9ff68341d4f3.html.

5. "Key Moments from President Trump's Interview Before the Super Bowl," *Washington Post*, February 3, 2020, https://www.washingtonpost.com/video/politics/key-moments -from-president-trumps-interview-before-the-super-bowl/2020/02/02/501dd685-893a-4700 -91ee-5ffd39c59beb_video.html.

6. Lily Kuo, "Coronavirus: Death Toll Passes Sars Virus as Dozens More Die in Wuhan," *Guardian*, February 3, 2020, https://www.theguardian.com/world/2020/feb/03 /coronavirus-dozens-more-deaths-chinese-province-centre-outbreak-hubei.

7. Milan Kundera, *The Book of Laughter and Forgetting* (New York: Penguin Books, 1980).

8. "A Mostly Ho-Hum January," *National Snow & Ice Data Center* (blog), February 4, 2020, https://nsidc.org/arcticseaicenews/2020/02; NASA, "Ice Sheets," Global Climate Change: Vital Signs of the Planet, June 2018, https://climate.nasa.gov/vital-signs/ice-sheets.

9. Jamie Gumbrecht, Madeline Holcombe, Nadia Kounang, and Michael Nedelman, "Report That Said Wuhan Coronavirus Can Spread Before Symptoms Was Flawed," CNN, February 5, 2020, https://www.cnn.com/2020/02/05/health/wuhan-coronavirus-flawed -report/index.html.

10. Jon Cartwright, "Fledgling Site Challenges ArXiv Server," *Physics World* 22, no. 8 (August 2009): 9.

11. Richard J. Abdill and Ran Blekhman, "Tracking the Popularity and Outcomes of All BioRxiv Preprints," ed. Emma Pewsey, Peter Rodgers, and Casey S. Greene, *eLife* 8 (April 24, 2019): e45133.

12. WHO, *Novel Coronavirus (2019-nCOV) Situation Report 12* (World Health Organization, February 1, 2020), https://apps.who.int/iris/handle/10665/330777.

13. Phil Helsel and Arata Yamamoto, "American with Coronavirus Died in Wuhan, China, Embassy Says," NBC News, February 7, 2020, https://www.nbcnews.com/news /world/american-coronavirus-died-wuhan-china-embassy-says-n1132946.

14. Madeleine Carlisle, "'An Appalling Abuse of the Public Trust.' Read Mitt Romney's Speech on Voting to Convict Donald Trump," *Time*, February 5, 2020, https://time.com /5778603/mitt-romney-speech-donald-trump.

15. Eric C. Schneider et al., "Mirror, Mirror 2017: International Comparison Reflects Flaws and Opportunities for Better U.S. Health Care," Commonwealth Fund, July 14, 2017, https://www.commonwealthfund.org/publications/fund-reports/2017/jul/mirror -mirror-2017-international-comparison-reflects-flaws-and.

16. Craig Palosky and Sue Ducat, "Premiums for Employer-Sponsored Family Health Coverage Rise 5% to Average $19,616; Single Premiums Rise 3% to $6,896," *KFF* (blog), October 3, 2018, https://www.kff.org/health-costs/press-release/employer-sponsored-family -coverage-premiums-rise-5-percent-in-2018.

17. Gary Claxton et al., *Employer Health Benefits 2019 Annual Survey* (San Francisco: Kaiser Family Foundation, 2019), https://www.kff.org/report-section/ehbs-2019-section-1 -cost-of-health-insurance.

18. Angie Drobnic Holan, "PolitiFact's Lie of the Year: 'Death Panels,'" *PolitiFact*, December 18, 2009, https://www.politifact.com/article/2009/dec/18/politifact-lie-year-death -panels.

19. Paul Starr, *The Social Transformation of American Medicine: The Rise of a Sovereign Profession and the Making of a Vast Industry* (New York: Basic Books, 1982).

20. Elisabeth Rosenthal, *An American Sickness: How Healthcare Became Big Business and How You Can Take It Back* (New York: Penguin Press, 2017), 8.

21. Gerard F. Anderson, Peter Hussey, and Varduhi Petrosyan, "It's Still the Prices, Stupid: Why the US Spends So Much on Health Care, and a Tribute to Uwe Reinhardt," *Health Affairs* 38, no. 1 (January 1, 2019): 87–95.

22. Edward P. Hoffer, "America's Health Care System Is Broken: What Went Wrong and How We Can Fix It, Parts 1–5," *American Journal of Medicine* (June–October 2019).

23. Robert P. Hudson, *Disease and Its Control: The Shaping of Modern Thought* (Westport, CT: Praeger, 1983), x.

24. Dominique Patton and David Stanway, "China's Hubei Province Sees Surge in Coronavirus Deaths on Switch to New Methodology," Reuters, February 13, 2020, https://www.reuters.com/article/us-china-health-hubei-toll-idUSKBN207010.

25. "SARS—Basics Factsheet," Centers for Disease Control and Prevention, February 8, 2019, https://www.cdc.gov/sars/about/fs-sars.html.

26. Cissy Zhou, Gigi Choy, and Zhuang Pinghui, "Coronavirus: China Reports 254 Deaths in a Day as Cases Surge After Including Clinically Diagnosed Patients," *South China Morning Post*, February 13, 2020, https://www.scmp.com/news/china/society/article/3050354/coronavirus-hubei-province-reports-sharp-spike-new-confirmed.

27. "Transcript for CDC Telebriefing: CDC Update on Novel Coronavirus," Centers for Disease Control and Prevention, February 12, 2020, https://www.cdc.gov/media/releases/2020/t0212-cdc-telebriefing-transcript.html.

28. Doi S., Yajima D., and Tsuru S., "Cruise Ship Put Under 2-Week Quarantine as 10 Cases Confirmed," *Asahi Shimbun Asia & Japan Watch*, February 5, 2020.

29. Wai Shing Leung et al., "Presumed COVID-19 Index Case on Diamond Princess Cruise Ship and Evacuees to Hong Kong," *Journal of Travel Medicine* (May 13, 2020).

30. Shimbun, "Cruise Ship with 3,711 on Board Put in Quarantine at Yokohama," *Asahi*, February 4, 2020, http://www.asahi.com/ajw/articles/13099539.

31. Ministry of Health, Labour and Welfare (Japan), press release, February 22, 2020, https://www.mhlw.go.jp/stf/houdou/houdou_list_202002.html.

32. Daniele Lepido and John Follain, "Venice Carnival Ends Early as Italy Virus Outbreak Spooks Europe," *Bloomberg*, February 23, 2020, https://www.bloomberg.com/news/articles/2020-02-23/venice-cancels-all-public-events-including-carnival.

33. Melissa Godin, "Italy Reports 17 Total COVID-19 Cases as Cluster Quadruples in One Day," *Time*, February 21, 2020, https://time.com/5788661/italy-coronavirus-cases.

34. Rush Limbaugh, "The Rush Limbaugh Show," February 24, 2020; Andrew Seifter, "Limbaugh on the NBA: 'Call It the TBA, the Thug Basketball Association . . . They're Going in to Watch the Crips and the Bloods,'" Media Matters for America, December 10, 2004. https://www.mediamatters.org/rush-limbaugh/limbaugh-nba-call-it-tba-thug-basketball-association-theyre-going-watch-crips-and.

35. Guy Debord, *Society of the Spectacle* (1967), trans. Ken Knabb (London: Rebel Press, 2005), 12.

36. Carl Sagan, *The Demon-Haunted World: Science as a Candle in the Dark* (New York: Ballantine, 1997), 241.

37. Laurie Garrett, "Trump Has Sabotaged America's Coronavirus Response," *Foreign Policy*, January 31, 2020.

38. Betsy McKay, "CDC to Scale Back Work in Dozens of Foreign Countries Amid Funding Worries," *Wall Street Journal*, January 19, 2018, https://www.wsj.com/articles/cdc-to-scale-back-work-in-dozens-of-foreign-countries-amid-funding-worries-1516398717.

39. Ricardo Alonso-Zaldivar and Jonathan Lemire, "Trump, US Officials Send Mixed Messages on Virus Risk Here," ABC News, February 25, 2020, https://abcnews.go.com/Health/wireStory/trump-defends-25b-coronavirus-request-dems-low-69196018.

40. Pam Belluck and Noah Weiland, "C.D.C. Officials Warn of Coronavirus Outbreaks in the U.S.," *New York Times*, February 25, 2020, https://www.nytimes.com/2020/02/25/health/coronavirus-us.html.

41. Jeanne Whalen and Abha Bhattarai, "U.S. Companies Face Crucial Test over China's Factory Shutdown," *Washington Post*, February 25, 2020, https://www.washingtonpost.com/business/2020/02/25/us-companies-so-far-are-surviving-chinas-factory-shutdown-next-few-weeks-are-crucial.

42. Bridget O'Brian, "Major American Companies Are Reeling from Coronavirus," CNN, February 25, 2020, https://www.cnn.com/2020/02/24/investing/coronavirus -outlook-companies/index.html.

43. "Investor Update on Quarterly Guidance," Apple Newsroom, February 17, 2020, https://www.apple.com/newsroom/2020/02/investor-update-on-quarterly-guidance.

44. Orange Wang, "China's Car Collapse Sign of Coronavirus Impact to Come," *South China Morning Post*, February 21, 2020, https://www.scmp.com/economy/china-economy /article/3051792/coronavirus-chinas-car-sales-collapse-officials-warn-sharp.

45. Rob McLean, Laura He, and Anneken Tappe, "Dow Plunges 1,000 Points, Posting Its Worst Day in Two Years as Coronavirus Fears Spike," CNN, February 24, 2020, https:// www.cnn.com/2020/02/23/business/stock-futures-coronavirus/index.html.

46. "Schumer Offers Detailed Proposal for $8.5 Billion in Emergency Coronavirus Funding," Senate Democrats, February 26, 2020, https://www.democrats.senate.gov /newsroom/press-releases/schumer-offers-detailed-proposal-for-85-billion-in-emergency -coronavirus-funding.

47. "Remarks by President Trump, Vice President Pence, and Members of the Coronavirus Task Force in Press Conference [2/26]," White House, February 27, 2020, https:// www.whitehouse.gov/briefings-statements/remarks-president-trump-vice-president-pence -members-coronavirus-task-force-press-conference.

48. Lena H. Sun and Yasmeen Abutaleb, "U.S. Workers Without Protective Gear Assisted Coronavirus Evacuees, HHS Whistleblower Says," *Washington Post*, February 27, 2020, https://www.washingtonpost.com/health/2020/02/27/us-workers-without-protective -gear-assisted-coronavirus-evacuees-hhs-whistleblower-says.

49. Geoffrey A. Fowler, Lenny Bernstein, and Laurie McGinley, "California Undertakes Extensive Effort to Trace Contacts of Woman with Coronavirus," *Washington Post*, February 27, 2020, https://www.washingtonpost.com/health/northern-californian-tests -positive-for-coronavirus-in-first-us-case-with-no-link-to-foreign-travel/2020/02/26 /b2088840-58fb-11ea-9000-f3cffee23036_story.html.

50. Factbase, "Donald Trump Holds a Political Rally in North Charleston, South Carolina—February 28, 2020," https://factba.se/transcript/donald-trump-speech-kag -rally-north-charleston-south-carolina-february-28-2020.

51. LaToya Harding, Louis Ashworth, and Josh White, "US Stocks Suffer Worst Week Since Financial Crisis After Seven Days of Losses," *Telegraph*, February 28, 2020, https:// www.telegraph.co.uk/business/2020/02/28/markets-live-latest-news-pound-euro-ftse-100 -live-updates.

52. Hale Stewart, "The Passive-Aggressive Investor for 2/24–2/28," *Seeking Alpha*, March 3, 2020, https://seekingalpha.com/article/4328985-passive-aggressive-investor-for -2-24minus-2-28.

53. Alice Hancock, Tanya Powley, and Chris Campbell, "Coronavirus Prompts a Crisis for the Travel Industry," *Financial Times*, February 28, 2020, https://www.ft.com/content /41b6a8ba-5a36-11ea-a528-ddof971febbc.

54. Erika Towne, "Third Case of COVID-19 Found in Santa Clara County," *Silicon Valley Voice*, February 29, 2020, https://www.svvoice.com/third-case-of-covid-19-found-in -santa-clara-county.

55. Caroline Chen et al., "Key Missteps at the CDC Have Set Back Its Ability to Detect the Potential Spread of Coronavirus," *ProPublica*, February 28, 2020, https://www .propublica.org/article/cdc-coronavirus-covid-19-test?token=loi8JndZRzf9U7hmG1DlFV 6RjLJo1zYf.

56. Adam Lynn, "First US Coronavirus Death Confirmed in Washington. State Health Officials Declare Emergency," *Olympian*, February 29, 2020, https://www.theolympian.com /news/state/washington/article240761641.html.

MARCH

1. Franklin Delano Roosevelt, "FDR's First Inaugural Address Declaring 'War' on the Great Depression," National Archives, August 15, 2016, https://www.archives.gov /education/lessons/fdr-inaugural.

2. OE24, "Neuer Hamsterkauf in Tirol sorgt für Lacher," *Österreich*, February 26, 2020, https://www.oe24.at/oesterreich/chronik/tirol/419016448.

3. Leon Festinger, *A Theory of Cognitive Dissonance* (Stanford, CA: Stanford University Press, 1957).

4. Michael R. Ent and Mary A. Gerend, "Cognitive Dissonance and Attitudes Toward Unpleasant Medical Screenings," *Journal of Health Psychology* 21, no. 9 (2016): 2075–84.

5. Robinson Meyer and Alexis C. Madrigal, "Exclusive: The Strongest Evidence Yet That America Is Botching Coronavirus Testing," *Atlantic*, March 6, 2020, https://www .theatlantic.com/health/archive/2020/03/how-many-americans-have-been-tested -coronavirus/607597.

6. James D. Walsh, "Inside the Desperate Scramble for N95 Masks," *Intelligencer*, March 5, 2020, https://nymag.com/intelligencer/2020/03/inside-the-desperate-scramble -for-n95-masks.html.

7. Trevor Bedford, "Cryptic Transmission of Novel Coronavirus Revealed by Genomic Epidemiology," *Bedford Lab* (blog), March 2, 2020, https://bedford.io/blog/ncov-cryptic -transmission.

8. Danny Vincent, "Coronavirus: A Cameroon Student on How He Recovered," *BBC News, Hong Kong*, February 17, 2020, https://www.bbc.com/news/world-africa-51502711.

9. Zambian Eye, "African Blood Resist Corovirus," *Zambian Eye*, February 15, 2020, https://zambianeye.com/african-blood-resisit-corovirus.

10. Jennifer Caudle, "5 Things You Shouldn't Believe About Coronavirus," Facebook, March 8, 2020, https://www.facebook.com/DrJenCaudle/videos/5-things-you-shouldnt -believe-about-coronavirus/203624910875632.

11. Kelly M. Hoffman et al., "Racial Bias in Pain Assessment and Treatment Recommendations, and False Beliefs about Biological Differences Between Blacks and Whites," *Proceedings of the National Academy of Sciences* 113, no. 16 (April 19, 2016): 4296–4301.

12. Isabella Rosario, "Viral Tweet Highlights Disbelief of Black Women's Pain by Doctors," *Medium*, October 29, 2018, https://medium.com/@isabellarosario/viral-tweet -highlights-disbelief-of-black-womens-pain-by-doctors-11107fbbcd89.

13. Sonja S. Hutchins et al., "Protection of Racial/Ethnic Minority Populations During an Influenza Pandemic," *American Journal of Public Health* 99, no. S2 (October 1, 2009): S261–70.

14. Joe Rogan, "Joe Rogan Experience #1439—Michael Osterholm," *PowerfulJRE*, March 10, 2020, available at https://www.youtube.com/watch?v=E3URhJxoNSw.

15. Bernadette Hogan, "NY AG Orders Televangelist to Quit Advertising Coronavirus Cures," *New York Post*, March 6, 2020, https://web.archive.org/web/20200306142558/https:// nypost.com/2020/03/06/ny-ag-letitia-james-orders-televangelist-jim-bakker-to-quit -advertising-coronavirus-cures.

16. Jason Wert, "FDA, FTC Sends Warning Letter to Jim Bakker Show," *Ozarks Independent* (blog), March 9, 2020, http://ozarksindependent.com/2020/03/09/fda-ftc-sends -warning-letter-to-jim-bakker-show.

17. Susan Sontag, *AIDS and Its Metaphors* (New York: Farrar, Straus and Giroux, 1989).

18. Edward W. Said, *Orientalism* (New York: Vintage, 1979), 3.

19. Annie Karni and Maggie Haberman, "In Rare Oval Office Speech, Trump Voices New Concerns and Old Themes," *New York Times*, March 12, 2020, https://www.nytimes .com/2020/03/12/us/politics/trump-coronavirus-address.html.

20. Carl Zimmer, "The French Disease, the Italian Disease, the Christian Disease—the New World Disease?" *Discover Magazine*, December 19, 2011, https://www.discover magazine.com/health/the-french-disease-the-italian-disease-the-christian-disease-the-new -world-disease.

21. Laura Spinney, *Pale Rider: The Spanish Flu of 1918 and How It Changed the World* (New York: PublicAffairs, 2017).

22. "Remarks by President Trump in Address to the Nation," White House, March 11, 2020, https://trumpwhitehouse.archives.gov/briefings-statements/remarks-president-trump -address-nation.

23. Howard Markel et al., "Nonpharmaceutical Interventions Implemented by US Cities During the 1918–1919 Influenza Pandemic," *JAMA* 298, no. 6 (August 8, 2007): 644–54.

24. US Census, "1920 Census Documents: Volume 1: Population, 1920. Number and Distribution of Inhabitants," https://www.census.gov/prod/www/decennial.html.

25. Michelle L. Holshue et al., "First Case of 2019 Novel Coronavirus in the United States," *New England Journal of Medicine* 382, no. 10 (March 5, 2020): 929–36.

26. Jamie Ducharme, "How News Coverage of Coronavirus in 2020 Compares to Ebola in 2018," *Time*, February 7, 2020, https://time.com/5779872/coronavirus-ebola-news -coverage.

27. Scott Cacciola and Sopan Deb, "N.B.A. Suspends Season After Player Tests Positive for Coronavirus," *New York Times*, March 11, 2020, https://www.nytimes.com/2020/03 /11/sports/basketball/nba-season-suspended-coronavirus.html.

28. "Travel Limits, Economic Fears Stoke Market Plunge," *New York Times*, March 12, 2020, https://www.nytimes.com/2020/03/12/business/stock-market-today.html.

29. Jessie Yeung et al., "March 12 Coronavirus News," CNN, March 12, 2020, https:// www.cnn.com/world/live-news/coronavirus-outbreak-03-12-20-intl-hnk/index.html.

30. Kelly Corbett, "Coronavirus Has Prompted Toilet Paper Gate and the Comeback of . . . Reusable Toilet Paper," *House Beautiful*, March 5, 2020, https://www.housebeautiful .com/lifestyle/a31225525/reusable-toilet-paper-coronavirus; Michael Corkery and Sapna Maheshwari, "Is There Really a Toilet Paper Shortage?" *New York Times*, March 13, 2020, https://www.nytimes.com/2020/03/13/business/toilet-paper-shortage.html; Julie Creswell, "'Where Do I Find Your Hand Sanitizer?' Sorry, We Have None," *New York Times*, February 29, 2020, https://www.nytimes.com/2020/02/29/business/coronavirus-hand-sanitizer .html; Emily Feng and Amy Cheng, "COVID-19 Has Caused a Shortage of Face Masks. But They're Surprisingly Hard to Make," NPR, March 16, 2020, https://www.npr.org /sections/goatsandsoda/2020/03/16/814929294/covid-19-has-caused-a-shortage-of-face -masks-but-theyre-surprisingly-hard-to-mak.

31. Zolan Kanno-Youngs, "Travelers from Coronavirus Hot Spots Say They Faced No Screening," *New York Times*, March 13, 2020, https://www.nytimes.com/2020/03/13/us /politics/coronavirus-travelers-screening.html.

32. "CDC Novel H1N1 Flu: The 2009 H1N1 Pandemic: Summary Highlights, April 2009-April 2010," Centers for Disease Control and Prevention, June 16, 2010, https://www .cdc.gov/h1n1flu/cdcresponse.htm.

33. "Declaration of a National Emergency with Respect to the 2009 H1N1 Influenza Pandemic," White House, April 6, 2009, https://obamawhitehouse.archives.gov/reality check/node/5697.

34. US Department of Health and Human Services, *An HHS Retrospective on the 2009 H1N1 Influenza Pandemic* (Washington, DC: HHS, June 15, 2012), 121.

35. Jackie Calmes and Donald G. McNeil Jr., "H1N1 Widespread in 46 States as Vaccines Lag," *New York Times*, October 24, 2009, https://www.nytimes.com/2009/10/25/us /politics/25flu.html.

36. Steve Liesman, "Federal Reserve Cuts Rates to Zero and Launches Massive $700 Billion Quantitative Easing Program," CNBC, March 15, 2020, https://www.cnbc.com/2020

/03/15/federal-reserve-cuts-rates-to-zero-and-launches-massive-700-billion-quantitative
-easing-program.html.

37. Ian Millhiser, "The Dow Jones Had Its Biggest Point Drop in History Monday,"
Vox, March 16, 2020, https://www.vox.com/2020/3/16/21182341/dow-jones-biggest-point
-drop-coronavirus-3000.

38. "National Survey: Americans Make Small Gains with Savings but More Carry
Credit Card Balances," *The Harris Poll* (blog), April 25, 2016, https://theharrispoll.com/the
-national-foundation-for-credit-counseling-nfcc-and-becu-the-nations-fourth-largest-not
-for-profit-credit-union-have-released-the-results-of-the-2016-financial-literacy-sur; "1 in
3 Americans Have Less Than $5,000 in Retirement Savings," Northwestern Mutual, May 8,
2018, https://news.northwesternmutual.com/2018-05-08-1-In-3-Americans-Have-Less
-Than-5-000-In-Retirement-Savings.

39. Timothy Bella, "Ohio Gov. Mike DeWine's Move to Close Primary Polls Because
of Coronavirus Spawns Confusion, Criticism," *Washington Post*, March 17, 2020, https://
www.washingtonpost.com/nation/2020/03/17/ohio-election-coronavirus.

40. Ian Swanson, "Trump Gives Himself 10 out of 10 on Coronavirus Response," *The
Hill*, March 16, 2020, https://thehill.com/homenews/administration/487883-trump-gives
-himself-10-out-of-10-on-coronavirus-response.

41. Dave Lawler, "China's Coronavirus Cover-up Was Among Worst in History, Congressman Says," *Axios*, March 18, 2020, https://www.axios.com/china-coronavirus-cover-up
-wuhan-pandemic-fa894bb8-998d-494b-8e7a-e834f86d2ea9.html.

42. Li Qingqing, "Pompeo Makes It a Habit of Blaming China, but Politicizing Virus
Is Not Good for the US," *Global Times*, March 1, 2020, https://www.globaltimes.cn/content
/1181192.shtml.

43. Xi Jinping, "Speech at the Meeting of the Standing Committee of the Political Bureau of the CPC Central Committee when Studying the Response to the New Coronavirus
Pneumonia," Qstheory.cn, February 3, 2020, https://translate.google.com/translate?sl=zh
-CN&tl=en&u=http%3A%2F%2Fwww.qstheory.cn%2Fdukan%2Fqs%2F2020-02%2F15
%2Fc_1125572832.htm.

44. Miao Zhonhan, "Wuhan Pneumonia: Wuhan Secretary Wants Citizens to Thank
the Communist Party for Citing a Rebound," CNA, March 7, 2020, https://www.cna.com
.tw/news/firstnews/202003070214.aspx.; James Griffiths, "Did Xi Jinping Know About the
Coronavirus Outbreak Earlier Than First Suggested?" CNN, February 17, 2020, https://
www.cnn.com/2020/02/17/asia/china-coronavirus-xi-jinping-intl-hnk/index.html.

45. Helen Davidson et al., "Trump Puts Pence in Charge of US Virus Response—As It
Happened," *Guardian*, February 27, 2020, https://www.theguardian.com/world/live/2020
/feb/26/coronavirus-latest-updates-who-mission-director-warns-world-is-simply-not-ready.

46. "43 Coronavirus Deaths and over 5,600 Cases in N.Y.C.," *New York Times*, March 20,
2020, https://www.nytimes.com/2020/03/20/nyregion/coronavirus-new-york-update.html.

47. Martha Quillin and Lucille Sherman, "As Coronavirus Keeps Spreading Across
NC, National Guard Activated and Citizens Stock Up," *News & Observer*, March 20, 2020,
https://www.newsobserver.com/news/coronavirus/article241363186.html.

48. Rachel Sandler, "States and Cities Begin to Close Bars and Restaurants amid
Coronavirus Outbreak," *Forbes*, March 15, 2020, https://www.forbes.com/sites/rachel
sandler/2020/03/15/states-begin-to-close-all-bars-and-restaurants-amid-coronavirus
-outbreak.

49. "House Democrats Introduce Families First Coronavirus Response Act," House
Ways and Means Committee—Democrats, March 11, 2020, https://waysandmeans.house
.gov/media-center/press-releases/house-democrats-introduce-families-first-coronavirus
-response-act.

50. Ali Griswold, "Gig Work in the Time of Coronavirus," *Oversharing*, March 5, 2020,
https://oversharing.substack.com; Eric Wittlake, "Three Reasons Marketing Is the First

Budget Cut—B2B Digital Marketing," January 29, 2013, http://b2bdigital.net/2013/01/29/b2b-marketing-budget.

51. Personal communication with Peacock. Real name withheld by request.

52. Carmine Gallo, "Marriott's CEO Demonstrates Truly Authentic Leadership in a Remarkably Emotional Video," *Forbes*, March 21, 2020, https://www.forbes.com/sites/carminegallo/2020/03/21/marriotts-ceo-demonstrates-truly-authentic-leadership-in-a-remarkably-emotional-video.

53. Gallo, "Marriott's CEO Demonstrates Truly Authentic Leadership in a Remarkably Emotional Video"; Ellen McGirt, "Marriott CEO's Authentic Message to Employees," Fortune.com, March 23, 2020, https://fortune.com/2020/03/23/marriott-ceos-authentic-message-to-employees.

54. Donald J. Trump (@realdonaldtrump), "Cure Worse Than Problem," Twitter, March 22, 2020, https://twitter.com/realdonaldtrump/status/1241935285916782593.

55. "US Surgeon General Jerome Adams on Coronavirus: 'This Week, It's Going to Get Bad,'" TODAY.com, March 23, 2020, https://www.today.com/video/us-surgeon-general-jerome-adams-on-coronavirus-this-week-it-s-going-to-get-bad-81091141801.

56. Matthew Perrone, "US Virus Testing Faces New Headwind: Lab Supply Shortages," ABC News, March 21, 2020, https://abcnews.go.com/Health/wireStory/us-virus-testing-faces-headwind-lab-supply-shortages-69710161.

57. Craig A. Spencer (@Craig_A_Spencer), "Thank You Everyone," Twitter, March 24, 2020, https://twitter.com/Craig_A_Spencer/status/1242302400762908685; tweets combined, edited, and printed with permission of Craig Spencer.

58. "Map: Coronavirus and School Closures," *Education Week*, March 6, 2020, https://www.edweek.org/ew/section/multimedia/map-coronavirus-and-school-closures.html.

59. Taylor Lorenz, Erin Griffith, and Mike Isaac, "From Zoom University to the Zoom Party," *New York Times*, March 17, 2020, https://www.nytimes.com/2020/03/17/style/zoom-parties-coronavirus-memes.html.

60. Martin Heidegger, *The Question Concerning Technology, and Other Essays* (New York: Harper Torchbooks, 1977).

61. Cal Newport, *Deep Work: Rules for Focused Success in a Distracted World* (New York: Grand Central Publishing, 2016).

62. Tyler Olson, "Trump Worries US Will See 'Suicides by the Thousands' if Coronavirus Devastates Economy," Fox News, March 24, 2020, https://www.foxnews.com/politics/trump-says-u-s-will-have-suicides-by-the-thousands-if-economic-slowdown-lasts-too-long.

63. Bess Levin, "Texas Lt. Governor: Old People Should Volunteer to Die to Save the Economy," *Vanity Fair*, March 24, 2020, https://www.vanityfair.com/news/2020/03/dan-patrick-coronavirus-grandparents; Ed Mazza, "'I'd Rather Die': Glenn Beck Urges Older Americans to Work Despite Coronavirus," *Huffington Post*, March 24, 2020, https://www.huffpost.com/entry/glenn-beck-coronavirus_n_5e7ab2d6c5b620022ab30851; Charles P. Pierce, "No Thanks, I Will Not Immolate Myself on the Altar of Your Stock Portfolio," *Esquire*, March 24, 2020, https://www.esquire.com/news-politics/politics/a31910755/coronavirus-republicans-sacrifice-old-people-stocks.

64. Lyn Kelly, "The Great Depression and the Real Story Behind the Jumpers of 1929," *History 101* (blog), February 14, 2020, https://www.history101.com/great-depression-truth-jumpers.

65. Holly Hedegaard, Sally C. Curtin, and Margaret Warner, "Increase in Suicide Mortality in the United States, 1999–2018, NCHS Data Brief, No. 362, April 2020," CDC, April 2020, https://www.cdc.gov/nchs/products/databriefs/db362.htm.

66. Jean M. Twenge et al., "Increases in Depressive Symptoms, Suicide-Related Outcomes, and Suicide Rates Among U.S. Adolescents After 2010 and Links to Increased New Media Screen Time," *Clinical Psychological Science* 6, no. 1 (November 14, 2017): 3–17.

67. N. Ferguson et al., *Report 9: Impact of Non-Pharmaceutical Interventions (NPIs) to Reduce COVID19 Mortality and Healthcare Demand* (Imperial College London, March 16, 2020), http://spiral.imperial.ac.uk/handle/10044/1/77482.

68. Ella Nilsen and Li Zhou, "The Senate Just Passed a $2 Trillion Coronavirus Stimulus Package. Here's What's in It," *Vox*, March 25, 2020, https://www.vox.com/2020/3/25/21192716/senate-deal-coronavirus-stimulus.

69. Manu Raju et al., "Senate Approves Historic $2 Trillion Stimulus Deal amid Growing Coronavirus Fears," CNN, March 25, 2020, https://www.cnn.com/2020/03/25/politics/stimulus-senate-action-coronavirus/index.html.

70. Jeremy Berke and Morgan McFall-Johnsen, "USA Now Has More COVID-19 Cases Than Any Other Country in the World," *ScienceAlert*, March 26, 2020, https://www.sciencealert.com/usa-is-now-the-centre-of-the-covid-19-outbreak-as-their-case-numbers-top-italy-s.

71. Michael Rothfeld et al., "13 Deaths in a Day: An 'Apocalyptic' Coronavirus Surge at an N.Y.C. Hospital," *New York Times*, March 25, 2020, https://www.nytimes.com/2020/03/25/nyregion/nyc-coronavirus-hospitals.html.

72. Jason Beaubien, "How South Korea Reined In the Outbreak Without Shutting Everything Down," NPR, March 26, 2020, https://www.npr.org/sections/goatsandsoda/2020/03/26/821688981/how-south-korea-reigned-in-the-outbreak-without-shutting-everything-down.

73. Alan Mauldin, "COVID-19 Suspected in Three Weekend Deaths in Dougherty County," *Albany Herald*, March 17, 2020, https://www.albanyherald.com/news/covid-19-suspected-in-three-weekend-deaths-in-dougherty-county/article_8b759eb6-6878-11ea-8de5-07fa83d6e0e6.html; Darran Todd, "UPDATE: Dougherty Co. Coronavirus Cases Linked to 2 Funerals," WALB News 10, March 17, 2020, https://www.walb.com/2020/03/17/watch-live-dougherty-co-address-latest-coronavirus.

74. Tom Engelhardt, *The End of Victory Culture: Cold War America and the Disillusioning of a Generation*, 2nd ed. (Amherst: University of Massachusetts Press, 2007), 9.

75. *Two Centuries of Law Guide Legal Approach to Modern Pandemic* (American Bar Association, April 2020), https://www.americanbar.org/news/abanews/publications/youraba/2020/youraba-april-2020/law-guides-legal-approach-to-pandemic.

76. Judy Woodruff, "Louisiana Governor: States Are Competing Against Each Other for Ventilators," *NewsHour*, PBS, March 25, 2020, https://www.pbs.org/newshour/show/louisiana-governor-states-are-competing-against-each-other-for-ventilators.

77. Olivia Solon and April Glaser, "'A Worldwide Hackathon': Hospitals Turn to Crowdsourcing and 3D Printing amid Equipment Shortages," NBC News, March 21, 2020, https://www.nbcnews.com/tech/innovation/worldwide-hackathon-hospitals-turn-crowdsourcing-3d-printing-amid-equipment-shortages-n1165026; Masks for Massachusetts, "Masks for Massachusetts," Facebook, March 28, 2020, https://www.facebook.com/Masks-for-Massachusetts-101109764870425/?ref=page_internal.

APRIL

1. "Read Florida Gov. DeSantis' Stay-at-Home Executive Order," *Orlando Sentinel*, April 1, 2020, https://www.orlandosentinel.com/coronavirus/os-ne-coronavirus-florida-stay-at-home-executive-order-20200401-2gzu3nenonaohaz6w5narcff3e-story.html.

2. Margaret Talev, "Axios-Ipsos Coronavirus Index: Rich Sheltered, Poor Shafted as Virus Rages," *Axios*, April 1, 2020, https://www.axios.com/axios-ipsos-coronavirus-index-rich-sheltered-poor-shafted-9e592100-b8e6-4dcd-aee0-a6516892874b.html.

3. SHADAC, "Per Person State Public Health Funding," State Health Access Data Assistance Center, University of Minnesota, 2017/2018/2019, http://statehealthcompare.shadac.org/map/117/per-person-state-public-health-funding#a/27/154.

4. Vann R. Newkirk II, "The Coronavirus's Unique Threat to the South," *Atlantic,* April 2, 2020, https://www.theatlantic.com/politics/archive/2020/04/coronavirus-unique -threat-south-young-people/609241.

5. Ryan Grim, "Rikers Island Prisoners Are Being Offered PPE and $6 an Hour to Dig Mass Graves," *The Intercept* (blog), March 31, 2020, https://theintercept.com/2020/03/31 /rikers-island-coronavirus-mass-graves.

6. Erin Cunningham and Dalton Bennett, "Coronavirus Burial Pits in Iran so Vast That They're Visible from Space," *Washington Post,* March 12, 2020, https://www.washingtonpost .com/graphics/2020/world/iran-coronavirus-outbreak-graves.

7. "New COVID-19 Forecasts: US Hospitals Could Be Overwhelmed in the Second Week of April by Demand for ICU Beds, and US Deaths Could Total 81,000 by July," Institute for Health Metrics and Evaluation, University of Washington, March 26, 2020, http:// www.healthdata.org/news-release/new-covid-19-forecasts-us-hospitals-could-be-overwhelmed -second-week-april-demand-icu.

8. Michael D. Shear, Michael Crowley, and James Glanz, "Coronavirus May Kill 100,000 to 240,000 in U.S. Despite Actions, Officials Say," *New York Times,* March 31, 2020, https://www.nytimes.com/2020/03/31/us/politics/coronavirus-death-toll-united-states.html.

9. Zak Faila, "April Will Be 'Horrible Month' for CT COVID-19 Cases," *Daily Voice,* March 31, 2020, https://dailyvoice.com/connecticut/fairfield/politics/april-will-be-horrible -month-for-ct-covid-19-cases-lamont-says-new-breakdown-of-cases/785876.

10. Elizabeth Cohen and John Bonifield, "New York Surgeon Writes Haunting Letter About Rationing Care for Patients Who Don't Have the Coronavirus," CNN, April 5, 2020, https://www.cnn.com/2020/04/05/health/rationing-care-patients-without-coronavirus /index.html.

11. HHS Office of Inspector General, *Hospital Experiences Responding to the COVID-19 Pandemic: Results of a National Pulse Survey March 23–27, 2020* (Washington, DC: Department of Health and Human Services, April 3, 2020), https://oig.hhs.gov/oei/reports/oei -06-20-00300.asp.

12. HHS Office of Inspector General, *Hospital Experiences Responding to the COVID-19 Pandemic.*

13. Yasmeen Abutaleb et al., "The U.S. Was Beset by Denial and Dysfunction as the Coronavirus Raged," *Washington Post,* April 4, 2020, https://www.washingtonpost.com /national-security/2020/04/04/coronavirus-government-dysfunction.

14. Geoff Baker, "Trump Administration Backs Off a Deal for Bothell's Ventec and GM to Produce 'up to 20,000' Ventilators a Month amid Coronavirus Crisis," *Seattle Times,* March 26, 2020, https://www.seattletimes.com/business/local-business/ventec-and-gm -hoping-to-produce-up-to-20000-ventilators-a-month-amid-coronavirus-crisis.

15. US Department of State, "Members of the Coronavirus Task Force Hold a Press Briefing," March 27, 2020, YouTube video, https://www.youtube.com/watch?v=MjbNW 07u3WA.

16. "Trump Berates Reporter for 'Threatening' Question During Briefing," CNN, YouTube video, https://www.youtube.com/watch?v=1uWT_L58MGc.

17. Justin Elliott, Annie Waldman, and Joshua Kaplan, "How New York City's Emergency Ventilator Stockpile Ended Up on the Auction Block," *ProPublica,* April 6, 2020, https://www.propublica.org/article/how-new-york-city-emergency-ventilator-stockpile -ended-up-on-the-auction-block?token=sYBNO6t1202JOb6ILFkA_eTWzPmpol3N.

18. Syra Madad et al., "Ready or Not, Patients Will Present: Improving Urban Pandemic Preparedness," *Disaster Medicine and Public Health Preparedness* (March 16, 2020): 1–4.

19. Jacob Jarvis, "Wuhan Lifts Coronavirus Lockdown After Months-Long Quarantine to Stem Covid-19 Spread," *London Evening Standard,* April 8, 2020, https://www.standard .co.uk/news/world/wuhan-coronavirus-china-lifts-lockdown-a4409706.html.

20. Felix Ringel, "Can Time Be Tricked? A Theoretical Introduction," *Cambridge Journal of Anthropology* 34, no. 1 (March 1, 2016): 22–31.

21. Laura Bear, "Doubt, Conflict, Mediation: The Anthropology of Modern Time," *Journal of the Royal Anthropological Institute* 20, no. S1 (2014): 3–30.

22. Jane I. Guyer, "Prophecy and the near Future: Thoughts on Macroeconomic, Evangelical, and Punctuated Time," *American Ethnologist* 34, no. 3 (2007): 409–21.

23. Summer Jentzen, "Tips for Homeschooling During the COVID-19 Lockdown," *Anxiety Mama* (blog), March 24, 2020, https://anxiety-mama.com/2020/03/24/tips-for -homeschooling-during-the-covid-19-lockdown.

24. Sharmilee M. Nyenhuis et al., "Race Is Associated with Differences in Airway Inflammation in Patients with Asthma," *Journal of Allergy and Clinical Immunology* 140, no. 1 (July 1, 2017): 257–265.e11.

25. Eric Levenson, "Why Black Americans Are at Higher Risk for Coronavirus," CNN, April 7, 2020, https://www.cnn.com/2020/04/07/us/coronavirus-black-americans -race/index.html.

26. Ray Sanchez, "Coronavirus in Black America: Living in the Eye of a 'Perfect Storm,'" CNN, April 11, 2020, https://www.cnn.com/2020/04/11/us/coronavirus-black -americans-deaths/index.html.

27. Dan Kopf, "Delivery Is the Fastest-Growing Job Industry in the US," *Quartz*, March 7, 2020, https://qz.com/1814110/delivery-jobs-are-the-fastest-growing-in-the-us.

28. Bureau of Labor Statistics, "Job Flexibilities and Work Schedules—2017–2018 Data from the American Time Use Survey," September 24, 2019, https://www.bls.gov/news .release/pdf/flex2.pdf.

29. Elise Gould and Heidi Shierholtz, "Not Everybody Can Work from Home: Black and Hispanic Workers Are Much Less Likely to Be Able to Telework," *Economic Policy Institute* (blog), March 19, 2020, https://www.epi.org/blog/black-and-hispanic-workers-are -much-less-likely-to-be-able-to-work-from-home.

30. Kate Bahn and Carmen Sanchez Cumming, "Four Graphs on U.S. Occupational Segregation by Race, Ethnicity, and Gender," *Equitable Growth* (blog), July 1, 2020, http:// www.equitablegrowth.org/four-graphs-on-u-s-occupational-segregation-by-race-ethnicity -and-gender.

31. N. Jamiyla Chisholm, "Mask Protection, but Not While Black," *Color Lines*, April 9, 2020, https://www.colorlines.com/articles/mask-protection-not-while-black; Damon Young, "Masking While Black: A Coronavirus Story," *Washington Post*, April 10, 2020, https://www .washingtonpost.com/outlook/2020/04/10/coronavirus-masks-black-america; Jeanie Stephens, "Video: Wood River Officer Made Men Leave Walmart Because They Wore Masks," *Alton Telegraph*, March 24, 2020, https://www.thetelegraph.com/news/article/Video-Wood -River-officer-has-men-leave-Walmart-15154393.php.

32. Alex Woodward, "'I Want to Stay Alive but I Also Want to Stay Alive': Video of Police Following Black Men Wearing Masks Raises Concern over Racial Profiling," *Independent*, April 9, 2020, https://www.independent.co.uk/news/world/americas/coronavirus-masks -racism-police-video-racial-profiling-walmart-video-a9458221.html.

33. "Miami Police Launch Investigation After Dr. Armen Henderson, Who Tests Homeless for COVID-19, Cuffed in Front of His Home," *CBS Miami* (blog), April 11, 2020, https://miami.cbslocal.com/2020/04/11/miami-police-internal-investigation-dr -armen-henderson-cuffed; Armen Henderson, "Doctor Handcuffed by Police as He Tosses Boxes to the Curb," *Miami Herald*, April 10, 2020, https://www.miamiherald.com/news /local/crime/article241932451.html.

34. Steve Peoples and Scott Bauer, "Wisconsin Primary Disproportionately Impacted Minority Voters," *Christian Science Monitor*, April 8, 2020, https://www.csmonitor.com/USA /Politics/2020/0408/Wisconsin-primary-disproportionately-impacted-minority-voters.

35. Scott Utterback, "Maryville Baptist Church's Easter Service Gets a Visit from the KSP," *Louisville Courier-Journal*, April 12, 2020, https://www.courier-journal.com/picture-gallery/news/local/2020/04/12/maryville-baptist-church-holds-in-person-easter-service/2979048001.

36. Keira Lombardo, "Smithfield Foods to Close Sioux Falls, SD Plant Indefinitely amid COVID-19," Smithfield Foods, press release, April 12, 2020, https://www.smithfield foods.com/press-room/company-news/smithfield-foods-to-close-sioux-falls-sd-plant -indefinitely-amid-covid-19.

37. Marissa Lute, "Gov. Noem, Mayor TenHaken Request Smithfield Foods Close Plant for 14 Days with More COVID-19 Cases per Capita in Sioux Falls Than Seattle or Chicago," *Keloland News*, April 11, 2020, https://www.keloland.com/news/healthbeat /coronavirus/south-dakota-gov-noem-sioux-falls-mayor-tenhaken-request-to-close-smith field-foods-for-14-days.

38. David Bacon, "Unions Come to Smithfield," *American Prospect*, December 17, 2008, https://prospect.org/api/content/de4ae676-5d2c-50cb-aaba-5ae73c1cd28e.

39. "UFCW Calls on CDC to Issue Mandatory Guidance for Frontline Workers During Coronavirus Outbreak," United Food and Commercial Workers International Union, April 8, 2020, http://www.ufcw.org/2020/04/08/cdcguidance.

40. Abha Bhattarai, "'It Feels like a War Zone': As More of Them Die, Grocery Workers Increasingly Fear Showing Up at Work," *Washington Post*, April 12, 2020, https://www .washingtonpost.com/business/2020/04/12/grocery-worker-fear-death-coronavirus.

41. Craig Mauger, "Michigan COVID-19 Cases Reach 28,000 with 1,900 Deaths," *Detroit News*, April 15, 2020. https://www.detroitnews.com/story/news/local/michigan/2020 /04/15/michigan-covid-19-cases-reach-28-000-1-900-deaths/5139228002.

42. Michigan Nurses Association, "Posts," Facebook, April 15, 2020, https://www .facebook.com/minurses/posts/statement-on-the-lansing-protest-against-the-stay-at-home -order-from-tina-ray-rn/10158131267658058.

43. Erin Bromage, "Where We Are Now?" *Erin Bromage: COVID-19 Musings* (blog), April 19, 2020, https://www.erinbromage.com/post/where-we-are-now.

44. Josh Rogin, State Department Cables Warned of Safety Issues at Wuhan Lab Studying Bat Coronaviruses," *Washington Post*, op-ed, April 14, 2020, https://www.washington post.com/opinions/2020/04/14/state-department-cables-warned-safety-issues-wuhan-lab -studying-bat-coronaviruses.

45. Roujian Lu et al., "Genomic Characterisation and Epidemiology of 2019 Novel Coronavirus: Implications for Virus Origins and Receptor Binding," *Lancet* 395, no. 10224 (February 22, 2020): 565–74.

46. Josephine Ma, "China's First Confirmed Covid-19 Case Traced Back to November 17," *South China Morning Post*, March 14, 2020, https://www.scmp.com/news/china/society /article/3074991/coronavirus-chinas-first-confirmed-covid-19-case-traced-back.

47. Lily Kuo, "Birth of a Pandemic: Inside the First Weeks of the Coronavirus Outbreak in Wuhan," *Guardian*, April 10, 2020, https://www.theguardian.com/world/2020/apr /10/birth-of-a-pandemic-inside-the-first-weeks-of-the-coronavirus-outbreak-in-wuhan.

48. Zolan Kanno-Youngs, "Travelers from Coronavirus Hot Spots Say They Faced No Screening," *New York Times*, March 13, 2020, https://www.nytimes.com/2020/03/13/us /politics/coronavirus-travelers-screening.html; Steve Eder et al., "430,000 People Have Traveled from China to U.S. Since Coronavirus Surfaced," *New York Times*, April 4, 2020, https://www.nytimes.com/2020/04/04/us/coronavirus-china-travel-restrictions.html.

49. Kristen V. Brown, "False Negatives Raise Doctors' Doubts About Coronavirus Tests," *Bloomberg*, April 11, 2020, https://www.bloomberg.com/news/articles/2020-04-11 /false-negative-coronavirus-test-results-raise-doctors-doubts.

50. Dominique Patton and David Stanway, "China's Hubei Province Sees Surge in Coronavirus Deaths on Switch to New Methodology," Reuters, February 13, 2020, https:// www.reuters.com/article/us-china-health-hubei-toll-idUSKBN207010.

51. Brad Plumer and Nadja Popovich, "Traffic and Pollution Plummet as U.S. Cities Shut Down for Coronavirus," *New York Times*, March 22, 2020, https://www.nytimes.com /interactive/2020/03/22/climate/coronavirus-usa-traffic.html.

52. Kathleen Schuster, "Coronavirus Lockdown Gives Animals Rare Break from Noise Pollution," *Deutsche Welle*, April 16, 2020, https://www.dw.com/en/coronavirus-lockdown -gives-animals-rare-break-from-noise-pollution/a-53106214; Helen Briggs, "How the Pandemic Is Putting the Spotlight on Wildlife Trade," BBC News, April 6, 2020, https://www .bbc.com/news/science-environment-52125309.

53. Laura Geggel, "Baby Leatherback Sea Turtles Thriving due to COVID-19 Beach Restrictions," *Live Science*, April 21, 2020, https://www.livescience.com/leatherback-sea -turtle-babies-thrive-covid-19-pandemic.html.

54. Emmanuel Felton, "The Coronavirus Meme About 'Nature Is Healing' Is So Damn Funny," *BuzzFeed News*, April 7, 2020, https://www.buzzfeednews.com/article/emmanuel felton/coronavirus-meme-nature-is-healing-we-are-the-virus; Martha Henriques, "Has Coronavirus Helped the Environment?" *BBC Future*, April 22, 2020, https://www.bbc.com /future/article/20200422-how-has-coronavirus-helped-the-environment.

55. "Remarks by President Trump, Vice President Pence, and Members of the Coronavirus Task Force in Press Briefing," White House, April 23, 2020, https://www.whitehouse .gov/briefings-statements/remarks-president-trump-vice-president-pence-members-corona virus-task-force-press-briefing-31.

56. "Improper Use of Disinfectants," RB.com, 2020, https://www.rb.com/media/news /2020/april/improper-use-of-disinfectants.

57. Elesa Zehndorfer, *Evolution, Politics and Charisma: Why Do Populists Win?* (New York: Routledge, 2019); Drew Westen, *The Political Brain: The Role of Emotion in Deciding the Fate of the Nation* (New York: PublicAffairs, 2008).

58. White House, "Remarks by President Trump, Vice President Pence, and Members of the Coronavirus Task Force in Press Briefing."

59. Ali Watkins et al., "Top E.R. Doctor Who Treated Virus Patients Dies by Suicide," *New York Times*, April 29, 2020, https://www.nytimes.com/2020/04/27/nyregion/new-york -city-doctor-suicide-coronavirus.html.

60. Ariana Eunjung Cha, "Young and Middle-Aged People, Barely Sick with Covid-19, Are Dying from Strokes," *Washington Post*, April 25, 2020, https://www.washingtonpost.com /health/2020/04/24/strokes-coronavirus-young-patients.

61. Emma Brown et al., "U.S. Deaths Soared in Early Weeks of Pandemic, Far Exceeding Number Attributed to Covid-19," *Washington Post*, April 27, 2020, https://www.washington post.com/investigations/2020/04/27/covid-19-death-toll-undercounted.

62. "The Ingraham Angle—Monday, April 8," Fox News, April 8, 2020, http://video .foxnews.com/v/6024216977001.

63. Jay Hancock, Phil Galewitz, and Elizabeth Lucas, "Furor Erupts: Billions Going to Hospitals Based on Medicare Billings, Not COVID-19," *Kaiser Health News* (blog), April 10, 2020, https://khn.org/news/furor-erupts-billions-going-to-hospitals-based-on-medicare -billings-not-covid-19.

64. Rosenthal, *An American Sickness*, 166–81.

65. Nick Miroff, Maria Sacchetti, and Tracy Jan, "Trump to Suspend Immigration to U.S. for 60 Days, Citing Coronavirus Crisis and Jobs Shortage, but Will Allow Some Workers," *Washington Post*, April 21, 2020, https://www.washingtonpost.com/immigration/coronavirus-trump -suspend-immigration/2020/04/21/464e2440-838d-11ea-ae26-989cfce1c7c7_story.html.

66. Christopher Weaver and Rebecca Ballhaus, "Coronavirus Testing Hampered by Disarray, Shortages, Backlogs," *Wall Street Journal*, April 19, 2020, https://www.wsj.com /articles/coronavirus-testing-hampered-by-disarray-shortages-backlogs-11587328441; German Lopez, "Why America Is Still Failing on Coronavirus Testing," *Vox*, April 10, 2020, https://www.vox.com/2020/4/10/21214218/trump-coronavirus-testing-social-distancing.

67. Maggie Fox, "Flu Killed 80,000 People This Past Season. Someone Infected All of Them," NBC News, September 27, 2018, https://www.nbcnews.com/health/health-news /doctors-speak-bluntly-about-record-80-000-flu-deaths-n914246.

68. World Health Organization, *International Guidelines for Certification and Classification (Coding) of COVID-19 as Cause of Death* (Geneva: WHO, April 16, 2020), https://www.who .int/classifications/icd/Guidelines_Cause_of_Death_COVID-19.pdf?ua=1.

69. "How CDC Estimates the Burden of Seasonal Influenza in the U.S.," Centers for Disease Control and Prevention, November 22, 2019, https://www.cdc.gov/flu/about /burden/how-cdc-estimates.htm.

70. Melissa A. Rolfes et al., "Annual Estimates of the Burden of Seasonal Influenza in the United States: A Tool for Strengthening Influenza Surveillance and Preparedness," *Influenza and Other Respiratory Viruses* 12, no. 1 (2018): 132–37.

71. Jeremy Samuel Faust, "Comparing COVID-19 Deaths to Flu Deaths Is like Comparing Apples to Oranges," *Scientific American Blog Network*, April 28, 2020, https://blogs .scientificamerican.com/observations/comparing-covid-19-deaths-to-flu-deaths-is-like -comparing-apples-to-oranges.

72. Angelo Fichera, "Social Media Posts Make Baseless Claim on COVID-19 Death Toll," *FactCheck* (blog), April 8, 2020, https://www.factcheck.org/2020/04/social-media-posts -make-baseless-claim-on-covid-19-death-toll.

73. Associated Press, "U.S. Online Alcohol Sales Jump 243% During Coronavirus Pandemic," MarketWatch, April 2, 2020, https://www.marketwatch.com/story/us-alcohol -sales-spike-during-coronavirus-outbreak-2020-04-01.

74. Dave Gilson, Laura Thompson, and Clara Jeffery, "A Timeline of Trump's 100 Days of Deadly Coronavirus Denial," *Mother Jones* (blog), April 29, 2020, https://www.mother jones.com/politics/2020/04/trump-coronavirus-timeline.

75. Matt Perez, "Trump Implies That the Coronavirus Will Be 'Eradicated' Without a Vaccine," *Forbes*, April 29, 2020, https://www.forbes.com/sites/mattperez/2020/04/29/trump -implies-that-the-coronavirus-will-be-eradicated-without-a-vaccine.

MAY

1. Mike Elk, "COVID-19 Strike Wave Interactive Map," *Payday Report* (blog), 2020, https://paydayreport.com/covid-19-strike-wave-interactive-map; Janine Jackson, "'This Many Strikes Says That Something Fundamentally Is Changing in the Country,'" *Fairness & Accuracy in Reporting* (blog), April 16, 2020, https://fair.org/home/this-many-strikes-says -that-something-fundamentally-is-changing-in-the-country.

2. Walter Einenkel, "Smithfield Pork Executives Deflect Blame for the South Dakota COVID-19 Outbreak on Immigrant Workers," AlterNet.org, April 22, 2020, https://www .alternet.org/2020/04/smithfield-pork-executives-deflect-blame-for-the-south-dakota-covid -19-outbreak-on-immigrant-workers.

3. Mike Elk, "With 23 UAW Members Dead, UAW Halts Big 3 Reopening Next Week—Payday Report," *Payday Report* (blog), April 24, 2020, https://paydayreport.com/with -23-uaw-members-dead-uaw-halts-automakers-reopening-next-week.

4. Chip Mitchell, "Nursing Home Workers in Illinois Move Toward Strike as Deadly Virus Spreads," *WBEZ Chicago*, April 27, 2020, https://www.wbez.org/stories/nursing-home -workers-in-illinois-move-toward-strike-as-deadly-virus-spreads/5c5e983c-fe3f-4e76-8855 -8551ee3a97a2.

5. Arise Chicago, "LSL Healthcare Production Workers Deliver Demand Letter," Facebook, May 1, 2020, https://www.facebook.com/watch/live/?v=1549147601927303&notif _id=1588348475106617&notif_t=live_video.

6. "Woman Jailed for Defying Lockdown," CNN, May 6, 2020, available at https:// www.youtube.com/watch?v=GNJUO61Kb00.

7. Margaret Peacock, *Innocent Weapons: The Soviet and American Politics of Childhood in the Cold War* (Chapel Hill: University of North Carolina Press, 2014), 5.

8. César Rodriguez and LMTonline.com/Laredo Morning Times, "Laredo Pair Allegedly Violated Coronavirus Stay-at-Home Order with Beauty Businesses," *Laredo Morning Times*, April 20, 2020, https://www.lmtonline.com/local/article/Laredo-pair-allegedly-violated-coronavirus-15212653.php.

9. "Video Shows Fatal Shooting of Ahmaud Arbery, Unarmed Black Man in Georgia," TMZ, May 5, 2020, https://www.tmz.com/2020/05/05/shooting-video-unarmed-black-man-killed-ahmaud-arbery-georgia-jogging.

10. "Venezuela Claims 2 Americans Were Captured in Failed Invasion," *New York Times*, May 5, 2020, https://www.nytimes.com/2020/05/05/world/americas/venezuela-invasion-americans-captured.html.

11. Frances Mulraney and Chris Jewers, "Two US 'Mercenaries' Are Arrested After Attempt 'to Kill' Maduro," *Daily Mail*, May 5, 2020, https://www.dailymail.co.uk/news/article-8287851/Two-mercenaries-arrested-failed-attempt-kill-Venezuelas-President-Maduro.html.

12. "Listen: Toilet Flushes as Supreme Court Holds Oral Arguments by Teleconference," NBC News, May 6, 2020, available at https://www.youtube.com/watch?v=xBobUt TvdCU.

13. Lucy van Dorp et al., "Emergence of Genomic Diversity and Recurrent Mutations in SARS-CoV-2," *Infection, Genetics and Evolution* (May 5, 2020).

14. "'They're Drunk on Power': Crenshaw Blasts Coronavirus Restrictions," May 7, 2020, Fox News, available at https://www.youtube.com/watch?v=g9nePRUD7Jg&feature =youtu.be.

15. Said, *Orientalism*.

16. "Why Is Massachusetts a Commonwealth?" Mass.gov, 2020, https://www.mass.gov /service-details/why-is-massachusetts-a-commonwealth.

17. Joshua Kaplan and Benjamin Hardy, "Early Data Shows Black People Are Being Disproportionally Arrested . . .," *ProPublica*, May 8, 2020, https://www.propublica.org /article/in-some-of-ohios-most-populous-areas-black-people-were-at-least-4-times-as -likely-to-be-charged-with-stay-at-home-violations-as-whites.

18. "Temporary Guidance—Road Closures or Restrictions on Tribal Lands," Department of Interior Bureau of Indian Affairs, April 8, 2020, https://turtletalk.files.wordpress .com/2020/05/bia-road-closure-guidance.pdf.

19. "What Workers Are Saying at a Meatpacking Plant Closed Due to Coronavirus Outbreak," NPR, April 17, 2020, https://www.npr.org/2020/04/17/837511566/what -workers-are-saying-at-a-meatpacking-plant-closed-due-to-coronavirus-outbrea.

20. Kristi Noem, "Letter from Kristi Noem to Oglala Sioux Tribe," South Dakota State News, May 8, 2020, https://news.sd.gov/newsitem.aspx?id=26770.

21. Harold Frazier, "Letter from Harold Frazier, Cheyenne River Sioux Tribe, to Kristi Noem," *Indianz*, May 8, 2020, https://www.indianz.com/covid19/2020/05/08/chairman -harold-frazier-cheyenne-river-sioux-tribe-2.

22. Thomas Beers et al., "Lessons of the 1918 Flu Pandemic and Today's Homeland Security," *JEMS* (blog), March 15, 2020, https://www.jems.com/exclusives/lessons-of-the -1918-flu-pandemic.

23. "Racial Disparities on Full Display—COVID-19 Is Disproportionately Affecting Communities of Color," Senate Democrats, April 30, 2020, https://www.democrats.senate .gov/dpcc/press-reports/dpcc-report-racial-disparities-on-full-displaycovid-19-is -disproportionately-affecting-communities-of-color.

24. Elizabeth Hlavinka, "COVID-19 Further Strains Care Disparities Among Native Americans," *Medpage Today*, May 21, 2020, https://www.medpagetoday.com/infectiousdisease /covid19/86633.

25. Kalen Goodluck, "The Erasure of Indigenous People in U.S. COVID-19 Data," *High Country News*, August 31, 2020, https://www.hcn.org/articles/indigenous-affairs-the-erasure-of-indigenous-people-in-us-covid-19-data.

26. Hlavinka, "COVID-19 Further Strains Care Disparities Among Native Americans."

27. Matthew Desmond, *Evicted: Poverty and Profit in the American City*, rep. ed. (New York: Broadway Books, 2017).

28. Dan Witters and Jim Harter, "Worry and Stress Fuel Record Drop in U.S. Life Satisfaction," Gallup.com, May 8, 2020, https://news.gallup.com/poll/310250/worry-stress-fuel-record-drop-life-satisfaction.aspx.

29. Aaron Rupar, "Trump's Latest Twitter Meltdown Featured QAnon and a Lot of 'OBAMAGATE,'" *Vox*, May 11, 2020, https://www.vox.com/2020/5/11/21254398/trump-tweets-mothers-day-obamagate-coronavirus.

30. Anna Nemtsova, "In Baku, the Trump Tower Dares Not Bear His Name," *Daily Beast*, March 16, 2020, https://www.thedailybeast.com/in-baku-the-trump-tower-dares-not-bear-his-name.

31. Rick Rojas, Richard Fausset, and Serge F. Kovaleski, "Georgia Killing Puts Spotlight on a Police Force's Troubled History," *New York Times*, May 8, 2020, https://www.nytimes.com/2020/05/08/us/glynn-county-police-ahmaud-arbery.html.

32. Marty Swant, "From 'Virtual Sleepover' to 'Accent Wall Dots,' Marketers Are Using Pinterest to Find COVID-19 Hobbies," *Forbes*, May 11, 2020, https://www.forbes.com/sites/martyswant/2020/05/11/marketers-are-using-pinterest-to-identify-the-covid-19-aesthetic.

33. Stephen Brown, Pauline Maclaren, and Lorna Stevens, "Marcadia Postponed: Marketing, Utopia and the Millennium," *Journal of Marketing Management* 12, no. 7 (October 1, 1996): 676; Robert V. Kozinets, "YouTube Utopianism: Social Media Profanation and the Clicktivism of Capitalist Critique," *Journal of Business Research* 98 (May 1, 2019): 66.

34. Susan M. Schoenbohm, "The Function and Questionable Purpose of Utopian Thought," *Soundings: An Interdisciplinary Journal* 91, no. 1/2 (2008): 22.

35. Bryan Koenig, "Mergers During COVID-19 Create New 'Failing Firm' Paradigm," *Law360*, May 11, 2020, https://www.law360.com/articles/1272292/mergers-during-covid-19-create-new-failing-firm-paradigm.

36. Ahiza Garcia-Hodges, "Some Tesla Factory Employees Say They're Being Pressured to Return to Work," NBC News, May 13, 2020, https://www.nbcnews.com/tech/tech-news/some-tesla-factory-employees-say-they-re-being-pressured-return-n1205866.

37. Blessed Are the Binary Breakers, https://www.blessedarethebinarybreakers.com, accessed June 15, 2021.

38. "The Economic Impact of Coronavirus on the Arts and Culture Sector," *Americans for the Arts*, March 17, 2020, https://www.americansforthearts.org/by-topic/disaster-preparedness/the-economic-impact-of-coronavirus-on-the-arts-and-culture-sector.

39. Stephanie M. Lee, "JetBlue's Founder Helped Fund a Stanford Study That Said the Coronavirus Wasn't That Deadly," *BuzzFeed News*, May 15, 2020, https://www.buzzfeednews.com/article/stephaniemlee/stanford-coronavirus-neeleman-ioannidis-whistleblower.

40. Lizandra Portal and Sabrina Lolo, "Woman Who Designed Florida's COVID-19 Dashboard Has Been Removed from Her Position," WPEC CBS News 12, May 18, 2020, https://cbs12.com/news/local/woman-who-designed-floridas-covid-19-dashboard-has-been-removed-from-her-position; Alessandro Marazzi Sassoon, "Coronavirus: As Florida Re-Opens, COVID-19 Data Chief Gets Sidelined and Researchers Cry Foul," *Florida Today*, May 18, 2020, https://www.floridatoday.com/story/news/2020/05/18/censorship-covid-19-data-researcher-removed-florida-moves-re-open-state/5212398002.

41. Jeffery Martin, "54,000 Fewer Americans Would Have Died If U.S. Went into Lockdown on March 1, Columbia University Estimates," *Newsweek*, May 21, 2020, https://www.newsweek.com/54000-fewer-americans-would-have-died-if-us-went-lockdown-march-1-columbia-university-1505592.

42. Sen Pei, Sasikiran Kandula, and Jeffrey Shaman, "Differential Effects of Intervention Timing on COVID-19 Spread in the United States," *MedRxiv*, May 29, 2020, https://doi.org/10.1101/2020.05.15.20103655.

43. H. Unwin et al., *Report 23: State-Level Tracking of COVID-19 in the United States* (London: Imperial College London, May 21, 2020), http://spiral.imperialac.uk/handle/10044/1/79231.

44. "Excess Deaths Associated with COVID-19," Centers for Disease Control and Prevention, May 20, 2020, https://www.cdc.gov/nchs/nvss/vsrr/covid19/excess_deaths.htm.

45. Charles E. Rosenberg, "What Is an Epidemic? AIDS in Historical Perspective," *Daedalus* 118, no. 2 (1989): 3.

46. Samuel K. Cohn, "Pandemics: Waves of Disease, Waves of Hate from the Plague of Athens to A.I.D.S.," *Historical Journal (Cambridge, England)* 85, no. 230 (November 1, 2012): 535–55.

47. Lydia Bourouiba, "Turbulent Gas Clouds and Respiratory Pathogen Emissions: Potential Implications for Reducing Transmission of COVID-19," *JAMA* 323, no. 18 (May 12, 2020): 1837–38.

48. "COVID-19 TV Habits Suggest the Days Are Blurring Together," Comcast, May 6, 2020, https://corporate.comcast.com/stories/xfinity-viewing-data-covid-19.

49. Rosenberg, "What Is an Epidemic?" 8.

50. Unwin et al., *Report 23*.

51. Flannery O'Connor, *Mystery and Manners: Occasional Prose*, ed. Sally Fitzgerald and Robert Fitzgerald (New York: Farrar, Straus and Giroux, 1970).

52. NCSL Elections Team, "All-Mail Elections (Aka Vote-By-Mail)," National Conference of State Legislatures, March 24, 2020, https://www.ncsl.org/research/elections-and-campaigns/all-mail-elections.aspx.

53. "Voter Fraud Map: Election Fraud Database," Heritage Foundation, May 26, 2020, https://www.heritage.org/voterfraud/search?state=VA.

54. Ari Berman, "A Voter-Fraud Witch Hunt in Kansas," *Nation*, June 11, 2015, https://www.thenation.com/article/archive/voter-fraud-witch-hunt-kansas; M. V. Hood and William Gillespie, "They Just Do Not Vote Like They Used To: A Methodology to Empirically Assess Election Fraud," *Social Science Quarterly* 93, no. 1 (January 12, 2012): 76–94; Christopher Ingraham, "7 Papers, 4 Government Inquiries, 2 News Investigations and 1 Court Ruling Proving Voter Fraud Is Mostly a Myth," *Washington Post*, July 9, 2014, https://www.washingtonpost.com/news/wonk/wp/2014/07/09/7-papers-4-government-inquiries-2-news-investigations-and-1-court-ruling-proving-voter-fraud-is-mostly-a-myth.

55. "Voter Turnout Data—National Turnout Rates, 1787–2018," US Elections Project, http://www.electproject.org/home/voter-turnout/voter-turnout-data.

56. "Voter Fraud: Debunking the Myths," *Stand Up Republic* (blog), April 22, 2020, https://standuprepublic.com/voter-fraud-debunking-the-myths.

57. Jeff Wagner, "'It's Real Ugly': Protesters Clash with Minneapolis Police After George Floyd's Death," *CBS Local*, May 26, 2020, https://minnesota.cbslocal.com/2020/05/26/hundreds-of-protesters-march-in-minneapolis-after-george-floyds-deadly-encounter-with-police.

58. John Grippe, "The Project Behind a Front Page Full of Names," *New York Times*, May 23, 2020, https://www.nytimes.com/2020/05/23/reader-center/coronavirus-new-york-times-front-page.html.

59. Seth Cohen, "Golfing as the U.S. Mourns 100,000 Dead? Trump's Ugly Memorial Day Message," *Forbes*, May 23, 2020, https://www.forbes.com/sites/sethcohen/2020/05/23/trump-golfs-as-us-mourns-100000-dead--the-presidents-ugly-memorial-day-message.

60. Tim Walz, "Gov. Tim Walz Press Conference Transcript on Minneapolis Riots," *Rev* (blog), May 29, 2020, https://www.rev.com/blog/transcripts/gov-tim-walz-press-conference-transcript-on-minneapolis-riots.

61. Tessa Duvall, Darcy Costello, and Phillip M. Bailey, "Senator Kamala Harris Demands Federal Investigation of Police Shooting of Breonna Taylor in Kentucky," *USA*

Today, May 13, 2020, https://www.usatoday.com/story/news/nation/2020/05/13/breonna
-taylor-not-target-louisville-police-investigation-when-shot/5181690002; Talis Shelbourne, "Breonna Taylor: Louisville EMT Killed in Botched Police Raid, Lawyer Says,"
Heavy.com, May 10, 2020, https://heavy.com/news/2020/05/breonna-taylor.

62. Mandy McLaren et al., "'No Justice, No Peace': 7 People Shot amid Downtown
Louisville Protests for Breonna Taylor," *Courier-Journal*, May 28, 2020, https://www.courier
-journal.com/story/news/2020/05/28/breonna-taylor-shooting-protesters-rally-downtown
-louisville/5280279002.

63. "Minneapolis Police Precinct and Businesses Set on Fire as Protests over George
Floyd's Death Rage On," May 29, 2020, CBS News Minneapolis, https://www.cbsnews.com
/news/george-floyd-protests-minneapolis-police-third-precinct.

64. Kenya Evelyn, "'We're Expendable': Black Americans Pay the Price as States Lift
Lockdowns," *Guardian*, May 25, 2020, https://www.theguardian.com/world/2020/may/25
/covid-19-lockdowns-african-americans-essential-workers.

65. "Police at Protests Are Concealing Their Identities," NowThis News.com, June 5,
2020, available at https://www.youtube.com/watch?v=6seudSyHW4w.

66. Author prefers to remain anonymous. Quote is from post in reply to "We Want to
Hear About Your Experience at the Black Lives Matter Protests," https://www.buzzfeed.com
/edwinj3, n.d.

67. Blake Stilwell, "Memorial Day by the Numbers: Casualties of Every American
War," Military.com, May 25, 2020, https://www.military.com/memorial-day/how-many-us
-militay-members-died-each-american-war.html.

68. Matthew Dessem, "Police Erupt in Violence Nationwide," *Slate*, May 31, 2020,
https://slate.com/news-and-politics/2020/05/george-floyd-protests-police-violence.html.

69. Elaine Godfrey, "The Congresswoman Pepper-Sprayed by Police," *Atlantic*, May
31, 2020, https://www.theatlantic.com/politics/archive/2020/05/congresswoman-pepper
-sprayed-joyce-beatty/612436.

70. "'These Cops Love You': Michigan Sheriff Joins George Floyd Protesters in Flint,"
Guardian News, May 31, 2020, available at https://www.youtube.com/watch?v=kDbKAkb8oLs.

71. Fannie Lou Hamer, "I'm Sick and Tired of Being Sick and Tired—Dec. 20, 1964,"
at *Archives of Women's Political Communication* (blog), December 20, 2019, https://awpc
.cattcenter.iastate.edu/2019/08/09/im-sick-and-tired-of-being-sick-and-tired-dec-20-1964.

72. Dessem, "Police Erupt in Violence Nationwide."

73. Frances Robles, "A Reporter's Cry on Live TV: 'I'm Getting Shot! I'm Getting
Shot!'" *New York Times*, May 30, 2020, https://www.nytimes.com/2020/05/30/us/minneapolis
-protests-press.html.

JUNE

1. Amanda Seitz, "Old Image Edited to Show White House Black Out," AP News,
June 1, 2020, https://apnews.com/afs:Content:8983690810; SoINeedAName, "Friday Fun:
He HATES Being Called 'Bunker Boy,'" *Politics Plus* (blog), June 5, 2020, https://www
.politicsplus.org/blog/2020/06/05/friday-fun-he-hates-being-called-bunker-boy.

2. Erin Banco, "Listen for Yourself: Trump's 'Unhinged' Rant to Governors on Protests," *Daily Beast*, June 1, 2020, https://www.thedailybeast.com/listen-to-trumps-unhinged
-rant-to-guvs.

3. Adam Jeffery, "Scenes of Protests Across the Country Demanding States Reopen the
Economy amid Coronavirus Pandemic," CNBC, April 18, 2020, https://www.cnbc.com
/2020/04/18/coronavirus-scenes-of-protests-across-the-country-demanding-states-reopen
-the-economy.html.

4. Aaron Morrison, "On the Spot Where George Floyd Died, His Brother Urges
Calm," AP News, June 1, 2020, https://apnews.com/article/virus-outbreak-us-news-ap-top
-news-mn-state-wire-tx-state-wire-20f27b81228c5a947528d9a4c5c88183.

5. Jonathan Allen, "Trump, Tear Gas in Lafayette Square: Memo from the Protest Front Lines," NBC News, June 2, 2020, https://www.nbcnews.com/politics/white-house/memo-front-lines-different-america-n1222066.

6. Sean Collins, "Trump's Push for 'Law and Order' Only Led to More Chaos in DC Monday Night," Vox, June 2, 2020, https://www.vox.com/2020/6/2/21277877/trump-law-and-order-protests-chaos-dc.

7. "Debs at Wysor Grand This Afternoon," advertisement, Muncie Sunday Star, March 25, 1917.

8. Gina Gerbasi, "Friends, I Am OK, but I Am, Frankly, Shaken," Facebook, June 1, 2020, https://www.facebook.com/gini.gerbasi/posts/10157575422089624.

9. Jordan Highsmith, "Confederate Monument Comes down in Linn Park," CBS 42 (blog), June 2, 2020, https://www.cbs42.com/alabama-news/confederate-monument-comes-down-in-linn-park; Audra D. S. Burch, "Birmingham Mayor Orders Removal of Confederate Monument in Public Park," New York Times, June 2, 2020, https://www.nytimes.com/2020/06/02/us/george-floyd-birmingham-confederate-statue.html.

10. Thomas Jefferson, "Founders Online: Proclamation on the Embargo, 19 April 1808," National Archives, April 19, 1808, http://founders.archives.gov/documents/Jefferson/99-01-02-7861.

11. H. N. Muller, "Smuggling into Canada: How the Champlain Valley Defied Jefferson's Embargo," Vermont History 38, no. 1 (Winter 1970): 5–21.

12. Domenico Montanaro, "What Is the Insurrection Act That Trump Is Threatening to Invoke?" NPR, June 1, 2020, https://www.npr.org/2020/06/01/867467714/what-is-the-insurrection-act-that-trump-is-threatening-to-invoke; Egan Millard, "Outraged Episcopal Leaders Condemn Tear-Gassing Clergy, Protesters for Trump Photo Op at Washington Church," Episcopal News Service, June 2, 2020, https://www.episcopalnewsservice.org/2020/06/02/episcopal-leaders-express-outrage-condemn-tear-gassing-protesters-for-trump-photo-op-at-washington-church.

13. Second Congress, Session 1, Chapter XXVIII, "The Militia Act of 1792," May 2, 1792, https://constitution.org/1-Activism/mil/mil_act_1792.htm.

14. Thomas Wentworth Higginson, "Nat Turner's Insurrection," Atlantic, November 7, 2011, https://www.theatlantic.com/magazine/archive/1861/08/nat-turners-insurrection/308736.

15. "R/Minneapolis—All Signs That the Destruction Tonight Were Organized and Largely Unrelated to the Protest," Reddit, June 2, 2020, https://www.reddit.com/r/Minneapolis/comments/gt9qsp/all_signs_that_the_destruction_tonight_were.

16. I must have heard this version of the story recounted to me ten times in the past five days.

17. Robert Evans and Jason Wilson, "The Boogaloo Movement Is Not What You Think," Bellingcat (blog), May 27, 2020, https://www.bellingcat.com/news/2020/05/27/the-boogaloo-movement-is-not-what-you-think.

18. Alex Goldenberg and Joel Finkelstein, Cyber Swarming, Memetic Warfare and Viral Insurgency: How Domestic Militants Organize on Memes to Incite Violent Insurrection and Terror Against Government and Law Enforcement (Network Contagion Research Institute, January 2020), https://ncri.io/reports/cyber-swarming-memetic-warfare-and-viral-insurgency-how-domestic-militants-organize-on-memes-to-incite-violent-insurrection-and-terror-against-government-and-law-enforcement.

19. James Bartholomew, "Easy Virtue," Spectator, April 18, 2015, https://www.spectator.co.uk/article/easy-virtue.

20. Victoria Albert, "Mother of George Floyd's 6-Year-Old Daughter Speaks Out: 'This Is What Those Officers Took,'" CBS News, June 2, 2020, https://www.cbsnews.com/news/george-floyd-mother-of-child-roxie-washington-speaks-out.

21. Mike Demond and Omar Fetouh, "GRAPHIC VIDEO: Two Buffalo Police Officers Suspended After Elderly Man Shoved and Injured," WBFO NPR Buffalo-Toronto, June 4,

2020, https://news.wbfo.org/post/graphic-video-two-buffalo-police-officers-suspended
-after-elderly-man-shoved-and-injured.

22. Greg Doucette and Jason E. Miller, "George Floyd Protest—Police Brutality Videos
on Twitter—Google Drive," 2020, https://docs.google.com/spreadsheets/u/1/d/1YmZeSxpz
52qT-1otkCjWOwOGkQqle7Wd1P7ZM1wMW0E/htmlview?pru=AAABcql6DI8
*mIHYeMnoj9XWUp3Svb_KZA.

23. Stacia Glenn, "'Can't Breathe': Tacoma Police Restraint of Manuel Ellis Caused His
Death, ME Reports," *News Tribune*, June 3, 2020, https://www.thenewstribune.com
/news/local/article243210681.html.

24. Abby Zimet, "The Criminalization of Blackness Itself: Let the Smearing Begin," *Common Dreams*, May 20, 2020, https://www.commondreams.org/further/2020/05/20
/criminalization-blackness-itself-let-smearing-begin.

25. Wesley Lowery, "Analysis: Aren't More White People Than Black People Killed by Police?
Yes, but No," *Washington Post*, July 11, 2016, https://www.washingtonpost.com/news/post-nation
/wp/2016/07/11/arent-more-white-people-than-black-people-killed-by-police-yes-but-no.

26. Samuel Sinyangwe and DeRay Mckesson, "Mapping Police Violence," Mapping
Police Violence, June 30, 2020, https://mappingpoliceviolence.org; Washington Post, "Fatal
Force: Police Shootings Database," *Washington Post*, August 10, 2020, https://www.washington
post.com/graphics/investigations/police-shootings-database; CPDP, "An Introduction to
the Citizens Police Data Project," Invisible Institute, https://invisible.institute/police-data,
accessed June 15, 2021.

27. Christian Davenport, Sarah A. Soule, and David A. Armstrong, "Protesting While
Black? The Differential Policing of American Activism, 1960 to 1990," *American Sociological
Review* 76, no. 1 (February 2011): 152–78.

28. James N. Miller, "Secretary Esper, You Violated Your Oath in Aiding Trump's Photo
Op. That's Why I'm Resigning," *Washington Post*, op-ed, June 2, 2020, https://www
.washingtonpost.com/opinions/2020/06/02/secretary-esper-you-violated-your-oath-aiding
-trumps-photo-op-thats-why-im-resigning.

29. Jeffrey Goldberg, "James Mattis Denounces President Trump, Describes Him as a
Threat to the Constitution," *Atlantic*, June 3, 2020, https://www.theatlantic.com/politics
/archive/2020/06/james-mattis-denounces-trump-protests-militarization/612640.

30. Erica Gonzales, "Obama to Young Black Americans: 'I Want You to Know That
You Matter,'" *Harper's Bazaar*, June 3, 2020, https://www.harpersbazaar.com/culture
/politics/a32759234/barack-obama-george-floyd-speech.

31. Edward-Isaac Dovere, "Why Obama Stepped In," *Atlantic*, June 4, 2020, https://
www.theatlantic.com/politics/archive/2020/06/obamas-minneapolis-race-speech/612646.

32. "A Conversation with President Obama: Reimagining Policing in the Wake of
Continued Police Violence," Obama Foundation, June 3, 2020, available at https://www
.youtube.com/watch?v=q_qB6SsErpA&feature=youtu.be.

33. Shubham Ghosh, "DC Mayor Muriel Bowser Takes on Trump, Sparks Third
Amendment Debate with Call to Remove Troops from Capital," *Meaww*, June 5, 2020,
https://meaww.com/washington-dc-mayor-muriel-bowser-sparks-third-amendment
-controversy-kicking-troops-out-trump.

34. Mark Segraves and NBC Washington Staff, "DC Mayor, President Trump Spar
over Federal Forces on City Streets," *NBC4 Washington* (blog), June 5, 2020, https://www
.nbcwashington.com/news/local/dc-police-inadvertently-gave-national-guard-police
-powers-as-mayor-asked-for-withdrawal/2323919.

35. Alisa Gumbs, "Washington, D.C. Mayor Muriel Bowser Trolls Trump in the Blackest
Way," *Black Enterprise*, June 5, 2020, https://www.blackenterprise.com/washington-d-c
-mayor-muriel-bowser-trolls-president-trump-in-the-blackest-way.

36. Julia Musto, "Trump Says He Went to White House Bunker for 'Inspection,' Hits
Back at Criticism of Church Visit," Fox News, June 3, 2020, https://www.foxnews.com

/media/trump-bunker-inspection-church-tear-gas; David Moye, "Trump Brutally Mocked for Saying He Went to Bunker Just to Inspect It," *Huffington Post*, June 3, 2020, https://www.huffpost.com/entry/trump-bunker-excuse-twitter-mock_n_5ed7c613c5b67887de3fa952.

37. Mary Papenfuss, "Comedy Gem Sarah Cooper Conquers Trump in Hilarious Tik-Tok Videos," *Huffington Post*, June 6, 2020, https://www.huffpost.com/entry/sarah-cooper-tik-tok-trump-spoofs_n_5edc5b97c5b6dcf35913c9a3.

38. Joe Biden, "On Winning a Majority of Delegates in the Democratic Presidential Primary," *Medium*, June 6, 2020, https://medium.com/@JoeBiden/on-winning-a-majority-of-delegates-in-the-democratic-presidential-primary-fc51510aeof8.

39. Josh Mitchell, "U.S. Unemployment Rate Fell to 13.3% in May," *Wall Street Journal*, June 6, 2020, https://www.wsj.com/articles/may-jobs-report-coronavirus-2020-11591310177.

40. US Bureau of Labor Statistics, "Table A-2. Employment Status of the Civilian Population by Race, Sex, and Age," June 6, 2020, https://www.bls.gov/news.release/empsit.to2.htm.

41. Katelyn Burns, "The Unemployment Rate Improved in May, but Left Black Workers Behind," *Vox*, June 6, 2020, https://www.vox.com/policy-and-politics/2020/6/6/21282611/black-workers-left-behind-unemployment.

42. Tyler Clifford, "Jim Cramer: The Pandemic Led to 'One of the Greatest Wealth Transfers in History,'" CNBC, June 4, 2020, https://www.cnbc.com/2020/06/04/cramer-the-pandemic-led-to-a-great-wealth-transfer.html.

43. Dan Burns, "U.S. Chapter 11 Bankruptcy Filings Surge in May," Reuters, June 4, 2020, https://www.reuters.com/article/us-health-coronavirus-bankruptcy-idUSKBN23B2K3.

44. Small Business Administration, *Paycheck Protection Program (PPP) Report, Approvals Through 05/16/2020* (US Small Business Administration, May 2020), https://content.sba.gov/sites/default/files/2020-05/PPP_Report_Net_200518_0.pdf; Emily Flitter, "Loan Money Runs Out While Small-Business Owners Wait in Line," *New York Times*, April 16, 2020, https://www.nytimes.com/2020/04/16/business/coronavirus-sba-loans-out-of-money.html; Danny Meyer and Randy Garutti, "Shake Shack Is Returning Its PPP Loan. Here's Why," *LinkedIn*, April 20, 2020, https://www.linkedin.com/pulse/shake-shack-returning-its-ppp-loan-heres-why-randy-garutti; Emily Stewart, "America's Monopoly Problem, Explained by Your Internet Bill," *Vox*, February 18, 2020, https://www.vox.com/the-goods/2020/2/18/21126347/antitrust-monopolies-internet-telecommunications-cheerleading.

45. President Truman's Committee on Civil Rights, *To Secure These Rights: The Report of President Truman's Committee on Civil Rights*, Harry S Truman Library & Museum: National Archives, October 29, 1947, https://www.trumanlibrary.gov/library/to-secure-these-rights.

46. Adam Harris, "Racism Won't Be Solved by Yet Another Blue-Ribbon Report," *Atlantic*, June 4, 2020, https://www.theatlantic.com/politics/archive/2020/06/george-floyd-racism-police-brutality/612565.

47. Michael McAdams, "Democrats Are Insane," NRCC, June 8, 2020, https://www.nrcc.org/2020/06/08/democrats-are-insane.

48. Scott Morefield, "Tucker Carlson Lays Out Theory on Who Is Funding Antifa," *We the People Daily*, June 5, 2020, https://wethepeopledaily.com/2020/06/05/tucker-carlson-lays-out-theory-on-who-is-funding-antifa.

49. Polly Mosendz and Jameelah D. Robinson, "While Crime Fell, the Cost of Cops Soared," *Bloomberg*, June 4, 2020, https://www.bloomberg.com/news/articles/2020-06-04/america-s-policing-budget-has-nearly-tripled-to-115-billion.

50. Morgan Whitaker, "GOP Declares War on 'War on Poverty,'" MSNBC, January 6, 2014, http://www.msnbc.com/politicsnation/gop-declares-war-the-war-poverty.

51. Mike Maciag, "The Daily Crisis Cops Aren't Trained to Handle," *Governing*, May 2016, https://www.governing.com/topics/public-justice-safety/gov-mental-health-crisis-training-police.html; Mark Meier, "Road Runners," Treatment Advocacy Center, May 2019, https://www.treatmentadvocacycenter.org/road-runners.

52. Jiachuan Wu et al., "Map of George Floyd Protests Around the World," NBC News, June 9, 2020, https://www.nbcnews.com/news/us-news/blog/2020-06-09-george-floyd-protests-n1228061/ncrd1228456#blogHeader.

53. Nature Journal, "Note from the Editors: Nature Joins #ShutDownSTEM," *Nature*, June 10, 2020.

54. Jasmine Roberts, "White Academia: Do Better," *Medium*, June 8, 2020, https://medium.com/the-faculty/white-academia-do-better-fa96cede1fc5.

55. "NASCAR Statement on Confederate Flag," Official Site of NASCAR, June 10, 2020, https://www.nascar.com/news-media/2020/06/10/nascar-statement-on-confederate-flag.

56. "On Capitol Hill, George Floyd's Brother Appeals for Changes to Policing," *NewsHour*, PBS, June 10, 2020, https://www.pbs.org/newshour/show/on-capitol-hill-george-floyds-brother-appeals-for-changes-to-policing.

57. Berkeley Lovelace Jr., "Dr. Anthony Fauci Says Coronavirus Turned 'Out to Be My Worst Nightmare' and It 'Isn't Over,'" CNBC, June 9, 2020, https://www.cnbc.com/2020/06/09/dr-anthony-fauci-says-coronavirus-turned-out-to-be-my-worst-nightmare-and-it-isnt-over.html.

58. Todd Gillman and Gromer Jeffers Jr., "At Dallas Talk on Police and Race, Trump Shrugs Off "Bad Apples' and Again Vows to 'Dominate the Streets,'" *Dallas News*, June 12, 2020, https://www.dallasnews.com/news/politics/2020/06/11/trump-snubs-dallas-top-law-enforcement-officials-all-black-for-talk-about-policing-and-race.

59. Patrick Svitek, "Donald Trump Cautions Against 'Falsely Labeling' Racists While in Dallas to Talk About George Floyd," *Texas Tribune*, June 11, 2020, https://www.texastribune.org/2020/06/11/donald-trump-dallas-texas-george-floyd.

60. John Bacon and Kristin Lam, "Ex-Fort Worth Police Officer Aaron Dean Charged with Murder After Shooting Atatiana Jefferson in Her Home," *USA Today*, October 14, 2019, https://www.usatoday.com/story/news/nation/2019/10/14/fort-worth-shooting-nephew-describes-moments-before-shooting/3973133002.

61. "President Trump Holds Economic Roundtable Discussion," June 11, 2020, C-SPAN, https://www.c-span.org/video/?472983-1/president-trump-holds-economic-roundtable-discussion.

62. Cornell Law School, "Charles C. Green et al. v. County School Board of New Kent County, Virginia et al.," Legal Information Institute, 1968, https://www.law.cornell.edu/supremecourt/text/391/430.

63. Virginia Museum of History et al., "School Busing," Virginia Museum of History & Culture, April 11, 2013, https://www.virginiahistory.org/collections-and-resources/virginia-history-explorer/civil-rights-movement-virginia/school-busing.

64. Dave Chappelle, *8:46*, Netflix Is a Joke, June 12, 2020, https://www.youtube.com/watch?v=3tR6mKcBbT4&feature=youtu.be.

65. Statista, "U.S. COVID-19 Case Rate by State," *Statista*, June 12, 2020, https://www.statista.com/statistics/1109004/coronavirus-covid19-cases-rate-us-americans-by-state.

66. "QuickFacts: Lowndes County, Alabama," US Census Bureau, 2010, https://www.census.gov/quickfacts/lowndescountyalabama.

67. Public School Review, "Top Lowndes County Public Schools," 2020, https://www.publicschoolreview.com/alabama/lowndes-county.

68. Melissa Brown, "An Era of Terror: Montgomery Family Remembers Father's Lynching, Legacy," *Montgomery Advertiser*, April 25, 2018, https://www.montgomeryadvertiser.com/story/news/2018/04/25/equal-justice-initiative-eji-alabama-lynchings-elmore-bolling/524675002.

69. Connor Sheets, "The Black Panther Party's Deep Alabama Roots," AL.com, February 28, 2016, https://www.al.com/news/2016/02/the_black_panther_partys_deep.html.

70. Laura Clawson, "Martin Luther King, Jr.: 'Our Struggle Is for Genuine Equality, Which Means Economic Equality,'" *Daily Kos*, January 21, 2013, https://www.dailykos.com

/story/2013/1/21/1180824/-Martin-Luther-King-Jr-Our-struggle-is-for-genuine-equality
-which-means-economic-equality; Michael K. Honey, "What Happened to Martin Luther
King Jr.'s Dream of Economic Justice?" *Time*, February 20, 2020, https://time.com/5783976
/martin-luther-king-jr-economic-justice.

71. Ed Pilkington, "A Journey Through a Land of Extreme Poverty: Welcome to
America," *Guardian*, December 15, 2017, https://www.theguardian.com/society/2017/dec
/15/america-extreme-poverty-un-special-rapporteur.

72. Phillip Rawls, "Judge: Bingo Witnesses Aimed to Suppress Black Voter Turnout,"
Tuscaloosa News, October 21, 2011, https://www.tuscaloosanews.com/article/20111021
/News/605313725.

73. Talis Shelbourne, "Rayshard Brooks: 5 Fast Facts You Need to Know," Heavy.com,
June 13, 2020, https://heavy.com/news/2020/06/rayshard-brooks-killed-by-atlanta-police.

74. Michelle Solomon, "10 Members of Hallandale Beach Police SWAT Team Resign,"
WPLG, June 13, 2020, https://www.local10.com/news/local/2020/06/13/entire-hallandale
-police-swat-teams-resigns.

75. Curtis Gilbert, Angela Caputo, and Geoff Hing, "Tasers Are Less Reliable Than
Their Maker Has Claimed. The Results Can Be Deadly," American Public Media, May 9,
2019, https://www.apmreports.org/episode/2019/05/09/when-tasers-fail.

76. Jodie Fleischer, "Family of Man Who Fell to Death After Taser Hit Sues County,
Officers," WSBTV, August 8, 2016, https://www.wsbtv.com/news/local/dekalb-county
/family-of-man-who-fell-to-death-after-tasering-sues-county-officers/419659793.

77. "Shock Tactics: Reuters Taser Tracker," Reuters, December 28, 2018, http://www
.reuters.com/investigates/special-report/usa-taser-tracker.

78. Steven Rice, "Does One Bad Apple Spoil the Bunch?" Education Committee of the
Botanical Society of America, Botany.org, March 2001, https://www.botany.org/bsa/misc
/mcintosh/badapple.html.

79. Martha Mendoza, "Deputy Killed in California Ambush by Travis-Based Air Force
Sergeant," *Air Force Times*, June 6, 2020, https://www.airforcetimes.com/news/your-air-force
/2020/06/07/deputy-killed-in-california-ambush-by-travis-based-air-force-sergeant.

80. AntiFash Gordon, "An @UR_Ninja Reporter Was Attacked Tonight in Philadelphia by a Vigilante Gang Armed with Baseball Bats," Threaderapp, June 13, 2020, https://
threadreaderapp.com/thread/1272024704610643970.html.

81. Jeff Gammage et al., "For Second Day, Group 'Protects' Christopher Columbus
Statue in South Philadelphia; Mayor Denounces 'Vigilantism,'" *Inquirer*, June 14, 2020,
https://www.inquirer.com/news/floyd-protest-columbus-statue-protesters-unrest-philadelphia
-police-20200614.html.

82. Mike Valerio, "National Museum of African American History & Culture Asks
Protesters for Lafayette Square Items," WUSA9, June 12, 2020, https://www.wusa9.com
/article/news/local/protests/smithsonian-museum-wants-objects-from-dc-protests-for
-history-collection/65-7fe2773f-ed7d-45bd-98c5-b3678df3f481.

83. "Montgomery City Council Meeting (6/16/20)," June 16, 2020, available at https://
www.youtube.com/watch?reload=9&v=73DkuZOy3T8&feature=youtu.be.

84. Steven Greenhouse, "In-House Audit Says Wal-Mart Violated Labor Laws," *New
York Times*, January 13, 2004, https://www.nytimes.com/2004/01/13/us/in-house-audit-says
-wal-mart-violated-labor-laws.html.

85. Catherine Ruetschlin and Dedrick Asante-Muhammad, "The Retail Race Divide,"
Demos.org, June 2, 2015, https://www.demos.org/research/retail-race-divide-how-retail
-industry-perpetuating-racial-inequality-21st-century.

86. Jamelle Bouie, "Why Juneteenth Matters," *New York Times*, June 18, 2020, https://
www.nytimes.com/2020/06/18/opinion/juneteenth-slavery-freedom.html.

87. "U.S. Sets Record for Daily New Cases as Virus Surges in South and West," *New York
Times*, June 24, 2020, https://www.nytimes.com/2020/06/24/world/coronavirus-updates.html.

88. Seth Cohen, "No Second Wave? Mike Pence's Reckless Anti-Science Optimism," *Forbes*, July 19, 2020, https://www.forbes.com/sites/sethcohen/2020/07/19/mike-pences -reckless-anti-science-optimism; Dylan Scott, "What Mike Pence Got Wrong About the New Coronavirus Spikes," *Vox*, June 17, 2020, https://www.vox.com/2020/6/17/21294392 /covid-19-coronavirus-us-cases-mike-pence-wsj.

89. Michael R. Pence, "There Isn't a Coronavirus 'Second Wave,'" US White House, June 16, 2020, https://www.whitehouse.gov/articles/vice-president-mike-pence-op-ed -isnt-coronavirus-second-wave.

90. Benjamin Swasey, "Trump Retweets Video of Apparent Supporter Saying 'White Power,'" NPR, June 28, 2020, https://www.npr.org/sections/live-updates-protests-for -racial-justice/2020/06/28/884392576/trump-retweets-video-of-apparent-supporter -saying-white-power.

91. Michael Grunwald, "The Future of the GOP Looks a Lot like This Fast-Growing Community in Florida," *Politico*, June 18, 2018, https://politi.co/2yk66FP.

92. Kim Bell and Rachel Rice, "Couple Points Guns at Protesters Marching to St. Louis Mayor's Home to Demand Resignation," *STLToday*, June 29, 2020, https://www.stltoday.com /news/local/crime-and-courts/couple-points-guns-at-protesters-marching-to-st-louis-mayor -s-home-to-demand-resignation/article_9edc57ed-c307-583f-9226-a44ba6ac9c03.html; Stefene Russell, "A Decades-Long Renovation Returns a Midwestern Palazzo to Its Origi- nal Glory," *STLmag*, August 16, 2018, https://www.stlmag.com/api/content/cffeeb48-a0e5 -11e8-86dd-120e7ad5cf50.

93. Shirin Ghaffary, "The Real Cost of Amazon," *Vox*, June 29, 2020, https://www.vox .com/recode/2020/6/29/21303643/amazon-coronavirus-warehouse-workers-protest-jeff -bezos-chris-smalls-boycott-pandemic.

94. Casey Newton, "How Amazon Is Growing Its Power During the Pandemic," *The Verge*, May 14, 2020, https://www.theverge.com/interface/2020/5/14/21257313/amazon -delivery-times-worker-raises-price-gouging-liability-pandemic.

JULY

1. "Business and Industry: Time Series/Trend Charts-44X72: Retail Trade and Food Services," US Census Bureau, https://www.census.gov/econ/currentdata/dbsearch?program =MRTS&startYear=2019&endYear=2020&categories=44511&dataType=MPCSM&geoLevel =US&notAdjusted=1&submit=GET+DATA&releaseScheduleId, accessed June 15, 2021; Liam O'Connell, "Monthly Food and Beverage Store Sales U.S. 2020," *Statista*, July 20, 2020, https://www.statista.com/statistics/805047/food-and-beverage-store-sales-us-by -month; USDA, "Summary Findings-Food Price Outlook 2020," US Department of Agri- culture, Economic Research Service, July 2020, https://www.ers.usda.gov/data-products /food-price-outlook/summary-findings.

2. Russell Redman, "Sales at Publix Jump 20% in Second Quarter," *Supermarket News*, August 3, 2020, https://www.supermarketnews.com/retail-financial/sales-publix-jump-20 -second-quarter.

3. George Petras and Paul Davidson, "The COVID Economy in 6 Charts: Rebounding from Recession Could Prove Tougher in Months Ahead," *USA Today*, July 26, 2020, https:// www.usatoday.com/in-depth/news/2020/07/26/covid-economy-unemployment-report-6 -charts/5471545002.

4. Sam Gillette, "Little Free Libraries Converted to Food Banks During Coronavirus Pandemic," People.com, March 20, 2020, https://people.com/food/little-free-libraries -converted-to-food-banks-during-coronavirus-pandemic.

5. Tami Luhby, "Food Banks Struggle as Demand Explodes," CNN, April 3, 2020, https:// www.cnn.com/2020/03/31/politics/food-banks-supplies-groceries-coronavirus/index.html.

6. Natalia Gurevich, "Cow Palace Shows Have Stopped, and Now It's Hosting Food Lines," Mission Local, July 29, 2020, https://missionlocal.org/2020/07/the-shows-have -stopped-at-the-cow-palace-now-it-is-host-to-one-of-the-citys-longest-food-lines.

7. Ben Pope, "SEE IT: United Center Packed with 774,840 Pounds of Food Destined for Chicago Food Pantries," *Chicago Sun-Times*, April 9, 2020, https://chicago.suntimes.com/coronavirus/2020/4/9/21215020/united-center-coronavirus-pandemic-greater-chicago-food-depository-blackhawks-bulls.

8. Jacob Carpenter, "HISD Ending Food Distribution Plan, Switching to Kids-Only Meal Pickup," *Houston Chronicle*, May 20, 2020, https://www.houstonchronicle.com/news/houston-texas/houston/article/HISD-ending-food-distribution-plan-switching-to-15281896.php.

9. William Wan and Heather Long, "'Cries for Help': Drug Overdoses Are Soaring During the Coronavirus Pandemic," *Washington Post*, July 1, 2020, https://www.washingtonpost.com/health/2020/07/01/coronavirus-drug-overdose.

10. Brianna Ehley, "Pandemic Unleashes a Spike in Overdose Deaths," *Politico*, June 29, 2020, https://www.politico.com/news/2020/06/29/pandemic-unleashes-a-spike-in-overdose-deaths-345183.

11. Kelly Kennedy, "Madison County Seeing a Spike in Overdoses, Deaths amid Pandemic," RocketCityNow.com, May 13, 2020, https://www.rocketcitynow.com/article/news/local/madison-county-seeing-a-spike-in-overdoses-deaths-amid-pandemic/525-021e43d6-44de-4c50-99ee-a326f2394a22.

12. Molly McCann Pineo and Rebecca M. Schwartz, "Commentary on the Coronavirus Pandemic: Anticipating a Fourth Wave in the Opioid Epidemic," *Psychological Trauma: Theory, Research, Practice, and Policy*, August 2020, https://pesquisa.bvsalud.org/global-literature-on-novel-coronavirus-2019-ncov/resource/en/covidwhomdl-32496102.

13. Yuhua Bao, Arthur Robin Williams, and Bruce R. Schackman, "COVID-19 Could Change the Way We Respond to the Opioid Crisis—for the Better," *Psychiatric Services* 71, no. 21 (August 12, 2020): appi.ps.202000226.

14. Rahi Abouk, Rosalie Liccardo Pacula, and David Powell, "Association Between State Laws Facilitating Pharmacy Distribution of Naloxone and Risk of Fatal Overdose," *JAMA Internal Medicine* 179, no. 6 (June 1, 2020): 805–11.

15. Julie Bruneau et al., "Management of Opioid Use Disorders: A National Clinical Practice Guideline," *CMAJ: Canadian Medical Association Journal* 190, no. 9 (March 5, 2018): E247–57.

16. Yuki Noguchi, "A New Addiction Crisis: Treatment Centers Face Financial Collapse," NPR, June 15, 2020, https://www.npr.org/sections/health-shots/2020/06/15/865006675/a-new-addiction-crisis-treatment-centers-face-financial-collapse.

17. "Medicare Telemedicine Health Care Provider Fact Sheet," Centers for Medicaid and Medicare Services, March 17, 2020, https://www.cms.gov/newsroom/fact-sheets/medicare-telemedicine-health-care-provider-fact-sheet.

18. Nora D. Volkow, "Collision of the COVID-19 and Addiction Epidemics," *Annals of Internal Medicine* 173, no. 1 (April 2, 2020): 61–62.

19. Sessi Kubawar Blanchard, "An Indiana Police Dept. No Longer Reversing Overdoses During Pandemic," *Filter* (blog), April 9, 2020, https://filtermag.org/cops-naloxone-coronavirus.

20. William C. Becker and David A. Fiellin, "When Epidemics Collide: Coronavirus Disease 2019 (COVID-19) and the Opioid Crisis," *Annals of Internal Medicine* 173, no. 1 (April 2, 2020): 59–60.

21. David Smith, "'I Think You Can Trust Me': Fauci Stands Firm as Trump Works to Undermine Him," *Guardian*, July 15, 2020, https://www.theguardian.com/us-news/2020/jul/15/dr-fauci-donald-trump-attacks-covid-19.

22. Peter Navarro, "Anthony Fauci Has Been Wrong About Everything with Me," *USA Today*, July 14, 2020, https://www.usatoday.com/story/opinion/todaysdebate/2020/07/14/anthony-fauci-wrong-with-me-peter-navarro-editorials-debates/5439374002.

23. Tamara Keith, "'He Shouldn't Be Doing That': Trump Weighs In on Navarro Op-Ed Attacking Fauci," NPR, July 15, 2020, https://www.npr.org/sections/coronavirus

-live-updates/2020/07/15/891327661/white-house-disavows-attack-on-fauci-from-trump
-trade-adviser.

24. "Mt. Lebanon's Joke & Murphy's Bad Advice," *Allegheny Institute for Public Policy* (blog), October 10, 2018, https://www.alleghenyinstitute.org/mt-lebanons-joke-murphys -bad-advice.

25. Gerard F. Anderson, Peter Hussey, and Varduhi Petrosyan, "It's Still the Prices, Stupid: Why the US Spends So Much on Health Care, and a Tribute to Uwe Reinhardt," *Health Affairs* 38, no. 1 (January 1, 2019): 87–95.

26. Associated Press, "Coronavirus Data Is Funneled away from CDC, Sparking Worries," *Los Angeles Times*, July 16, 2020, https://www.latimes.com/world-nation/story/2020 -07-16/coronavirus-data-is-funneled-away-from-cdc-sparking-worries.

27. NPR (@NPR) "BREAKING: John Lewis, an icon of the civil rights movement, has died at 80. He began his nearly 60-year career in public service leading sit-ins at segregated lunch counters in the Jim Crow-era South. He went on to become a force in Democratic politics. https://T.Co/AJyydTtXnI," Twitter, July 17, 2020, https://twitter.com/NPR /status/1284339170052313091.

28. Colin Dwyer, "C.T. Vivian, Civil Rights Leader and Champion of Nonviolent Action, Dies at 95," NPR, July 17, 2020, https://www.npr.org/2020/07/17/892223763/c-t -vivian-civil-rights-leader-and-champion-of-nonviolent-action-dies-at-95.

29. Cameron McWhirter, *Red Summer: The Summer of 1919 and the Awakening of Black America* (New York: Henry Holt, 2011), 15.

30. Equal Justice Initiative, *Lynching in America: Targeting Black Veterans* (Montgomery, AL: Equal Justice Initiative, October 2017), https://eji.org/wp-content/uploads/2019/10 /lynching-in-america-targeting-black-veterans-web.pdf.

31. BlackPast, (1919) W. E. B. Du Bois, "Returning Soldiers," editorial from The Crisis, April 7, 2019, https://www.blackpast.org/african-american-history/w-e-b-dubois -returning-soldiers-editorial-from-the-crisis-may-1919.

32. Eric Arnesen, "'Red Summer: The Summer of 1919 and the Awakening of Black America' by Cameron McWhirter," *Chicago Tribune*, November 18, 2011, https://www .chicagotribune.com/entertainment/books/ct-xpm-2011-11-18-sc-ent-books-red-summer -mcwhirter-20111118-story.html.

33. Matthew Wills, "The Mob Violence of the Red Summer," *JSTOR Daily*, May 14, 2019, https://daily.jstor.org/the-mob-violence-of-the-red-summer.

34. See the full catalog of CSA monuments at "Whose Heritage? Public Symbols of the Confederacy," Southern Poverty Law Center, February 1, 2019, https://www.splcenter .org/20190201/whose-heritage-public-symbols-confederacy.

35. Olivia B. Waxman, "The Forgotten March That Started the National Civil Rights Movement Took Place 100 Years Ago," *Time*, July 28, 2017, https://time.com/4828991/east -saint-louis-riots-1917.

36. "World-Wide Ship Strike, Plan of Reds," *New York Tribune*, July 17, 1919.

37. Sara Bullard, ed., *The Ku Klux Klan: A History of Racism & Violence*, 5th ed. (Montgomery, AL: Southern Poverty Law Center, 1997).

38. Alex Riggens and Teri Figueroa, "Video Shows Undercover San Diego Police Arresting Protester, Rushing Her into Unmarked Van," *Los Angeles Times*, June 6, 2020, https://www.latimes.com/california/story/2020-06-06/video-undercover-san-diego-police -arresting-protester-unmarked-van.

39. David Edwards, "Columbus 'Paramilitary' Police with Assault Weapons Jump Out of Unmarked Vans to Abduct Protester," *Raw Story*, June 25, 2020, https://www.rawstory .com/2020/06/columbus-paramilitary-police-with-assault-weapons-jump-out-of-unmarked -vans-to-abduct-protester.

40. Anna Akhmatova, "'Epilogue,' from Requiem (1935–1940)," *Brooklyn Quarterly*, March 19, 2014, http://brooklynquarterly.org/epilogue-from-requiem-1935-1940.

41. Kaitlin Flanigan, "Timeline: 50 Days of Portland Protests," *KOIN CBS 6* (blog), July 18, 2020, https://www.koin.com/news/protests/timeline-50-days-of-portland-protests.

42. Jonathan Levinson and Conrad Wilson, "Federal Law Enforcement Use Unmarked Vehicles to Grab Protesters Off Portland Streets," OPB, July 16, 2020, https://www.opb.org/news/article/federal-law-enforcement-unmarked-vehicles-portland-protesters.

43. "DHS Official on Reports of Federal Officers Detaining Protesters in Portland, Ore.," *All Things Considered*, NPR, July 17, 2020, https://www.npr.org/2020/07/17/892393079/dhs-official-on-reports-of-federal-officers-detaining-protesters-in-portland-ore.

44. Tatiana Cozzarelli, "Trump's Federal Police Are Kidnapping and Brutalizing Protesters in Portland," *Truthout*, July 18, 2020, https://truthout.org/articles/trumps-federal-police-are-kidnapping-and-brutalizing-protesters-in-portland; David A. Graham, "America Gets an Interior Ministry," *Atlantic*, July 21, 2020, https://www.theatlantic.com/ideas/archive/2020/07/americas-interior-ministry/614389.

45. Josh Marshall, "Cuccinelli: Totally Legal and Totally Cool How CBP and ICE Now Control Your City," *Talking Points Memo*, July 18, 2020, https://talkingpointsmemo.com/edblog/cuccinelli-totally-legal-and-totally-cool-how-cpb-and-ice-now-control-your-city.

46. Megan R. Gerber, "The Things They Carry: Veterans and the COVID-19 Pandemic," *Journal of General Internal Medicine* (July 28, 2020): 1–2.

47. Jodie G. Katon et al., "Adverse Childhood Experiences, Military Service, and Adult Health," *American Journal of Preventive Medicine* 49, no. 4 (October 2015): 573–82.

48. "COVID-19 National Summary—VA Access to Care," Veterans Administration, July 28, 2020, https://www.accesstocare.va.gov/Healthcare/COVID19NationalSummary.

49. Danielle Zoellner, "Portland's Wall of Moms Protest Group Describe the Abuse They've Received from Federal Officers," *Independent*, July 23, 2020, https://www.independent.co.uk/news/world/americas/portland-wall-of-moms-protest-federal-officers-trump-a9635066.html.

50. Steve Vladeck and Robert Chesney, "The National Security Law Podcast: Portland Trailblazing," *Lawfare*, July 21, 2020, https://www.lawfareblog.com/national-security-law-podcast-portland-trailblazing.

51. "Justice Department Releases $61 Million in Awards to Support Efforts to Combat Violent Crime in Seven U.S. Cities," US Department of Justice, May 11, 2020, https://www.justice.gov/opa/pr/justice-department-releases-61-million-awards-support-efforts-combat-violent-crime-seven-us.

52. "Attorney General William P. Barr Announces Launch of Operation Legend," US Department of Justice, July 8, 2020, https://www.justice.gov/opa/pr/attorney-general-william-p-barr-announces-launch-operation-legend.

53. "Operation Legend," Federal Bureau of Investigation, 2020, https://www.fbi.gov/wanted/operation-legend.

54. Matt Zapotosky and Annie Gowen, "Trump's 'Operation Legend' Was Supposed to Combat Crime. It's Produced One Arrest, and Some See a Political Stunt," *Washington Post*, July 23, 2020, https://www.washingtonpost.com/national-security/trumps-operation-legend-was-supposed-to-combat-crime-its-produced-one-arrest-and-some-see-a-political-stunt/2020/07/23/cf03eba6-cd09-11ea-91f1-28aca4d833a0_story.html.

55. Piper McDaniel, "Portland Protests Draw Thousands, Intense Federal Response, Gas Friday," *OregonLive*, July 25, 2020, https://www.oregonlive.com/portland/2020/07/protesters-in-portland-prepared-friday-for-looming-confrontation-with-federal-officers-live-updates.html.

56. Tuck Woodstock, "No Matter How Many Meals We Serve, They're Still Going to Attack Us," *Bon Appétit*, July 29, 2020, https://www.bonappetit.com/story/riot-ribs-pdx.

57. E. D. Mondainé, "Portland's Protests Were Supposed to Be About Black Lives. Now, They're White Spectacle," *Washington Post*, op-ed, July 23, 2020, https://www.washingtonpost.com/opinions/2020/07/23/portlands-protests-were-supposed-be-about-black-lives-now-theyre-white-spectacle.

58. Mike Baker and Hallie Golden, "Seattle Protests: Fires and Tear Gas as Thousands March Through City," *New York Times*, July 25, 2020, https://www.nytimes.com/2020/07/25/us/protests-seattle-portland.html.

59. Lucy Tompkins, "Here's What You Need to Know About Elijah McClain's Death," *New York Times*, June 30, 2020, https://www.nytimes.com/article/who-was-elijah-mcclain.html.

60. Stephen Goin, "LMPD Announces Safety Plan Ahead of Black Armed Group Action, Counter Protests," WAVE3 NBC Louisville, July 23, 2020, https://www.wave3.com/2020/07/23/lmpd-announces-safety-plan-ahead-black-armed-group-action-counter-protests.

61. Chris Kenning et al., "Louisville Protests: NFAC, Three Percenters Demonstrate Downtown," *Louisville Courier-Journal*, July 25, 2020, https://www.courier-journal.com/story/news/local/2020/07/25/louisville-protests-nfac-three-percenters-expected-demonstrate/3288198001.

62. "GSS General Social Survey," NORC, July 30, 2020, http://www.gss.norc.org.

63. Marc Hetherington and Jonathan M. Ladd, "Destroying Trust in the Media, Science, and Government Has Left America Vulnerable to Disaster," *Brookings* (blog), May 1, 2020, https://www.brookings.edu/blog/fixgov/2020/05/01/destroying-trust-in-the-media-science-and-government-has-left-america-vulnerable-to-disaster.

64. Kelly McBride, "NPR Let the US Attorney General Tell a Falsehood On the Air," NPR, July 16, 2020, https://www.npr.org/sections/publiceditor/2020/07/16/890401446/npr-let-the-us-attorney-general-tell-a-falsehood-on-the-air.

65. Sarah N. Lynch and Jan Wolfe, "U.S. Attorney General Barr Fends Off Democrats' Attacks over Protests," Reuters, July 29, 2020, https://af.reuters.com/article/worldNews/idAFKCN24T1AP.

66. Will Steakin and Libby Cathey, "Trump Suggests Delaying November Election, Something He Doesn't Have the Power to Do," ABC News, July 30, 2020, https://abcnews.go.com/Politics/trump-suggests-delaying-november-election/story?id=72074375.

67. Dara Lind, "'Defendant Shall Not Attend Protests': In Portland, Getting Out of Jail Requires Relinquishing Constitutional Rights," *ProPublica*, July 28, 2020, https://www.propublica.org/article/defendant-shall-not-attend-protests-in-portland-getting-out-of-jail-requires-relinquishing-constitutional-rights?token=Z8oNpH3ypdpU2VX97FRFIzEJC6NBjm2A.

68. Catherine Herridge, (@CBS_Herridge), "#Whistleblower #PortlandProtest," Twitter, September 14, 2020, https://twitter.com/CBS_Herridge/status/1305642555854524419.

69. Shane Harris, "DHS Compiled 'Intelligence Reports' on Journalists Who Published Leaked Documents," *Washington Post*, July 30, 2020, https://www.washingtonpost.com/national-security/dhs-compiled-intelligence-reports-on-journalists-who-published-leaked-documents/2020/07/30/5be5ec9e-d25b-11ea-9038-af089b63ac21_story.html.

70. Jacques Ellul, *Propaganda: The Formation of Men's Attitudes*, trans. Konrad Kellen and Jean Lerner (New York: Vintage, 1973).

71. Rachel Siegel and Andrew Van Dam, "U.S. Economy Contracted at Fastest Quarterly Rate on Record from April to June as Coronavirus Walloped Workers, Businesses," *Washington Post*, July 30, 2020, https://www.washingtonpost.com/business/2020/07/30/gdp-q2-coronavirus; Andrew Van Dam, "Did a Third of the Economy Really Vanish in Just Three Months?" *Washington Post*, July 30, 2020, https://www.washingtonpost.com/business/2020/07/30/did-third-economy-really-vanish-just-three-months.

72. Dirk VanderHart and Conrad Wilson, "Oregon Gov. Kate Brown Announces 'Phased' Removal of Federal Officers from Portland," *OPB*, July 29, 2020, https://www.opb.org/article/2020/07/29/oregon-portland-deal-announced-federal-officers-phased-removal.

AUGUST

1. Laurie Garrett, "America's Schools Are a Moral and Medical Catastrophe," *Foreign Policy* (blog), July 24, 2020, https://foreignpolicy.com/2020/07/24/americas-schools-are-a-moral-and-medical-catastrophe.

2. Young Joon Park et al., "Early Release—Contact Tracing During Coronavirus Disease Outbreak, South Korea, 2020," *Emerging Infectious Disease Journal* 26, no. 10 (July 16, 2020).

3. Gilad Edelman, "'Covid Parties' Are Not a Thing," *Wired*, July 2, 2020, https://www.wired.com/story/covid-parties-are-not-a-thing.

4. Soo Kim, "Kentucky Bar Defies Mask Order: 'We Are Americans—We're Going to Do What We Want,'" *Newsweek*, July 14, 2020, https://www.newsweek.com/kentucky-bar -defies-mask-order-we-are-americanswere-going-do-what-we-want-1517533.

5. Joanne Guthrie and Katherine Ralston, "USDA ERS—School Breakfast Program," USDA, October 1, 2020, https://www.ers.usda.gov/topics/food-nutrition-assistance/child -nutrition-programs/school-breakfast-program.

6. Peter S. Goodman, Patricia Cohen, and Rachel Chaundler, "European Workers Draw Paychecks. American Workers Scrounge for Food," *New York Times*, July 3, 2020, https://www .nytimes.com/2020/07/03/business/economy/europe-us-jobless-coronavirus.html.

7. Alex Henderson, "Betsy DeVos Accused of Diverting Coronavirus Relief Funds from Poor Students to Wealthy Private Schools: 'As Immoral as It Is Illegal,'" AlterNet.org, July 23, 2020, https://www.alternet.org/2020/07/betsy-devos-accused-of-diverting-coronavirus -relief-funds-from-poor-students-to-wealthy-private-schools-as-immoral-as-it-is-illegal; Arianna MacNeill, "Pressley to DeVos on Opening Schools Safely: 'I Wouldn't Trust You to Care for a House Plant,'" MSN, July 13, 2020, https://www.msn.com/en-us/news/us /pressley-to-devos-on-opening-schools-safely-i-wouldn-e2-80-99t-trust-you-to-care-for-a -house-plant/ar-BB16EqJM?fbclid=IwAR2_vvaICqVOKVOKyARZzLVTrP574Q05AY8gm -sQA4r8pNSqGNcnMjNbXxw.

8. Jeneen Interlandi, "Why We're Losing the Battle with Covid-19," *New York Times*, July 14, 2020, https://www.nytimes.com/2020/07/14/magazine/covid-19-public-health-texas.html; Marty Schladen, "Ohio Democrats Frustrated by Reluctance Toward Mask Order Enforce- ment," *ColumbusUnderground.com* (blog), July 13, 2020, https://www.columbusunderground .com/ohio-democrats-frustrated-by-reluctance-toward-mask-order-enforcement-ocj1.

9. "Trump's Brutal Interview with Chris Wallace," *The Daily Show with Trevor Noah*, Comedy Central, July 20, 2020, available at https://www.youtube.com/watch?v=5coxkg X4itQ; "President Trump Exclusive Interview," with Jonathan Swan, *AXIOS on HBO*, August 3, 2020, available at https://www.youtube.com/watch?v=zaaTZkqsaxY&feature=emb_logo.

10. Gwenda Blair, "How Norman Vincent Peale Taught Donald Trump to Worship Himself," *Politico*, October 6, 2015, https://politi.co/2HiMQss.

11. Walter C. Langer, *A Psychological Analysis of Adolph Hitler, His Life and Legend* (Wash- ington, DC: Office of Strategic Services/CIA, 1943), https://www.cia.gov/library/readingroom /document/cia-rdp78-02646r000600240001-5.

12. Michael Lind, "This Is What the Future of American Politics Looks Like," *Politico Magazine*, May 22, 2016, https://www.politico.com/magazine/story/2016/05/2016-election -realignment-partisan-political-party-policy-democrats-republicans-politics-213909.

13. "Shortage of Coins in Circulation Causes Concerns for Small Businesses and Con- sumers," *CBS Evening News*, July 11, 2020, available at https://www.youtube.com/watch?v =lO5YsgnegdI; "Fed Chair Powell: Fed Plans to Work with U.S. Mint and Create Task Force to Address Coin Shortage," CNBC, July 29, 2020, available at https://www.youtube .com/watch?v=oamBAcdZaqo.

14. "Statement from the U.S. Coin Task Force on the Coin Circulation Issue," US Federal Reserve, July 24, 2020, https://www.frbservices.org/news/communications/072420 -cash-us-coin-task-force-coin-circulation-issue.html.

15. "The Fed—Why Do U.S. Coins Seem to Be in Short Supply?" US Federal Reserve, August 7, 2020, https://www.federalreserve.gov/faqs/why-do-us-coins-seem-to-be-in-short -supply-coin-shortage.htm; Kelly Anne Smith, "Is There Really a Coin Shortage?" *Forbes*, July 20, 2020, https://www.forbes.com/sites/advisor/2020/07/20/is-there-really-a-coin-shortage.

16. Tim Congdon, "Get Ready for the Return of Inflation," *Wall Street Journal*, op-ed, April 23, 2020, https://www.wsj.com/articles/get-ready-for-the-return-of-inflation -11587659836.

17. David Beckworth, "Inflation: A Misguided Fear," *National Review* (blog), May 6, 2020, https://www.nationalreview.com/2020/05/inflation-a-misguided-fear; Neil Irwin, "Should We Fear Post-Pandemic Inflation?" *New York Times*, May 28, 2020, https://www.nytimes.com/2020 /05/28/upshot/should-we-fear-inflation.html; Gary Smith, "Inflation Is the Least of Our Worries!" *Mind Matters*, June 29, 2020, https://mindmatters.ai/2020/06/inflation-is-the -least-of-our-worries.

18. Catherine Thorbecke, "'Nothing Compares': Unemployment Filings Top 1 Million for 20th Straight Week," ABC News, August 6, 2020, https://abcnews.go.com/Business /compares-unemployment-filings-top-million-20th-straight-week/story?id=71942446.

19. L. Frazier and Deborah Cohen, eds., *Gender and Sexuality in 1968: Transformative Politics in the Cultural Imagination* (New York: Palgrave Macmillan US, 2009).

20. Gerd-Rainer Horn, *The Spirit of '68: Rebellion in Western Europe and North America, 1956–1976* (New York: Oxford University Press, 2007).

21. Adam Hilton, "Searching for a New Politics: The New Politics Movement and the Struggle to Democratize the Democratic Party, 1968–1978," *New Political Science* 38, no. 2 (April 2, 2016): 141–59.

22. This Day in American History, "Today, 1968—Democratic Convention Besieged by Protesters," Facebook, August 20, 2020, https://www.facebook.com/watch/?v=6488451324 89290.

23. Ed Kilgore, "The Origins of the 'Police Riot,'" *Intelligencer*, June 9, 2020, https:// nymag.com/intelligencer/2020/06/remembering-the-walker-report-and-the-first-police -riot.html.

24. Judy Tzu-Chun Wu, "The U.S. 1968: Third-Worldism, Feminisms, and Liberal- ism," *American Historical Review* 123, no. 3 (June 1, 2018): 710–16.

25. Matt Stevens, "Joe Biden Accepts Presidential Nomination: Full Transcript," *New York Times*, August 20, 2020, https://www.nytimes.com/2020/08/20/us/politics/biden -presidential-nomination-dnc.html.

26. Russell Berman, "Barack Obama Is Scared," *Atlantic*, August 20, 2020, https://www .theatlantic.com/politics/archive/2020/08/obama-trump-biden-dnc/615436.

27. Eddie Rivera, "One Officer's Camera Off During Shooting, Other Officer's Foot- age to Be Released Today; Demonstrations Continue," *PasadenaNow.com*, August 19, 2020, https://www.pasadenanow.com/main/protests-ramp-up-in-pasadena-over-fatal-police -shooting.

28. Timothy B. Lee, "Detroit Police Chief Cops to 96-Percent Facial Recognition Er- ror Rate," *Ars Technica*, June 30, 2020, https://arstechnica.com/tech-policy/2020/06/detroit -police-chief-admits-facial-recognition-is-wrong-96-of-the-time; Kate Cox, "Cops in Miami, NYC Arrest Protesters from Facial Recognition Matches," *Ars Technica*, August 19, 2020, https://arstechnica.com/tech-policy/2020/08/cops-in-miami-nyc-arrest-protesters from-facial-recognition-matches.

29. Danielle Schulkin, "White Supremacist Infiltration of US Police Forces: Fact- Checking National Security Advisor O'Brien," *Just Security*, June 1, 2020, https://www .justsecurity.org/70507/white-supremacist-infiltration-of-us-police-forces-fact-checking -national-security-advisor-obrien.

30. "Video: Video Captures Fatal Police Shooting of Trayford Pellerin," ABC News, August 23, 2020, https://abcnews.go.com/US/video/video-captures-fatal-police-shooting -trayford-pellerin-72555713; Chandler Thornton and Dakin Andone, "Louisiana Officials Are Investigating the Police Shooting of a 31-Year-Old Black Man," CNN, August 24, 2020, https://www.cnn.com/2020/08/22/us/trayford-pellerin-louisiana-police-shooting /index.html.

31. Megan Wyatt, "Trayford Pellerin, Who Died at Hands of Lafayette Police, Had Lengthy Criminal History," *Acadiana Advocate*, August 25, 2020, https://www.theadvocate .com/acadiana/news/crime_police/article_788584e6-e687-11ea-8665-076eb1a4c875.html.

32. John McWhorter, "Racist Police Violence Reconsidered," *Quillette* (blog), June 11, 2020, https://quillette.com/2020/06/11/racist-police-violence-reconsidered.

33. Seren Morris, "Tropical Storms Marco and Laura Are Both Forecast to Hit Louisiana This Week," *Newsweek*, August 24, 2020, https://www.newsweek.com/tropical-storms -marco-laura-path-tracker-hurricane-louisiana-1527113.

34. Rong-Gong Lin II, Alex Wigglesworth, and Susanne Rust, "Over 1 Million California Acres Have Burned Since July as Monster Fires Rage in Bay Area," *Los Angeles Times*, August 22, 2020, https://www.latimes.com/california/story/2020-08-22/more-than-a-million -acres-have-burned-in-california-since-july-as-monster-fires-rage-around-bay-area.

35. Les Steed, "Incredibly Rare 'FIRENADO' Touches Down During Wild California Blaze," *Sun*, August 16, 2020, https://www.thesun.co.uk/news/12418815/rare-firenado -rotating-columns-fire-whirls-wild-california-nevada-blaze.

36. Kasha Patel, "Smoke Shrouds the U.S. West After More Than 10,000 Lightning Strikes Ignite Hundreds of Wildfires Across California," *SciTechDaily* (blog), August 21, 2020, https://scitechdaily.com/smoke-shrouds-the-u-s-west-after-more-than-10000 -lightning-strikes-ignite-hundreds-of-wildfires-across-california.

37. Kellen Browning et al., "Scope of California Wildfires Is Staggering," *New York Times*, August 24, 2020, https://www.nytimes.com/2020/08/24/us/california-fires.html.

38. Emily Wilder, "Arizona Wildfires So Far in 2020 Burn More Than 2018 and 2019 Combined," *Arizona Republic*, August 17, 2020, https://www.azcentral.com/story/news/local /arizona-weather/2020/08/17/nearly-700-000-acres-burned-2020-wildfires/3367619001.

39. Paul Tullis, "The Burning Problem of America's Sugar Cane Growers," *Claims Journal*, March 30, 2020, https://www.claimsjournal.com/news/southeast/2020/03/30 /296280.htm.

40. Oliver Milman and Gina Lachman, "How the Climate Crisis Is Already Harming America—Photo Essay," *Guardian*, August 20, 2020, https://www.theguardian.com/us-news /2020/aug/20/climate-crisis-environment-america.

41. Jessica McBride, "Kyle Rittenhouse Named as Accused Kenosha Shooter," Heavy .com, August 26, 2020, https://heavy.com/news/2020/08/kyle-rittenhouse; Meg Jones, "After Teen Is Charged with Killing 2 at Protests over Jacob Blake Shooting, Turmoil in Kenosha Spreads and Reaches New Heights," *Milwaukee Journal Sentinel*, August 26, 2020, https:// www.jsonline.com/story/news/crime/2020/08/26/illinois-teen-charged-homicide-kenosha -protest-case/5633334002.

42. Susan B. Glasser, "The Malign Fantasy of Donald Trump's Convention," *New Yorker*, August 28, 2020, https://www.newyorker.com/news/letter-from-trumps-washington /the-malign-fantasy-of-donald-trumps-convention; Dorothy Wickenden, "Trump's Convention and the Allure of the Politics of Fear," *New Yorker*, August 27, 2020, https://www .newyorker.com/podcast/political-scene/trumps-convention-and-the-allure-of-the-politics -of-fear.

43. I am paraphrasing: David Frum, "The Platform the GOP Is Too Scared to Publish," *Atlantic*, August 25, 2020, https://www.theatlantic.com/ideas/archive/2020/08/new -gop-platform-authoritarianism/615640.

SEPTEMBER

1. Robert Channick, "Pepsi Pulls This Controversial Kendall Jenner Ad After Widespread Backlash," *Chicago Tribune*, April 5, 2017, https://www.chicagotribune.com/business /ct-pepsi-kendall-jenner-protest-video-backlash-0406-biz-20170405-story.html.

2. Pierre Bourdieu, *Language and Symbolic Power* (Cambridge, MA: Harvard University Press, 1991).

3. John McWhorter, "Academics Are Really, Really Worried About Their Freedom," *Atlantic*, September 1, 2020, https://www.theatlantic.com/ideas/archive/2020/09/academics-are-really-really-worried-about-their-freedom/615724.

4. Zaid Jilani, "Don't Blame Police Racism for America's Violence Epidemic," *Quillette* (blog), July 27, 2019, https://quillette.com/2019/07/27/dont-blame-police-racism-for-americas-violence-epidemic.

5. The Fifth Column, "188: On Anti-Racism II w/ Glenn Loury, John McWhorter, Coleman Hughes, Thomas Chatterton Williams," *The Fifth Column* (podcast), July 1, 2020, https://shows.acast.com/wethefifth/episodes/188-on-anti-racism-and-covid.

6. John McWhorter, "The Dehumanizing Condescension of 'White Fragility,'" *Atlantic*, July 15, 2020, https://www.theatlantic.com/ideas/archive/2020/07/dehumanizing-condescension-white-fragility/614146.

7. McWhorter, "Academics Are Really, Really Worried About Their Freedom."

8. Barbara M. Benedict, *Framing Feeling: Sentiment and Style in English Prose Fiction, 1745–1800* (New York: AMS Press, 1994), 11.

9. Michael Ignatieff, "The Nightmare from Which We Are Trying to Awake," in *The Warrior's Honor: Ethnic War and the Modern Conscience* (London: Chatto & Windus, 1998), 166–90.

10. Ibram X. Kendi, *Stamped from the Beginning: The Definitive History of Racist Ideas in America*, repr. ed. (New York: Bold Type Books, 2017).

11. Ignatieff, "The Nightmare from Which We Are Trying to Awake," 166–90.

12. Michael Sainato, "'They Set Us Up': US Police Arrested over 10,000 Protesters, Many Non-Violent," *Guardian*, June 8, 2020, https://www.theguardian.com/us-news/2020/jun/08/george-floyd-killing-police-arrest-non-violent-protesters.

13. Jack Fink, "Some Technology-Related Glitches Mark Dallas ISD's First Day of School Online," CBS DFW, September 8, 2020, https://dfw.cbslocal.com/2020/09/08/technology-glitches-dallas-isd-first-day-school-online; Hannah Natanson, "Back to School, but Not Back to Normal: Students and Teachers in Northern Virginia Launch Online Learning," *Washington Post*, September 8, 2020, https://www.washingtonpost.com/local/education/back-to-school-but-not-back-to-normal-students-and-teachers-in-northern-virginia-launch-online-learning/2020/09/07/f05cea94-efa7-11ea-99a1-71343d03bc29_story.html; Sarah Schulte and Alexis McAdams, "Chicago Public School Students, Teachers Return to Virtual Learning Tuesday," *ABC7 Chicago*, September 8, 2020, https://abc7chicago.com/6413638.

14. Perry Stein, "As Neighborhood Public School Buildings Remain Closed, Charters Begin Offering in-Person Learning for Small Groups," *Washington Post*, September 8, 2020, https://www.washingtonpost.com/local/education/as-neighborhood-public-school-buildings-remain-closed-charters-begin-offering-in-person-learning-for-small-groups/2020/09/08/308ff3b4-ee99-11ea-ab4e-581edb849379_story.html.

15. "COVID-19 Resources for Schools, Students, and Families," US Department of Education, 2020, https://www.ed.gov/coronavirus.

16. H. L. and Evolving Ed, "Defining the Teacher's Role in Hybrid Education," *Schoology Exchange* (blog), September 4, 2020, https://www.schoology.com/blog/defining-teacher%E2%80%99s-role-hybrid-education.

17. Richard Armitage and Laura B. Nellums, "Considering Inequalities in the School Closure Response to COVID-19," *Lancet Global Health* 8, no. 5 (May 1, 2020): e644; Wim Van Lancker and Zachary Parolin, "COVID-19, School Closures, and Child Poverty: A Social Crisis in the Making," *Lancet Public Health* 5, no. 5 (May 1, 2020): e243–44.

18. Robert Costa and Philip Rucker, "Woodward Book: Trump Says He Knew Coronavirus Was 'Deadly' and Worse Than the Flu While Intentionally Misleading Americans," *Washington Post*, September 9, 2020, https://www.washingtonpost.com/politics/bob-woodward-rage-book-trump/2020/09/09/0368fe3c-efd2-11ea-b4bc-3a2098fc73d4_story.html.

19. Eviction Lab, "Milwaukee, Wisconsin: Eviction Tracking System," *Eviction Lab*, September 11, 2020, https://evictionlab.org/eviction-tracking/milwaukee-wi.

20. "Local Area Unemployment Statistics," Bureau of Labor Statistics, September 11, 2020, https://data.bls.gov/timeseries/LAUMT553334000000004?amp%253bdata_tool =XGtable&output_view=data&include_graphs=true.

21. Desmond, *Evicted*.

22. Jeff Karabanow, *Being Young and Homeless: Understanding How Youth Enter and Exit Street Life* (New York: Peter Lang, 2004).

23. National Alliance to End Homelessness, *State of Homelessness: 2020 Edition* (NAEH, September 11, 2020), https://endhomelessness.org/homelessness-in-america/homelessness -statistics/state-of-homelessness-2020.

24. Marjorie Hope and James Young, *The Faces of Homelessness* (Lexington, MA: Lexington Books, 1986).

25. Jonathan Kozol, *Rachel and Her Children: Homeless Families in America* (New York: Crown, 1988).

26. Nino Abdaladze et al., "COVID's Invisible Victims," *Cronkite News—Arizona PBS*, August 24, 2020, https://cronkitenews.azpbs.org/wp-content/uploads/2020/08/DSC_8331 -Edited-800x500-1.jpg.

27. Bob Brigham, "Americans Are So Frightened by RBG's Death That 'No. No. No.' Trended Nationwide on Twitter," *Raw Story*, September 18, 2020, https://www.rawstory .com/2020/09/americans-are-so-frightened-by-rbgs-that-no-no-no-trended-nationwide -on-twitter.

28. Aaron Mak, "The Reasons Conservatives Say They Need to Replace RBG Before the Election," *Slate*, September 19, 2020, https://slate.com/news-and-politics/2020/09 /ruth-bader-ginsburg-conservative-media.html.

29. Eitan Hersh, *Politics Is for Power: How to Move Beyond Political Hobbyism, Take Action, and Make Real Change* (New York: Scribner, 2020).

30. Steven Smith, "The Senate Syndrome," *Issues in Governance Studies*, no. 35 (June 2010): 132–58.

31. Vann R. Newkirk II, "Five Decades of White Backlash," *Atlantic*, January 15, 2018, https://www.theatlantic.com/politics/archive/2018/01/trump-massive-resistance-history -mlk/550544.

32. Michael Grunwald, *The New New Deal: The Hidden Story of Change in the Obama Era* (New York: Simon & Schuster, 2012).

33. Michael Grunwald, "The Party of No: New Details on the GOP Plot to Obstruct Obama," *Time*, August 23, 2012, https://swampland.time.com/2012/08/23/the-party-of-no -new-details-on-the-gop-plot-to-obstruct-obama.

34. Jerry Dillon, "Should Pseudoephedrine (PSE) Be Moved from Behind the Counter to Prescription-Only?" (Martin School of Public Administration, University of Kentucky, 2011), https://martin.uky.edu/sites/martin.uky.edu/files/Capstone_Projects/Capstones _2011/Dillon.pdf.

35. Sarah Elizabeth Richards, "Why Our Minds Can't Make Sense of COVID-19's Enormous Death Toll," *Science*, September 22, 2020, https://www.nationalgeographic.com /science/2020/09/why-minds-brains-cannot-make-sense-coronavirus-enormous-death-toll.

36. Indiana Department of Child Services, *Assessment Decisions Summary by Child* (July 2020), https://www.in.gov/dcs/files/AssessmentDecisions20207.pdf.

37. Eli Rapoport et al., "Reporting of Child Maltreatment During the SARS-CoV-2 Pandemic in New York City from March to May 2020," *Child Abuse & Neglect* (September 9, 2020).

38. Samantha Schmidt and Hannah Natanson, "With Kids Stuck at Home, ER Doctors See More Severe Cases of Child Abuse," *Washington Post*, April 30, 2020, https://www .washingtonpost.com/education/2020/04/30/child-abuse-reports-coronavirus.

39. Richard Winton, "'We Do Not Want Another Gabriel Fernandez' Coronavirus Leads to 'Alarming' Drop in Child Abuse Reports," *Los Angeles Times*, April 21, 2020, https://www.latimes.com/california/story/2020-04-21/coronavirus-child-abuse-reports-decline; Matt Stout, "Reports of Child Abuse and Neglect Are Plummeting Across New England," *Boston Globe*, April 9, 2020, https://www.bostonglobe.com/2020/04/09/nation/reports-child-abuse-neglect-are-plummeting-across-new-england-thats-not-good-thing; Kylie Storm, "Falling Child-Abuse Reports in Los Angeles Have Experts Worried," *Crosstown*, August 10, 2020, https://xtown.la/2020/08/10/child-abuse-los-angeles-covid-19.

40. Candy Woodall, "Covid-19 in Pa.: Child Abuse Doctors See a Disturbing Trend as the Pandemic Continues," *York Daily Record*, August 29, 2020, https://www.ydr.com/story/news/2020/08/29/covid-19-pa-child-abuse-doctors-see-disturbing-trend/3342976001.

41. Bridget M. Kuehn, "Surge in Child Abuse, Harm During COVID-19 Pandemic Reported," *JAMA* 324, no. 7 (August 18, 2020): 621.

42. Indiana Department of Child Services, *Assessment Decisions Summary by Child*, July 2020.

43. Indiana Department of Child Services, *Assessment Decisions Summary by Child*, July 2019, https://www.in.gov/dcs/files/AssessmentDecisions201907.pdf.

44. Jai Sidpra et al., "Rise in the Incidence of Abusive Head Trauma During the COVID-19 Pandemic," *Archives of Disease in Childhood* (June 30, 2020); Rapoport et al., "Reporting of Child Maltreatment During the SARS-CoV-2 Pandemic in New York City from March to May 2020."

45. "Child Abuse, Neglect Data Released," US Department of Health and Human Services, Administration for Children and Families, January 15, 2020, https://www.acf.hhs.gov/media/press/2020/child-abuse-neglect-data-released.

46. David Leonhardt, "18 Revelations from a Trove of Trump Tax Records," *New York Times*, September 27, 2020, https://www.nytimes.com/2020/09/27/us/trump-taxes-takeaways.html.

47. Ryan Ellis, "New York Times' Trump Tax Return 'Bombshell' Is a Joke," *Federalist*, September 28, 2020, https://thefederalist.com/2020/09/28/new-york-times-trump-tax-return-bombshell-is-a-joke.

48. Andrea Bernstein and Ilya Marritz, "Trump's Taxes, Finally," *Trump, Inc.* (podcast), September 28, 2020, https://www.propublica.org/series/trump-inc.

49. Rachel Augustine Potter, "How Trump Uses a Crisis: Repeal Rules While Nobody Is Looking," *Washington Post*, June 9, 2020, https://www.washingtonpost.com/outlook/2020/06/09/how-trump-uses-crisis-repeal-rules-while-nobody-is-looking.

50. Isabel Togoh, "Why Last Night's Debate Is Already Considered the Worst in Presidential History," *Forbes*, September 30, 2020, https://www.forbes.com/sites/isabeltogoh/2020/09/30/why-last-nights-debate-is-already-considered-the-worst-in-presidential-history.

51. "Undecided Voters Left Disappointed, Frustrated by First Presidential Debate: Pollster Frank Luntz," Fox News, September 30, 2020, https://www.foxnews.com/media/biden-trump-debate-undecided-voters-react; Dan McLaughlin, "Everybody Loses, Which Helps Biden," *National Review* (blog), September 30, 2020, https://www.nationalreview.com/corner/everybody-loses-which-helps-biden; Bruce Wolpe, "The Worst Debate in Modern American History: How Hope Was Mugged in the Trump-Biden Clash," *Sydney Morning Herald*, September 30, 2020, https://www.smh.com.au/world/north-america/the-worst-debate-in-modern-american-history-how-hope-was-mugged-in-the-trump-biden-clash-20200930-p56on9.html.

52. Mark Cronin, "A Guide to Trump's Reality TV Debate Techniques," *Columbia Journalism Review*, September 28, 2020, https://www.cjr.org/opinion/a-guide-to-trumps-reality-tv-debate-techniques.php; John F. Harris, "An Epic Moment of National Shame: The Debate Was an Embarrassment for the Ages," *Politico*, September 30, 2020, https://www.politico.com/news/magazine/2020/09/30/presidential-debate-national-shame-423521.

53. Clarissa-Jan Lim, "The First Debate Between Trump and Biden Was a Stressful, Chaotic Trash Fire," *BuzzFeed News*, September 29, 2020, https://www.buzzfeednews.com /article/clarissajanlim/trump-biden-debate-twitter-reactions.

54. "Trump Tells Proud Boys: 'Stand Back and Stand By,'" Associated Press, September 29, 2020, available at https://www.youtube.com/watch?v=qIHhB1ZMV_0.

55. Ben Collins and Brandy Zadrozny, "Proud Boys Say They Are 'Standing Down and Standing By' After Trump's Debate Callout," NBC News, September 29, 2020, https://www .nbcnews.com/tech/tech-news/proud-boys-celebrate-after-trump-s-debate-call-out-n1241512; Adam Gabbatt, "Trump's Refusal to Condemn White Supremacy Fits Pattern of Extremist Rhetoric," *Guardian*, September 30, 2020, https://www.theguardian.com/us-news/2020/sep /30/trump-white-supremacy-extremist-rhetoric; Jordan Valinsky, "Amazon Removes 'Stand Back and Stand By' Merchandise," CNN, October 1, 2020, https://www.cnn.com/2020/10 /01/business/amazon-removal-stand-back-stand-by/index.html.

56. Ed Kilgore, "Trump Closes Debate by Threatening Election Night Chaos," *Intelligencer*, September 30, 2020, https://nymag.com/intelligencer/2020/09/trump-biden-debate -threatening-election-night-chaos.html.

57. Associated Press, "Another GOP Challenge Tries to Block Absentee Ballot Order," WILX10.com, September 30, 2020, https://www.wilx.com/2020/09/30/another-gop -challenge-tries-to-block-absentee-ballot-order; Anita Kumar, "Trump Readies Thousands of Attorneys for Election Fight," *Politico*, September 27, 2020, https://www.politico.com /news/2020/09/27/trump-legal-network-election-day-fight-422035.

58. Zoë Richards, "After Trump's Debate Tantrum, Commentators Question Whether Others Should Go Forward," *Talking Points Memo*, September 30, 2020, https://talking pointsmemo.com/news/after-trumps-debate-tantrum-some-question-whether-others -should-go-forward.

OCTOBER

1. Peter Baker and Maggie Haberman, "Trump Tests Positive for the Coronavirus," *New York Times*, October 2, 2020, https://www.nytimes.com/2020/10/02/us/politics/trump -covid.html.

2. Mark Landler, Mike Ives, and Carlos Tejada, "News That the President Has Contracted the Virus Shakes the World," *New York Times*, October 2, 2020, https://www.nytimes .com/live/2020/10/02/world/covid-19-coronavirus.

3. Jeff Mason, "Trump Starts 'Quarantine Process' After Aide Hope Hicks Tests Positive for Coronavirus," Reuters, October 1, 2020, https://www.reuters.com/article/health -coronavirus-usa-hicks-int-idUSKBN26N0FV.

4. Zolan Kanno-Youngs and Michael S. Schmidt, "Trump's Secret Service Has Struggled with Outbreak at Training Center," *New York Times*, October 2, 2020, https://www .nytimes.com/2020/10/02/us/politics/secret-service-coronavirus-trump.html.

5. Jessica McBride, "Amy Coney Barrett Tested Negative for COVID-19 After Concern It Spread at Nomination Event," Heavy.com, October 2, 2020, https://heavy.com/news /amy-coney-barrett-covid-19-coronavirus.

6. Sarah Evanega et al., *Coronavirus Misinformation: Quantifying Sources and Themes in the COVID-19 "Infodemic"* (Ithaca, NY: Cornell Alliance for Science, Department of Global Development, October 1, 2020, https://allianceforscience.cornell.edu/wp-content/uploads /2020/09/Evanega-et-al-Coronavirus-misinformationFINAL.pdf.

7. Kate Kelland and Ludwig Burger, "Older, Overweight and Male: Trump's COVID Risk Factors Make Him Vulnerable," Reuters, October 2, 2020, https://www.reuters.com /article/health-coronavirus-usa-trump-risk-int-idUSKBN26N23I.

8. Pedro Bordalo et al., "Older People Are Less Pessimistic About the Health Risks of Covid-19," National Bureau of Economic Research Working Paper Series, July 2020, http://www.nber.org/papers/w27494.pdf.

9. Chantal Da Silva, "Boris Johnson Saw Uptick in Popularity After He Contracted Coronavirus. Will Trump See the Same?" *CBC*, October 2, 2020, https://www.cbc.ca/news /world/boris-coronavirus-impact-1.5747877.

10. Barry Sussman, "Shooting Gives Reagan Boost in Popularity," *Washington Post*, April 2, 1981, https://www.washingtonpost.com/archive/politics/1981/04/02/shooting -gives-reagan-boost-in-popularity/9515e340-f295-42e7-89c4-c96ed0ab7a44.

11. Beatrice Peterson, "Why Trump Loves 'Evita,' and What It Says About His Presidency," ABC News, December 1, 2018, https://abcnews.go.com/Politics/trump-loves-evita -presidency/story?id=59350378.

12. Tomas Eloy Martinez, "The Woman Behind the Fantasy," *Time*, January 20, 1997, https://web.archive.org/web/20011221053805/http://www.time.com/time/magazine/1997 /int/970120/cinema.the_woman.html.

13. Tim Miller, "The Weirdest 90 Seconds in Presidential History," *The Bulwark*, October 5, 2020, https://thebulwark.com/the-weirdest-90-seconds-in-presidential-history.

14. Patti LuPone (@PattiLuPone), Twitter, October 5, 2020, https://twitter.com /PattiLuPone/status/1313285830476259334.

15. Jen Christensen, "Regeneron's Antibody Cocktail for Coronavirus: Early Data Shows Promising Results," CNN, September 29, 2020, https://www.cnn.com/2020/09/29 /health/regeneron-covid-19-early-antibody-treatment-results/index.html.

16. Paul R. La Monica, "Trump Has Ties to Drugmaker Regeneron—and Now Its Stock Is Surging," CNN, October 5, 2020, https://www.cnn.com/2020/10/05/investing /trump-regeneron/index.html.

17. Antonio Regalado, "Trump's Antibody Treatment Was Tested Using Cells Originally Derived from an Abortion," *MIT Technology Review*, October 7, 2020, https://www .technologyreview.com/2020/10/07/1009664/trumps-antibody-treatment-was-tested-using -cells-from-an-abortion.

18. Meghan Brenan, "One in Four Americans Consider Abortion a Key Voting Issue," *Gallup.com*, July 7, 2020, https://news.gallup.com/poll/313316/one-four-americans-consider -abortion-key-voting-issue.aspx.

19. "Coronavirus Disease 2019 (COVID-19)—Transmission," Centers for Disease Control and Prevention, October 6, 2020, https://www.cdc.gov/coronavirus/2019-ncov /prevent-getting-sick/how-covid-spreads.html.

20. Will Feuer, "CDC Revises Coronavirus Guidance to Acknowledge That It Spreads Through Airborne Transmission," CNBC, October 5, 2020, https://www.cnbc.com/2020 /10/05/cdc-revises-coronavirus-guidance-to-acknowledge-that-it-spreads-through-airborne -transmission.html; Azeen Ghorayshi and Stephanie M. Lee, "The CDC Finally Acknowledged That the Coronavirus Can Spread Through Air," *BuzzFeed News*, October 5, 2020, https://www.buzzfeednews.com/article/azeenghorayshi/cdc-airborne-update-masks -ventilation.

21. David Gorski, "In the Age of the COVID-19 Pandemic, Can We Trust the CDC and FDA Any More?" *Science-Based Medicine*, September 14, 2020, https://sciencebased medicine.org/can-we-trust-the-cdc-and-fda-any-more.

22. Dan Diamond, "Trump Officials Interfered with CDC Reports on Covid-19," *Politico*, September 11, 2020, https://www.politico.com/news/2020/09/11/exclusive-trump -officials-interfered-with-cdc-reports-on-covid-19-412809.

23. Robert J. McCarthy, "Michael Caputo Receives 'Metastatic Head and Neck Cancer' Diagnosis," *Buffalo News*, September 24, 2020, https://buffalonews.com/news/michael -caputo-receives-metastatic-head-and-neck-cancer-diagnosis/article_e1bcb148-fe77-11ea -862a-d375b2b7683d.html.

24. Sharon LaFraniere, "Trump Health Aide Pushes Bizarre Conspiracies and Warns of Armed Revolt," *New York Times*, September 14, 2020, https://www.nytimes.com/2020/09 /14/us/politics/caputo-virus.html.

25. Andrew O'Reilly, "Trump HHS Spokesperson Michael Caputo Deletes Twitter Account After Late-Night Rant," Fox News, September 14, 2020, https://www.foxnews.com /politics/trump-hhs-spokesperson-deletes-twitter-account-after-late-night-rant.

26. Bloomberg Quicktake, "Trump Says a Coronavirus Vaccine Could Be Ready in October at a White House Briefing," September 7, 2020, available at https://youtu.be/YDDvNsEupbw.

27. Sara Murray and Kevin Liptak, "Trump Has Personally Pressured Drug Company CEOs Repeatedly to Speed Vaccine," CNN, October 6, 2020, https://www.cnn.com/2020 /10/06/politics/trump-pfizer-vaccine/index.html.

28. "Biopharma Leaders Unite to Stand with Science," Business Wire, September 8, 2020, https://www.businesswire.com/news/home/20200908005282/en/Biopharma -Leaders-Unite-to-Stand-with-Science; Shawn Radcliffe, "9 Pharma Companies Promise COVID-19 Vaccine Safety in Open Letter," *Healthline*, September 9, 2020, https://www .healthline.com/health-news/9-pharma-companies-join-to-release-open-letter-promising -covid-19-vaccine-safety.

29. Gorski, "In the Age of the COVID-19 Pandemic, Can We Trust the CDC and FDA Any More?"

30. Carole Levine, "Single Moms Hit Hard by Economic Impact of COVID-19," *Nonprofit Quarterly*, June 23, 2020, https://nonprofitquarterly.org/single-moms-hit-hard-by -economic-impact-of-covid-19.

31. Tim Henderson, "Single Mothers Hit Hard by Job Losses," *Pew Charitable Trust*, May 26, 2020, https://pew.org/2zWmlKx.

32. Oliver Armantier, Gizem Kosar, and Rachel Pomerantz, "The Disproportionate Effects of COVID-19 on Households with Children," Federal Reserve Bank of New York, August 13, 2020, https://libertystreeteconomics.newyorkfed.org/2020/08/the-disproportionate -effects-of-covid-19-on-households-with-children.html.

33. "NBC News to Host Town Hall with Trump on Thursday," NBC News, October 14, 2020, https://www.nbcnews.com/politics/2020-election/nbc-news-host-town-hall-trump -thursday-n1243300.

34. Nellie Andreeva, "Top Actors & Showrunners Ask NBC to Move Donald Trump Town Hall from Slot Opposite ABC's Joe Biden Special," *Deadline* (blog), October 15, 2020, https://deadline.com/2020/10/donald-trump-town-hall-actors-showrunners-ask-nbc-move -slot-opposite-abc-joe-biden-mariska-hargitay-j-j-abrams-ryan-murphy-greg-berlanti-ava -duvernay-seth-macfarlane-damon-lindelof-kenya-1234597879; Nicole Lyn Pesce, "Dueling Trump and Biden Town Halls Spur NBC Protests," *MSN*, October 15, 2020, https:// www.msn.com/en-us/entertainment/news/dueling-trump-and-biden-town-halls-spur-nbc -protests/ar-BB1a1E6k.

35. Christopher Rosen, "Jimmy Kimmel Rips NBC for Hosting Trump Town Hall Opposite ABC's Biden Event," *Vanity Fair*, October 15, 2020, https://www.vanityfair.com /hollywood/2020/10/kimmel-trump-nbc-town-hall.

36. Matthew Yglesias, "The Delightful Boringness of Joe Biden," *Vox*, October 15, 2020, https://www.vox.com/2020/10/15/21518718/biden-town-hall-abc.

37. Meg Cunningham and Quinn Scanlan, "5 Key Takeaways from Joe Biden's Town Hall with ABC News," ABC News, October 16, 2020, https://abcnews.go.com/Politics /key-takeaways-joe-bidens-town-hall-abc-news/story?id=73641281.

38. Evan Brechtel, "Trump Advisor Compares Biden Town Hall to 'Mr. Rogers' and People Fired Back with the Same Response," *Second Nexus*, October 16, 2020, https:// secondnexus.com/fred-rogers-joe-biden-schlapp; Susan B. Glasser, "The Presidential Town Halls Were Mister Rogers Versus Nasty Uncle Trump," *New Yorker*, October 16, 2020, https://www.newyorker.com/news/letter-from-trumps-washington/mister-rogers-versus -nasty-uncle-trump.

39. Rebecca Morin, "After Town Hall Wraps Up, Biden Sticks Around to Take Questions from Audience," *USA Today*, October 15, 2020, https://www.usatoday.com/story/news

/politics/elections/2020/10/15/town-hall-biden-sticks-around-after-take-more-questions
-voters/3673340001.

40. Meaghan Ellis, "NBC's Savannah Guthrie Praised for Explosive Trump Town Hall for Two Big Reasons," AlterNet.org, October 16, 2020, https://www.alternet.org/2020/10 /savannah-guthrie-town-hall; Emily Stewart, "Savannah Guthrie Delivered the Trump Interview We've Been Wanting for Years," *Vox*, October 15, 2020, https://www.vox.com /policy-and-politics/2020/10/15/21518763/savannah-guthrie-trump-town-hall-nbc-miami.

41. Meaghan Ellis, "Trump Brags About Good Town Hall Reviews—But Ratings Signal a Town Hall Win for Biden," *Raw Story*, October 16, 2020, https://www.rawstory .com/2020/10/trump-brags-about-good-town-hall-reviews-but-ratings-signal-a-town -hall-win-for-biden; Jeffery Martin, "Town Hall YouTube Views Suggest Biden Hit Trump Where It Hurts Him Most—Ratings," *Newsweek*, October 15, 2020, https://www .newsweek.com/youtube-views-suggest-biden-hit-trump-where-it-hurts-him-mostratings -1539635.

42. "Sexual Assault Evidence Kit Backlog Reduction Project," City of Albuquerque, October 19, 2020, https://www.cabq.gov/police/sexual-assault-evidence-kit-backlog/sexual -assault-evidence-kit-backlog.

43. Mary Spicuzza, "'People Are Dying Every Night': Staff at Overwhelmed Wisconsin Hospital Urge People to Take Coronavirus Seriously," *Milwaukee Journal Sentinel*, October 19, 2020, https://www.jsonline.com/story/news/2020/10/19/aspirus-wausau-hospital-staff -urge-wisconsin-take-covid-seriously/3669849001.

44. Lauren Hughes and Roberto Silva, "In Rural America, Resentment over COVID-19 Shutdowns Is Colliding with Rising Case Numbers," *The Conversation*, October 26, 2020, http://theconversation.com/in-rural-america-resentment-over-covid-19-shutdowns-is -colliding-with-rising-case-numbers-148310; Katie Moore, "As This Rural Kansas County Sees Surge in COVID-19 Cases, Governor Urges Mask Mandate," *Kansas City Star*, October 20, 2020, https://www.kansascity.com/news/state/kansas/article246581368.html.

45. Elie Dolgin, "Core Concept: The Pandemic Is Prompting Widespread Use—and Misuse—of Real-World Data," *Proceedings of the National Academy of Sciences*, October 21, 2020.

46. "Great Barrington Declaration and Petition," 2020, https://gbdeclaration.org.

47. Apoorva Mandavilli and Sheryl Gay Stolberg, "A Viral Theory Cited by Health Officials Draws Fire from Scientists," *New York Times*, October 20, 2020.

48. David Gorski, "The Great Barrington Declaration: COVID-19 Deniers Follow the Path Laid down by Creationists, HIV/AIDS Denialists, and Climate Science Deniers," *Science-Based Medicine*, October 12, 2020, https://sciencebasedmedicine.org/great -barrington-declaration; Christopher Leonard, *Kochland: The Secret History of Koch Industries and Corporate Power in America* (New York: Simon & Schuster, 2019); Nancy MacLean, *Democracy in Chains: The Deep History of the Radical Right's Stealth Plan for America* (New York: Viking, 2017).

49. Gary Claxton et al., "How Many Adults Are at Risk of Serious Illness If Infected with Coronavirus? Updated Data," *KFF* (blog), April 23, 2020, https://www.kff.org/corona virus-covid-19/issue-brief/how-many-adults-are-at-risk-of-serious-illness-if-infected-with -coronavirus.

50. "John Snow Memorandum," 2020, https://www.johnsnowmemo.com.

51. Nisreen A. Alwan et al., "Scientific Consensus on the COVID-19 Pandemic: We Need to Act Now," *Lancet* 396, no. 10260 (October 15, 2020): e71–72.

52. Cameron Joseph and Rob Arthur, "The US Eliminated Nearly 21,000 Election Day Polling Locations for 2020," *Vice*, October 22, 2020, https://www.vice.com/en/article /pkdenn/the-us-eliminated-nearly-21000-election-day-polling-locations-for-2020.

53. Statistical Atlas, "The Demographic Statistical Atlas of the United States—Miami— Median Household Income," Statistical Atlas, October 26, 2020, https://statisticalatlas.com /county/Florida/Miami-Dade-County/Race-and-Ethnicity.

54. Ovetta Wiggins et al., "Citing a History of Voter Suppression, Black Marylanders Turn Out to Vote in Person," *Washington Post*, October 26, 2020, https://www.washington post.com/local/md-politics/maryland-early-voting-prince-georges-trust/2020/10/25/847c5afc -1537-11eb-ad6f-36c93e6e94fb_story.html; Statistical Atlas, "The Demographic Statistical Atlas of the United States—Maryland," Statistical Atlas, October 26, 2020, https://statistical atlas.com/state/Maryland/Race-and-Ethnicity.

55. "More Than 10-Hour Wait and Long Lines as Early Voting Starts in Georgia," *Guardian*, October 13, 2020, http://www.theguardian.com/us-news/2020/oct/13/more-than -10-hour-wait-and-long-lines-as-early-voting-starts-in-georgia.

56. US Elections Project, "2020 General Election Early Vote Statistics," October 26, 2020, https://electproject.github.io/Early-Vote-2020G/index.html.

NOVEMBER

1. Nathaniel Meyersohn, Alexis Benveniste, and Chauncey Alcorn, "From Tiffany to Target, Stores Are Boarding Up Windows in Case of Election Unrest," CNN, November 3, 2020, https://www.cnn.com/2020/11/02/business/retail-election-security/index.html; Christopher Maag, "Wilkes-Barre: In a City Up for Grabs, Fear of Violence May Be an Illusion," North Jersey Media Group, October 31, 2020, https://www.northjersey.com/story/news /columnists/christopher-maag/2020/10/31/battleground-city-fear-election-violence-trumps -reality/6068039002.

2. John T. Bennett, "Three-Quarters of Americans Fear Post-Election Violence and Riots, Independent Reveals," *Independent*, October 21, 2020, https://www.independent.co .uk/news/world/americas/us-election-2020/election-results-2020-riots-trump-biden -b1700559.html.

3. Daniel L. Byman and Colin P. Clarke, "Why the Risk of Election Violence Is High," *Brookings* (blog), October 27, 2020, https://www.brookings.edu/blog/fixgov/2020/10/27 /why-the-risk-of-election-violence-is-high.

4. Matt Zapotosky and Devlin Barrett, "Justice Dept., FBI Planning for the Possibility of Election Day Violence, Voting Disruptions," *Washington Post*, October 2, 2020, https:// www.washingtonpost.com/national-security/fbi-election-poll-watchers/2020/10/02/6d482f48 -0414-11eb-a2db-417cddf4816a_story.html.

5. Donald J. Trump (@realdonaldtrump), Twitter, November 1, 2020.

6. Stefan Becket et al., "Pivotal States Too Close to Call as Race Hangs in the Balance," CBS, November 3, 2020, https://www.cbsnews.com/live-updates/election-night-2020-live -coverage.

7. Corbin Carson, "The Rocky History of Martin Luther King Jr. Day in Arizona," KTAR.com, January 20, 2020, https://ktar.com/story/1903240/history-martin-luther-king -jr-day-arizona.

8. Yochai Benkler, Robert Faris, and Hal Roberts, *Network Propaganda: Manipulation, Disinformation, and Radicalization in American Politics* (New York: Oxford University Press, 2018).

9. Michael Gerson, "Some White Evangelicals Are Difficult to Recognize as Christians at All," *Washington Post*, op-ed, August 15, 2019, https://www.washingtonpost.com/opinions /how-we-christians-order-our-outrage-says-a-lot-about-us/2019/08/15/a5a0c2e2-bf91-11e9 -a5c6-1e74f7ec4a93_story.html; Rev. Michael McBride, "The Last Holdouts: White Evangelical Christians, Why Can't You See?" *The Root*, August 18, 2019, https://www.theroot com/the-last-holdouts-white-evangelical-christians-why-ca-1837304983; Emma Green, "The Unofficial Racism Consultants to the White Evangelical World," *Atlantic*, July 5, 2020, https://www.theatlantic.com/politics/archive/2020/07/white-evangelicals-black-lives -matter/613738.

10. J. D. Vance, *Hillbilly Elegy: A Memoir of a Family and Culture in Crisis* (New York: Harper, 2016).

11. Matthew 25:31–46.

12. Tara Isabella Burton, "The Biblical Story the Christian Right Uses to Defend Trump," *Vox*, March 5, 2018, https://www.vox.com/identities/2018/3/5/16796892/trump -cyrus-christian-right-bible-cbn-evangelical-propaganda.

13. Gerson, "Some White Evangelicals Are Difficult to Recognize as Christians at All"; McBride, "The Last Holdouts: White Evangelical Christians, Why Can't You See?"; Green, "The Unofficial Racism Consultants to the White Evangelical World."

14. Donald J. Trump (@realdonaldtrump), Twitter, November 4, 2020, https://twitter .com/realDonaldTrump/status/1324139647111409667.

15. Todd Spangler, "Biden Takes Lead in Michigan as Vote Count Continues in Largest Counties," *Holland Sentinel*, November 4, 2020, https://www.hollandsentinel.com/news /20201104/biden-takes-lead-in-michigan-as-vote-count-continues-in-largest-counties.

16. Kristen Jordan Shamus and Tresa Baldas, "Chaos Erupts at TCF Center as Republican Vote Challengers Cry Foul in Detroit," *Detroit Free Press*, November 4, 2020, https:// www.freep.com/story/news/politics/elections/2020/11/04/tcf-center-challengers-detroit -michigan/6164715002.

17. Andrew Kirell, "Pro-Trump 'Count the Vote' Protesters in Arizona Chant 'Fox News Sucks,'" *The Daily Beast*, November 5, 2020, https://www.thedailybeast.com/pro -trump-count-the-vote-protesters-in-arizona-chant-fox-news-sucks.

18. "'Stop the Count!': Trump Supporters Protest Polling Centers," Reuters, editorial, November 5, 2020, https://reut.rs/3p11kmP.

19. "Remarks by President Trump on the Election," White House, November 5, 2020, https://www.whitehouse.gov/briefings-statements/remarks-president-trump-election; Addy Baird et al., "There Have Been No Widespread Problems Counting Votes, So Trump Is Making Up a Bunch of Lies," *BuzzFeed News*, November 5, 2020, https://www.buzzfeednews .com/article/addybaird/trump-lies-presidential-election-fraud.

20. Tom Jones, "Networks Pulled Away from President Trump's Shocking Press Conference," *Poynter* (blog), November 6, 2020, https://www.poynter.org/newsletters/2020 /networks-pulled-away-from-president-trumps-shocking-press-conference.

21. Peter Baker and Maggie Haberman, "In Torrent of Falsehoods, Trump Claims Election Is Being Stolen," *New York Times*, November 5, 2020, https://www.nytimes.com /2020/11/05/us/politics/trump-presidency.html.

22. Dennis Perkins, "Stephen Colbert: 'Donald Trump Is a Fascist,'" *AV Club*, November 6, 2020, https://news.avclub.com/an-emotional-stephen-colbert-ditches-his -monologue-to-c-1845592126.

23. Carla K. Johnson, Hannah Fingerhut, and Pia Deshpande, "Counties with Worst Virus Surges Overwhelmingly Voted Trump," AP News, November 5, 2020, https://apnews .com/article/counties-worst-virus-surges-voted-trump-d671a483534024b5486715da6edb6ebf.

24. Brian Slodysko, "Explainer: Why AP Called the 2020 Election for Joe Biden," *US News & World Report*, November 7, 2020, https://www.usnews.com/news/politics/articles /2020-11-07/explainer-why-ap-called-the-2020-election-for-joe-biden.

25. Faith Karimi, "For Stacey Abrams, Revenge Is a Dish Best Served Blue," CNN, November 7, 2020, https://www.cnn.com/2020/11/07/us/stacey-abrams-georgia-voter -suppression-trnd/index.html.

26. Libby Nelson, "'Grab 'Em by the Pussy': How Trump Talked About Women in Private Is Horrifying," *Vox*, October 7, 2016, https://www.vox.com/2016/10/7/13205842 /trump-secret-recording-women; Lauren Dubois, "What Is Four Seasons Total Landscaping? Donald Trump Canceled Conference Location Confuses," *International Business Times*, November 7, 2020, https://www.ibtimes.com/what-four-seasons-total-landscaping-donald -trump-canceled-conference-location-3078130; Mikael Thalen, "Trump Team Roasted for Seemingly Booking the Wrong 'Four Seasons' and Ending Up at Landscaping Business," *The Daily Dot*, November 7, 2020, https://www.dailydot.com/debug/trump-four-seasons -landscaping.

27. Philip Bump, "It Was Perhaps Inevitable It Would End When Trump Was on the Golf Course," *Washington Post*, November 7, 2020, https://www.washingtonpost.com /politics/2020/11/07/it-was-perhaps-inevitable-it-would-end-when-trump-was-golf-course.

28. Rachel Kiley, "Viral Photo Shows Trump Watching Americans Celebrate His Loss," *The Daily Dot*, November 7, 2020, https://www.dailydot.com/unclick/viral-photo -trump-loss.

29. Reese Oxner, "Texas Reports More Than 1 Million Coronavirus Cases, According to John Hopkins," NPR, November 11, 2020, https://www.npr.org/2020/11/11/933952445 /texas-surpasses-1-million-coronavirus-cases-according-to-johns-hopkins-universit; Shawn Shinneman, "Texas Hits 1 Million COVID-19 Cases—More Than Any Other State," *Texas Monthly*, November 11, 2020, https://www.texasmonthly.com/news/texas-one-million -covid-19-cases.

30. J. David Goodman, "As Hospitalizations Soar, El Paso Brings in New Mobile Morgues," *New York Times*, November 11, 2020, https://www.nytimes.com/2020/11/10/us /coronavirus-hospitalizations-el-paso-texas.html; Staff, "El Paso Inmates Help Move Bodies to Medical Examiner's Office," KFOX, November 14, 2020, https://kfoxtv.com/news/local /el-paso-inmates-help-move-bodies-to-medical-examiners-office.

31. Zeynep Tufekci, "It's Time to Hunker Down," *Atlantic*, November 14, 2020, https://www.theatlantic.com/health/archive/2020/11/lock-yourself-down-now/617106.

32. Daniel W. Johnson, "I'm Sorry This Post Is So Dark, but We Need to Get the Word Out About the COVID-19 Situation in Nebraska," *Nebraska Medicine*, November 11, 2020, https://www.nebraskamed.com/COVID/please-inform-your-family.

33. Gregory Lemos and Christina Maxouris CNN, "More than 900 Mayo Clinic Staff Members Diagnosed with Covid-19 in Midwest over Two Weeks," CNN, November 19, 2020, https://www.cnn.com/2020/11/19/us/mayo-clinic-900-staff-positive-covid/index.html.

34. Paul John Scott, "900 on Mayo Clinic Staff Have Contracted Coronavirus in Last Two Weeks," *Twin Cities* (blog), November 18, 2020, https://www.twincities.com/2020/1 /17/over-900-mayo-staff-have-gotten-covid-19-in-past-two-weeks.

35. Ed Yong, "'No One Is Listening to Us,'" *Atlantic*, November 13, 2020, https:// www.theatlantic.com/health/archive/2020/11/third-surge-breaking-healthcare-workers /617091.

36. Daniel Funke, "The 'Million MAGA March' Did Not Have 1 Million or More At-tendees," *PolitiFact*, November 16, 2020, https://www.politifact.com/factchecks/2020/nov/16 /kayleigh-mcenany/million-maga-march-did-not-have-more-1-million-att; Samira Sadeque, "Million Maga March: Trump Fans Rage Against Dying of the Light," *Guardian*, November 15, 2020, https://www.theguardian.com/us-news/2020/nov/15/million-maga-march-trump -supporters; Krystie Lee Yandoli, "Trump Supporters Who Refuse to Admit He Lost the Election Went to Protest in Washington DC," *BuzzFeed News*, November 14, 2020, https:// www.buzzfeednews.com/article/krystieyandoli/trump-supporters-million-maga-march-dc.

37. Matt Keeley, "Man Stabbed as Violence Erupts After 'Million MAGA March' in Washington D.C.," *Newsweek*, November 14, 2020, https://www.newsweek.com/man -stabbed-violence-erupts-after-million-maga-march-washington-dc-1547530; Jemima McEvoy, "'Million Maga March' Ends in Stabbing, Arrests After Trump Supporters and Counter Protesters Brawl," *Forbes*, November 15, 2020, https://www.forbes.com/sites /jemimamcevoy/2020/11/15/million-maga-march-ends-in-stabbing-arrests-after-trump -supporters-and-counter-protesters-brawl.

38. Tamar Lapin, "Police Release More Details About Million MAGA March Arrests, Stabbing," *New York Post* (blog), November 17, 2020, https://nypost.com/2020/11/16/police -release-more-details-about-million-maga-march-arrests.

39. Tyler G. Anbinder, *Nativism and Slavery: The Northern Know Nothings and the Politics of the 1850s* (New York: Oxford University Press, 1994); Evan Taparata, "An Anti-Immigrant Political Movement That Sparked an Election Day Riot—150 Years Ago," *The World from*

PRX, March 5, 2016, https://www.pri.org/stories/2016-03-05/anti-immigrant-political-movement-sparked-election-day-riot-150-years-ago; Kevin W., "'Bloody Monday'/American (Know-Nothing) Party Historical Marker," Historical Marker Database/HMdb.org, August 1, 2020, https://www.hmdb.org/m.asp?m=25914.

40. Harriet Alexander, "Another One Back from the Dead! Widow, 94, Who Trump Said Was 'Dead Voter' Says She Voted for Biden," *Daily Mail*, November 14, 2020, https://www.dailymail.co.uk/news/article-8949723/Another-one-dead-Widow-94-Trump-said-dead-voter-says-voted-Biden.html; Frances Mulraney, "Federal Agencies Say Election 'The Most Secure in American History,'" *Mail Online*, November 13, 2020, https://www.dailymail.co.uk/news/article-8944631/Federal-agencies-overseeing-election-security-say-secure-American-history.html; Tina Nguyen and Mark Scott, "How 'SharpieGate' Went from Online Chatter to Trumpworld Strategy in Arizona," *Politico*, November 5, 2020, https://www.politico.com/news/2020/11/05/sharpie-ballots-trump-strategy-arizona-434372.

41. Ross Jones (@rossjonesWXYZ), Twitter, November 4, 2020.

42. Eric Geller and Natasha Bertrand, "Top Cyber Official Expecting to Be Fired as White House Frustrations Hit Agency Protecting Elections," *Politico*, November 12, 2020, https://www.politico.com/news/2020/11/12/cyber-official-chris-krebs-likely-out-436342.

43. "Rumor Control," Cybersecurity & Infrastructure Security Agency, October 28, 2020, https://www.cisa.gov/rumorcontrol.

44. Chris Kahn, "Half of Republicans Say Biden Won Because of a 'Rigged' Election: Reuters/Ipsos Poll," Reuters, November 18, 2020, https://www.reuters.com/article/us-usa-election-poll-idUSKBN27Y1AJ.

DECEMBER

1. Sarai Martinez-Suazo, "Timeline of US Naturalization Law/Civics Exam," University of Virginia School of Medicine, June 2015, https://med.virginia.edu/family-medicine/wp-content/uploads/sites/285/2017/02/Sarai-Martinez-Suazo-US-Naturalization_Web.pdf.

2. "128 Civics Questions and Answers with MP3 Audio (2020 Version)," US Citizenship and Immigration Services, December 15, 2020, https://www.uscis.gov/citizenship-resource-center/the-2020-version-of-the-civics-test/128-civics-questions-and-answers-with-mp3-audio-2020-version.

3. Reuters Staff, "'No Choice Except to Flee': After Back-to-Back Hurricanes, Central Americans Go North," NBC News, December 4, 2020, https://www.nbcnews.com/news/latino/no-choice-except-flee-after-back-back-hurricanes-central-americans-n1249993.

4. Martin Bagot and Martin Fricker, "'Super-Gran' Margaret Keenan's Coronavirus Jab Sets UK on Road to Normality," *Mirror*, December 8, 2020, https://www.mirror.co.uk/news/uk-news/uk-super-gran-first-receive-23137329.

5. Emily Crane and Frances Mulraney, "Thanksgiving COVID Surge: 2,534 Americans Die and 215k Test Positive," *Mail Online*, December 9, 2020, https://www.dailymail.co.uk/news/article-9033147/Experts-say-just-start-Thanksgiving-COVID-19-surge-213K-test-positive.html.

6. Olga Khazan, "Americans Aren't Actually Quarantining," *Atlantic*, December 8, 2020, https://www.theatlantic.com/politics/archive/2020/12/states-coronavirus-travel-restrictions-quarantine-hawaii/617321.

7. AP Staff, "Hospitals Desperate to Hire Nurses and Doctors amid Pandemic Surge," CBS News, December 3, 2020, https://www.cbsnewcom/news/nurses-needed-hospitals-covid-pandemic.

8. "CDC Novel H1N1 Flu/The 2009 H1N1 Pandemic," Centers for Disease Control and Prevention, June 16, 2010, https://www.cdc.gov/h1n1flu/cdcresponse.htm.

9. Rebecca Heilweil, "How Quickly Can the US Distribute a Covid-19 Vaccine? Here Are the Four Biggest Logistical Challenges," *Vox*, December 7, 2020, https://www.vox.com/recode/22151473/vaccine-covid-19-pfizer-glass-syringes-needles-freezers.

10. Sarah Foster, "Survey: 42% of U.S. Households Say Income Hasn't Recovered from Initial Coronavirus Hit," *Bankrate*, December 9, 2020, https://www.bankrate.com /surveys/coronavirus-income-reduction.

11. "Unemployment Insurance Weekly Claims (Week Ending 12/5/20)," US Department of Labor, December 10, 2020, https://www.dol.gov/ui/data.pdf.

12. Brett Wilkins, "'Hunger Like They've Never Seen It Before': US Food Banks Struggle as 1 in 6 Families with Children Don't Have Enough to Eat," *Common Dreams*, November 27, 2020, https://www.commondreams.org/news/2020/11/27/hunger-theyve -never-seen-it-us-food-banks-struggle-1-6-families-children-dont-have.

13. "Impact of the Coronavirus on Food Insecurity," Feeding America, April 22, 2020, https://www.feedingamerica.org/sites/default/files/2020-04/Brief_Impact%20of%20Covid %20on%20Food%20Insecurity%204.22%20%28002%29.pdf.

14. Amirio Freeman, "The Impact of the Coronavirus on Food Insecurity," *Feeding America Action* (blog), October 30, 2020, https://www.feedingamericaaction.org/the-impact -of-coronavirus-on-food-insecurity.

15. Marcelino Benito, "'It Can Get a Lot Worse': Food Insecurity in Houston Growing Problem as COVID-19 Cases Climb," KHOU 11, November 23, 2020, https://www.khou .com/article/news/health/coronavirus/food-insecurity-in-houston-growing-problem/285 -24369f03-43c3-433d-9c0b-314ab6e667e9.

16. Mark Felix, "A Growing Number of Americans Are Going Hungry," *Washington Post*, November 25, 2020, https://www.washingtonpost.com/graphics/2020/business /hunger-coronavirus-economy.

17. World Health Organization, *The WHO Pandemic Phases* (Geneva: WHO, 2009), https://www.ncbi.nlm.nih.gov/books/NBK143061.

18. Orion Rummler, "The Major Police Reforms Enacted Since George Floyd's Death," *Axios*, October 1, 2020, https://www.axios.com/police-reform-george-floyd-protest -2150b2dd-a6dc-4a0c-a1fb-62c2e999a03a.html.

19. Luis Ferré-Sadurní, Jeffery C. Mays, and Ashley Southall, "Defying Police Unions, New York Lawmakers Ban Chokeholds," *New York Times*, June 8, 2020, https://www.nytimes .com/2020/06/08/nyregion/floyd-protests-police-reform.html; T. C. R. Staff, "California Bans Chokeholds, Shuts Juvenile Halls in New Reform Package," *The Crime Report*, October 1, 2020, https://thecrimereport.org/2020/10/01/california-bans-chokeholds-shuts -juvenile-halls-in-new-reform-package.

20. Daniel Beekman, "Seattle City Council Bans Police Use of Tear Gas and Chokeholds as Protests for Black Lives Continue," *Seattle Times*, June 15, 2020, https://www .seattletimes.com/seattle-news/politics/seattle-city-council-bans-police-use-of-tear-gas -and-chokeholds-as-protests-for-black-lives-continue; Julie Zauzmer and Fenit Nirappil, "D.C. Toughens Officer Hiring and Discipline, as Wave of Police Reform Sweeps the U.S.," *Washington Post*, June 9, 2020, https://www.washingtonpost.com/local/dc-politics /dc-council-police-reform/2020/06/09/c77ae6b0-aa49-11ea-a9d9-a81c1a491c52_story.html.

21. Michael D'Onofrio, "Philly City Council Passes Police Reforms, Shelves Others for the Summer," *Pennsylvania Capital-Star* (blog), June 26, 2020, https://www.penncapital-star .com/civil-rights-social-justice/philly-city-council-passes-police-reforms-shelves-others -for-the-summer.

22. James Benedetto, "Tuscaloosa Bans Biased Policing, Use of Chokeholds," *Tuscaloosa Thread*, September 29, 2020, https://tuscaloosathread.com/tuscaloosa-bans-biased-policing -use-of-chokeholds; Karina Zaiets, Janie Haseman, and Jennifer Borresen, "Cities and States across the US Announce Police Reform Following Demands for Change," *USA Today*, June 19, 2020, https://www.usatoday.com/in-depth/news/2020/06/18/2020-protests-impact-city -and-state-changes-policing/5337751002.

23. Bill Atkinson, "Breonna Taylor's Aunt Tells Virginia Bill-Signing Ceremony Her Niece 'Still Needs Justice,'" *Progress-Index*, December 7, 2020, https://www.progress-index

.com/story/news/2020/12/07/virginia-ceremoniously-signs-breonnas-law-into-existence
/3857957001.

24. Catie Edmondson, "House Passes Sweeping Policing Bill Targeting Racial Bias and Use of Force," *New York Times*, June 26, 2020, https://www.nytimes.com/2020/06/25/us/politics/house-police-overhaul-bill.html.

25. David Morgan, "U.S. Drive for Police Reform Hamstrung by Deadlock in Congress," Reuters, June 23, 2020, https://www.reuters.com/article/us-minneapolis-police-congress-idUSKBN23U2BL.

26. Chrystie F. Swiney, "The Counter-Associational Revolution: The Rise, Spread, and Contagion of Restrictive Civil Society Laws in the World's Strongest Democratic States," *Fordham International Law Journal* 43, no. 2 (January 1, 2019): 399.

27. Alleen Brown, "Powerful Petrochemical Lobbying Group Advanced Anti-Protest Legislation Amid Pandemic," *The Intercept*, June 7, 2020, https://theintercept.com/2020/06/07/pipeline-petrochemical-lobbying-group-anti-protest-law; ICNL, "US Protest Law Tracker," *International Center for Not-For-Profit Law* (blog), 2020, 2016, http://www.icnl.org/usprotestlawtracker.

28. Marty Schladen, "Bill in Ohio House Would Impose Harsh New Penalties on Protesters," *Columbus Underground* (blog), November 17, 2020, https://www.columbusunderground.com/bill-in-ohio-house-would-impose-harsh-new-penalties-on-protesters-ocj1.

29. Natalie Allison, "Tennessee Legislature Cracks Down on Protesters, Making It a Felony to Camp Overnight Outside Capitol," *Tennessean*, August 12, 2020, https://www.tennessean.com/story/news/politics/2020/08/12/tennessee-passes-law-targeting-protesters-makes-capitol-camping-felony/3354879001; Andy Sher, "Tennessee Lawmakers Pass Controversial Bills Discouraging COVID-19 Lawsuits, Targeting Protesters," *Chattanooga Times Free Press*, August 12, 2020, https://www.timesfreepress.com/news/local/story/2020/aug/12/controversial-provision-removed-protest-bill/529664.

30. Adam Schnelting, "Bill Information for HB56," Missouri House of Representatives, December 1, 2020, https://house.mo.gov/bill.aspx?bill=HB56&year=2021&code=R.

31. Chris Gelardi, "Detroit Is Suing Black Lives Matter Protesters for 'Civil Conspiracy,'" *The Intercept*, December 21, 2020, https://theintercept.com/2020/12/21/detroit-black-lives-matter-lawsuit.

32. Bethany Bruner, "Unarmed Black Man Fatally Shot by Columbus Police Officer Responding to Noise Complaint," *Columbus Dispatch*, December 22, 2020, https://www.dispatch.com/story/news/local/2020/12/22/one-killed-after-police-shooting-northwest-side/4004989001; Michael Levenson, "Philadelphia Releases Body-Camera Video of Fatal Police Shooting of Black Man," *New York Times*, November 4, 2020, https://www.nytimes.com/2020/11/04/us/philadelphia-walter-wallace-video.html; Laurie Ure, Rebekah Riess, and Hollie Silverman, "A Sheriff's Deputy Killed a Black Man Entering His Own Home in Columbus, Ohio. His Family Wants Answers," CNN, December 8, 2020, https://www.cnn.com/2020/12/08/us/ohio-police-shooting-casey-goodson/index.html.

33. Allison Klein, "Historic D.C. Black Churches Attacked During Pro-Trump Rallies Saturday," *Washington Post*, December 13, 2020, https://www.washingtonpost.com/local/social-issues/historic-black-churches-attacked-during-pro-trump-rallies-saturday/2020/12/13/d897bfb0-3d54-11eb-8bc0-ae155bee4aff_story.html.

34. Tamar Lapin, "Trump Pardons 26, Including Paul Manafort, Roger Stone and Charles Kushner," *New York Post* (blog), December 24, 2020, https://nypost.com/2020/12/23/trump-pardons-paul-manafort-roger-stone-and-charles-kushner.

35. Joseph Neff and Keri Blakinger, "Michael Cohen and Paul Manafort Got to Leave Federal Prison Due to COVID-19. They're the Exception," Marshall Project, May 21, 2020, https://www.themarshallproject.org/2020/05/21/michael-cohen-and-paul-manafort-got-to-leave-federal-prison-due-to-covid-19-they-re-the-exception.

36. Keri Blakinger and Joseph Neff, "Thousands of Sick Federal Prisoners Sought Compassionate Release. 98 Percent Were Denied," Marshall Project, October 7, 2020, https://www.themarshallproject.org/2020/10/07/thousands-of-sick-federal-prisoners-sought -compassionate-release-98-percent-were-denied.

37. Beth Schwartzapfel and Katie Park, "1 in 5 Prisoners in the U.S. Has Had COVID-19," Marshall Project, December 18, 2020, https://www.themarshallproject.org /2020/12/18/1-in-5-prisoners-in-the-u-s-has-had-covid-19.

38. Marty Roney, "Alabama Sheriff 'Big John' Williams' Killing a 'Huge Misunder- standing,' Defense Lawyer Says," *Montgomery Advertiser*, August 27, 2020, https://www .montgomeryadvertiser.com/story/news/2020/08/27/alabama-sheriff-big-john-williams -killing-capital-murder-william-chase-johnson-lowndes-county/5631891002.

39. Kaiser Foundation, "Poverty Rate by Race/Ethnicity," *KFF* (blog), October 23, 2020, https://www.kff.org/other/state-indicator/poverty-rate-by-raceethnicity.

40. "Fatal Shooting of Unarmed Black Man in Columbus, Ohio," CNN, December 24, 2020, https://www.cnn.com/2020/12/23/us/columbus-ohio-mayor-calls-for-firing-of -officer/index.html.

41. Edward E. Baptist, *The Half Has Never Been Told: Slavery and the Making of American Capitalism* (New York: Basic Books, 2016).

42. "President Trump's July 3 Mount Rushmore Speech," *Newsmax*, July 4, 2020, https://www.newsmax.com/us/mount-rushmore-speech-transcript-july-3/2020/07/04/id /975688.

43. " Martin Luther King Jr.: The Legacy," *Washington Post*, 1998, https://www .washingtonpost.com/wp-srv/national/longterm/mlk/legacy/legacy.htm.

44. James Baldwin, *No Name in the Street*, repr. ed. (New York: Vintage, 2007).

EPILOGUE

1. Russ Bynum, "'Only in America': Warnock's Rise from Poverty to US Senator," AP News, January 6, 2021, https://apnews.com/article/raphael-warnock-senate-georgia -0c1e250f03cf1c4dbd8b9fe4d65d91f0.

2. Grace Panetta and Sinéad Baker, "Ossoff and Warnock Win Georgia Runoffs, Hand- ing Democrats Control of the US Senate," *Business Insider*, January 6, 2021, https://www .businessinsider.com/georgia-senate-runoffs-loeffler-warnock-ossoff-perdue-live-results -2021-1.

3. Donald Trump, "Donald Trump Speech 'Save America' Rally Transcript January 6," *Rev* (blog), January 6, 2021, https://www.rev.com/blog/transcripts/donald-trump-speech -save-america-rally-transcript-january-6.

4. Igor Bobic (@igorbobic), Twitter, January 6, 2021, https://twitter.com/igorbobic /status/1346911809274478594.

5. Kate Conger, Mike Isaac, and Sheera Frenkel, "Twitter and Facebook Lock Trump's Accounts After Violence on Capitol Hill," *New York Times*, January 6, 2021, https://www .nytimes.com/2021/01/06/technology/violence-election-capitol-hill-social-media.html.

6. Rick Perlstein, "This Is Us: Why the Trump Era Ended in Violence," *New Republic*, January 20, 2021, https://newrepublic.com/article/160975/trump-era-always-going-end -violence.

PHOTO INSERT CREDITS

1. Wikimedia Commons, Navy Medicine, Washington, DC
2. Lucas Jackson/Reuters
3. Mario Tama/Getty Images
4. Marcus Yam/Los Angeles Times via Getty Images
5. Giles Clarke/Getty Images
6. Brett Carlson/Getty Images
7. Seth Herald/Reuters Reuters
8. Lucas Jackson/Reuters
9. Sean Rayford/Getty Images
10. Noah Riffe/Anadolu Images
11. Eze Amos/Getty Images
12. Noah Berger/AP Photo
13. Andrew Caballero-Reynolds/AFP via Getty Images

INDEX